PSYCHIATRIC NURSING

Case studies, nursing diagnoses, and care plans

D1082248

Edited by

Luc Reginald Pelletier, MSN, RN, CS
Formerly, Nursing Coordinator/Adult Psychiatry
UCLA Neuropsychiatric Hospital
Los Angeles, California

Assistant Clinical Professor
UCLA School of Nursing
Los Angeles, California

Clinical Applications Analyst
Hospital Information System
UCLA Neuropsychiatric Institute and Hospital
Los Angeles, California

BSN, Fairfield University
MSN, Yale University

Springhouse Corporation
Springhouse, Pennsylvania

Publisher: Keith Lassner
Senior Acquisitions Editor: Susan L. Taddei
Art Director: John Hubbard
Editorial Services Manager: David Moreau
Senior Production Manager: Deborah C. Meiris

Special thanks to Stanley Loeb, Bernadette Glenn, and Carol Robertson, who assisted in the preparation of this volume.

The editor, authors, and publisher have endeavored to ensure that the drug information set forth in this book is in accordance with current recommendations and clinical practice at the time of publication. However, in view of ongoing research, changes in government regulations, and the dynamic flow of information relating to drug therapy and drug interactions, the reader is urged to read the package insert for each drug for any changes in indications, warnings, and dosage recommendations. This is particularly important when the recommended psychopharmacologic agent is a new or infrequently used drug. The identifying data and clinical information presented herein has been disguised substantially by each contributing author and the editor. The cases are composites of actual clients. Any resemblance of the case to a real-life person is purely coincidental. The clinical procedures described and recommended in this publication are based on research and consultation with nursing, medical, and legal authorities. To the best of our knowledge, these procedures reflect currently accepted practice; nevertheless, they can't be considered absolute and universal recommendations. For individual application, all recommendations must be considered in light of the patient's clinical condition and, before administration of new or infrequently used drugs, in light of latest package-insert information. The authors and the publisher disclaim responsibility for any adverse effects resulting directly or indirectly from the suggested procedures, from any undetected errors, or from the reader's misunderstanding of the text.

Printed in the United States of America.

Library of Congress Cataloging-in-Publication Data
Psychiatric nursing.

Includes bibliographies and index.
1. Psychiatric nursing. I. Pelletier, Luc Reginald.
[DNLM: 1. Nursing Assessment. 2. Patient Care Planning. 3. Psychiatric Nursing.
WY 160 P9724]
RC440.P754 1987 610.73'68 87-7108
ISBN 0-87434-090-X

To Mary Beth Goulet-Connolly, Alene W. Polio, Barbara R. Garson, and Frank Lambert Muzzy

What I must do is all that concerns me, not what the people think. This rule, especially arduous in intellectual life, may serve for the whole distinction between greatness and meanness. It is the harder because you will always find those who think they know what is your duty better than you know it. It is easy in the world to live after the world's opinion; it is easy in solitude to live after our own, but the great man is he who in the midst of the crowd keeps with perfect sweetness the independence of solitude.

—Emerson
   First Essays, *Self Reliance*

Contents

I. Introduction

II. Nursing of Clients in Inpatient Psychiatric Settings

III. Nursing of Clients in the Home and Clinic

IV. Nursing of Clients in Outpatient Psychiatric Settings

Consultant

Elizabeth C. Poster, PhD, RN
Assistant Director of Nursing Service
UCLA Neuropsychiatric Hospital

Assistant Clinical Professor
UCLA School of Nursing
UCLA School of Medicine
Los Angeles, California

Contributors

Billie Dixon Barringer, MA, RN
Assistant Professor
Northeast Louisiana University
Monroe, Louisiana

Ellen Bowen, MN, RN
Formerly,
Clinical Specialist/Adolescent Unit
UCLA Neuropsychiatric Hospital
Los Angeles, California

Dessye-Dee Clark, MSN, RN
Clinical Nurse Specialist
Child Psychiatry
UCLA Neuropsychiatric Hospital
Los Angeles, California

Ann Cousins, MSN, RN, CS
Clinical Nurse Specialist
Harvard Community Health Plan
Cambridge, Massachusetts

Ellen C. Drever, MS, RN, CS
Psychiatric Clinical Nurse Specialist
Behavioral Neuroscience Unit—Adults
UCSF-Langley Porter Psychiatric
    Institute
San Francisco, California

Johanna Ehlhardt, BSN, RN
Clinical Nurse III/Adult Psychiatry
UCLA Neuropsychiatric Hospital
Los Angeles, California

Kathleen J. Faude, MN, RN, CS
Nursing Coordinator/Geriatic
    Psychiatry
UCLA Neuropsychiatric Hospital
Los Angeles, California

Stephen William Foster, PhD, MSN, RN
Clinical Nurse Specialist
San Francisco General Hospital
Research Associate, Department of
    Anthropology
University of California, Berkeley
Berkeley, California

Barbara R. Garson, MSN, RN, CS
Coordinator of Inpatient Services and
    Director of Mental Health Nursing
Greater Lynn Community Mental
    Health Center
Atlanticare Medical Center
Lynn, Massachusetts

**Susan Abbott Gierszewski, MS, RN,
    PHN**
Community Health Nurse
Region of Peel Health Department
Mississauga, Ontario
Canada

Diane L. Grimaldi, MS, RN, CS
Team Coordinator/Psychiatric
    Outpatient Department
Cambridge Hospital
Lecturer in Psychiatry
The Departments of Psychiatry,
    Cambridge Hospital and Harvard
    Medical School
Private Psychotherapy Practice
Cambridge, Massachusetts

Jill Ione Lomax, MN, RN
Clinical Nurse III/Adult Psychiatry
UCLA Neuropsychiatric Hospital
Los Angeles, California

Geoffry W. McEnany, MS, RN
Clinical Nurse Specialist/Program
  Evaluation and Research Coordinator
Psychiatric Nursing Division,
Department of Psychiatry
San Francisco General Hospital
Assistant Clinical Professor
UCSF School of Nursing
San Francisco, California

Marcia Pearson Miller, MS, RN
Psychiatric Clinical Nurse Specialist
Psychiatric Home Care Program
Northern California Visiting Nurses
  Association
Albany, California

Diane Moreau, MN, RN, CNA
Nursing Coordinator/Adolescent
  Psychiatry
UCLA Neuropsychiatric Hospital
Los Angeles, California

Deidre O'Connor Rea, MSN, RN
Advanced Registered Nurse Practitioner
Director, Department of Clinical
  Specialists/Evaluation Coordinators
Fair Oaks Hospital at Boca/Delray
Delray Beach, Florida

Sarah A. Roumanis, RN
Head Nurse, General Adult Unit
Yale–New Haven Medical Center
Courtesy Faculty, Clinical Instructor
Yale University School of Nursing
New Haven, Connecticut

Jill Shapira, MN, RN, C, ANP
Clinical Nurse Specialist
West Los Angeles—Veteran's
  Administration Medical Center
Brentwood Division
Assistant Clinical Professor

Carole J. Singer, MSN, RN, CS
Psychiatric Clinical Nurse Specialist
Instructor, Northeastern University
  College of Nursing
Boston, Massachusetts
Private Psychotherapy Practice
Lexington, Massachusetts

Joanne Thompson, MSN, RN
Clinical Nurse Specialist
Outpatient Child Division
UCLA Neuropsychiatric Hospital
Los Angeles, California

Foreword

Although recent moves have been made to deinstitutionalize the mentally ill in America, the majority of clients with psychiatric disorders continues to receive treatment in inpatient settings, such as free-standing private hospitals and psychiatric units of general hospitals. Recent economic constraints, in the form of reduced reimbursement for medical care, have had an impact on the client needing psychiatric services. This, in turn, has affected the severity of the client's illness before he reaches the hospital or clinic. Clients admitted to various settings these days generally display more acute symptomatology and require rapid, skilled nursing interventions. Now, more than ever, the psychiatric nurse needs the skills, the knowledge, and the ability to treat short-term problems in the acute care setting. Those clients treated in outpatient clinics and the home also require the services of a psychiatric nurse who is armed with knowledge about interpersonal relations, psychopathology, medication management, and family dynamics.

Regardless of the mental health delivery setting, psychiatric nurses assist multidisciplinary team members in rendering care to severely ill clients. They do so by incorporating psychiatric–mental health nursing concepts derived from nursing science and the social sciences, as well as from medicine (e.g., psychiatry). They deliver nursing care within the context of a psychotherapeutic relationship that employs the nursing process.

Although all nursing programs provide the student nurse with basic psychiatric nursing concepts, the majority of learning takes place in the clinical arena, where the student is stimulated to integrate knowledge with clinical practice. The clinical experience also molds skills and abilities for use in future client contacts. Student nurses as well as new graduates learn psychiatric nursing techniques by entering into relationships with clients, clinical preceptors, nursing personnel, and other mental health practitioners.

The case study method of data presentation is a quite effective format for imparting clinical knowledge. Rather than merely relating facts and theoretical information, this method gives the reader the *experience* of clinical decision-making—which fosters an investigative approach in formulating and understanding the cases presented. Thus, the reader learns by *doing*. With this process comes the realization that decision-making under real circumstances is not always an exact science and that it does not always produce the desired effect. In essence, this process makes the reader's education more of a personal experience—an intense, absorbing, exciting involvement in academic and personal growth.

The diagnostic reference used throughout the book has been taken from the latest North American Nursing Diagnosis Association (NANDA) listing (see pages 18-19). Because NANDA is the national clearinghouse for nursing diagnosis development and refinement, the editor has made only minimal changes to the listing.

This book has evolved from the editor's desire to examine case studies that illustrate the state-of-the-art in psychiatric–mental health nursing. Accordingly, each chapter presents a different case study and details the process of describing, identifying, formulating, diagnosing, planning, intervening, and evaluating the care of a client with unique psychophysiological responses to a major psychiatric illness.

The book is divided into three sections. Sections I and II present case studies that illustrate the nurse generalist's work with clients. The case studies in Section III represent the work of the nurse specialist who engages in psychotherapy. In their practice, nurse specialists more frequently use medical terminology (*DSM-III*), in addition to conceptualizing responses in terms of nursing diagnosis. Thus, this section of the book illustrates this expanded role for nurses.

In all, the cases provide the reader with data to simulate the process of clinical decision-making. The experience gained in completing a nursing care plan for each client will prepare the reader to deal with similar clients in an actual practice setting. By refining diagnostic and intervention skills, the nurse will be more able to effect positive changes in such clients.

Acknowledgments

Whether they know it or not, many individuals and groups have been an integral part of this venture. Most important, I wish to acknowledge the thoughtful efforts of the contributing authors. The case studies reflect their sensitive, clinically expert work with clients and truly represent the state-of-the-art of psychiatric–mental health nursing.

Writings, lectures, and personal conversations with the following nurses have influenced my basic understanding of professional nursing and guide me in my pursuit to teach others. Those who have helped me define the healing art of nursing include Doris Banchik, Luther Christman, Donna Diers, Jacqueline Flaskerud, Sharon Gedan, Martha Harrell, Colleen Hewes, Hildegard Peplau, Elizabeth Poster, Jane Ryan, Barbara Sideleau, Bertha Unger, and Duane Walker.

In addition, many clinical nurses have inspired me throughout the years in this field. I acknowledge the staff of the general unit at Yale–New Haven Hospital, and most especially thank those nurses on 2 West/Adult Psychiatry at the UCLA Neuropsychiatric Hospital with whom I worked for three years. I also thank the nursing staff at the Center for Mental Health, San Fernando Community Hospital.

I would also like to thank Susan Taddei from Springhouse Book Company, who provided editorial guidance throughout the project, and Bo Tendis, who typed the manuscript.

My thanks also to Lynda Juall Carpenito for her consultation regarding nursing diagnoses.

Finally, I commend all those nurses who have revealed themselves through their healing art in the passionate experience of caring for others.

Introduction

Developing The Nurse-Client Relationship

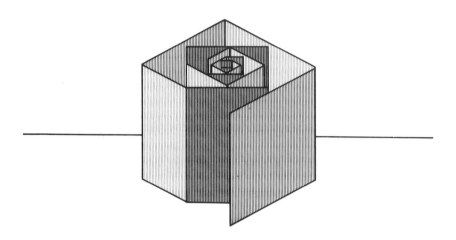

Luc R. Pelletier

Interpersonal relations are the specialized skills that nurses use to treat clients in psychiatric–mental health nursing settings. Hildegard Peplau was the first nurse to spell out the nature and uses of these highly developed skills within a systematic, theoretical framework for psychiatric or "psychodynamic" nursing. Although Peplau wrote her most famous work, *Interpersonal Relations in Nursing*, in 1952, her concepts remain relevant and timely. Influenced primarily by Sullivanian and learning theorists, she carefully examined the effect of the client's *intra*personal experience on *inter*personal functioning. For example, inner beliefs and perceptions influence outward or interpersonal relations. Peplau conceptualized the development of a nurse-client relationship as a continuum from separate individual strangers to partners working together to solve a particular problem. Her framework used the nursing process to help describe the therapeutic process as "a vehicle through which the patient is enabled to clarify and reconstruct feelings, thoughts and ideas already held" (see Figure 1.1). Inherent in this interpersonal process is the need for nurses to be aware of their own values, judgments, and theoretical orientations when working with clients. This chapter focuses on the development and progress of the therapeutic relationship.

Continued on page 4

CONTINUUM OF THE NURSE-CLIENT RELATIONSHIP

Figure 1.1

This figure illustrates the process of melding the client's personal goals with the nurse's professional goals.

CLIENT: NURSE:
Personal Goals   Professional Goals

Entirely separate goals and interests. Both are strangers to each other.

Individual preconceptions on the meaning of the problem and the roles of each in the problematic situation.

Partially mutual understanding of the nature of the problem.

Mutual understanding of the nature of the problem, roles of the nurse and client, and requirements of nurse and client in the solution of the problem. Common goals.

Collaborative efforts directed towards solving the problem together, productively.

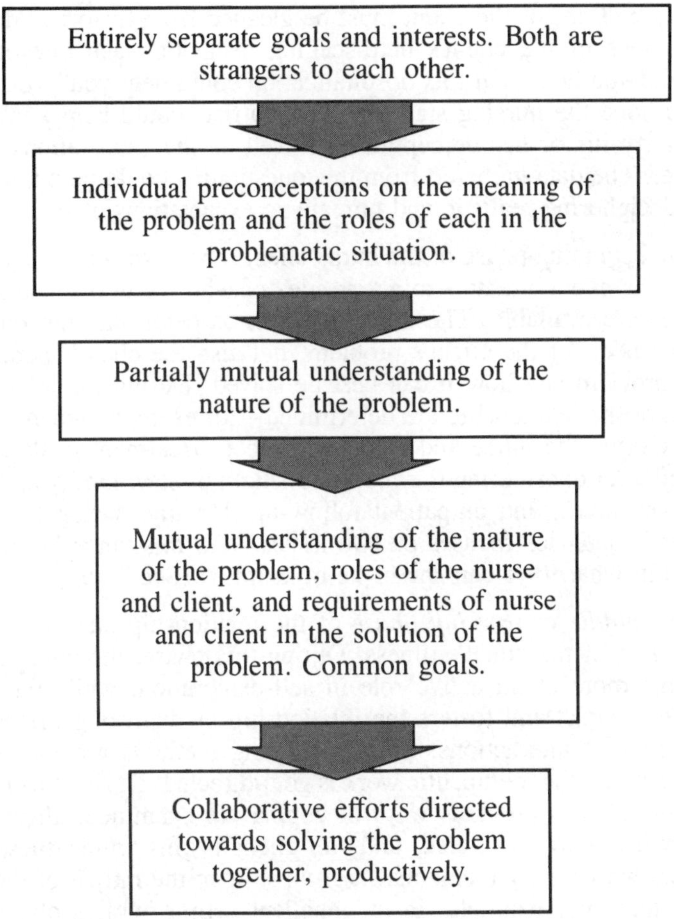

CLIENT: NURSE

Source: Adapted from Peplau, H. *Interpersonal Relations in Nursing*. New York: G.P. Putnam's Sons, 1952, p. 10.

DEVELOPMENTAL PHASES

Every nurse-client relationship passes through several distinct phases of development. The *beginning phase* is characterized by questioning and knowledge-seeking by both client and nurse. The nurse assesses the client's present state of well-being or illness and the potential for growth. An accurate physical and psychosocial history must be gathered to provide baseline data regarding the client's premorbid functioning at home, in school, and in the workplace. Such data is crucial to a later evaluation of the effectiveness of nursing interventions (expected outcomes).

Expectations of the client must be gleaned from historical data. In examinations of the client's help-seeking behavior, such questions as "How did you hope that this hospitalization could help you?" or "How did you hope the nursing staff and psychiatrists could help you?" can help clarify his or her perceptions, as well as the expectations of the caregiver. The data gathered from this questioning could be put to good use in deciphering realistic and unrealistic expectations of the client.

The beginning phase of the nurse-client relationship is fraught with testing. The client attempts to get an idea of who the nurse is and what resources are available. The nurse attempts to determine not only the clinical aspects of the client's problem, but also the client's perception of that problem and how it can best be solved. During this phase, the logistics of the relationship are determined—for example, where, when, and how often the nurse and client will meet. Treatment goals are established after considering the proposed length of stay, family and community resources, and outpatient follow-up. Usually, during this time, the client's behavior focuses on two issues: Will this nurse be here for me, and in what ways can she or he be helpful? (See Figure 1.2.)

The *middle* or *working phase* of the relationship has as its focus the meaning of the client's illness. During this phase, the client begins to assume more of an active role in self-exploration, while the nurse maintains contact and fosters the relationship by analyzing the content and process of interactions. Problem-solving methods are maintained and, in general, the therapeutic work is goal-directed. During this middle phase, the client's previous ways of coping are examined: alternatives are introduced by the nurse, and the client begins trying these new behaviors with family members, in groups, or in the milieu of the psychiatric unit. For example, in an inpatient setting with a client who recently slashed both wrists, the nurse explores alternatives in help-seeking behavior; the client offers to seek out the nurse the next time he feels suicidal (see Figure 1.3).

Continued on page 8

NURSING ASSESSMENT, THE BEGINNING PHASE OF THE NURSE-CLIENT RELATIONSHIP

Figure 1.2

Assessment involves the nurse's inquiry into various aspects of the client's life: biopsychological, spiritual, physical, and sociocultural. At admission, the nurse, client, and family together plan the course of treatment and discharge disposition.

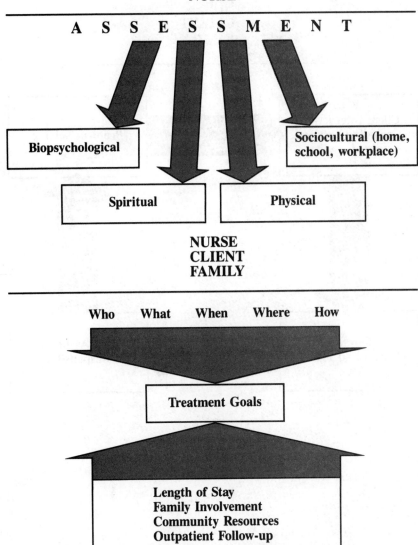

THE MIDDLE PHASE OF THE NURSE-CLIENT RELATIONSHIP

Figure 1.3

This diagram illustrates the process of the nurse and client/family exploring ineffective means of coping and instituting more effective coping strategies.

**NURSE
CLIENT
FAMILY**

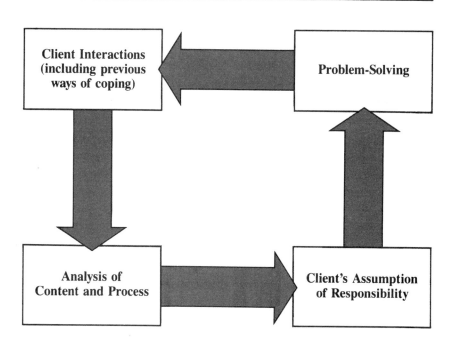

TERMINATION PHASE OF THE NURSE-CLIENT RELATIONSHIP

Figure 1.4

From admission to discharge, the therapeutic relationship travels through three phases, ending in termination. Reminiscing about this process is crucial as the client plans his life away from the treatment setting.

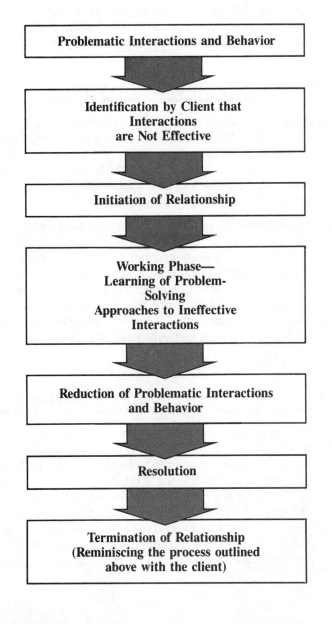

Problematic Interactions and Behavior

Identification by Client that
Interactions
are Not Effective

Initiation of Relationship

Working Phase—
Learning of Problem-
Solving
Approaches to Ineffective
Interactions

Reduction of Problematic Interactions
and Behavior

Resolution

Termination of Relationship
(Reminiscing the process outlined
above with the client)

The final phase, *termination*, marks the culmination of the nurse-client relationship in all settings: inpatient, outpatient, and the home. Although, by this phase of the relationship, the client should be more spontaneous and independent and more able to take control of the situation, termination may still arouse feelings of separation, loss, dissolution, inadequacy, or abandonment in the client. The nurse's major task at this time is to assist the client in internalizing the relationship. This can be done through reminiscing about the nature of the relationship: how it started, the major issues addressed, the process of resolution, and plans for the future. For the termination process to flow smoothly, the nurse must also encourage the client to express related feelings and then must take the time to explore these feelings (see Figure 1.4).

AUTOGNOSIS (SELF-AWARENESS)

Diagnosis consists of evaluating subjective and objective data, then naming the problem to be addressed. Therefore, a crucial component of the nurse-client relationship is the nurse's ability to examine the information presented and synthesize it into understandable and usable categories. Self knowledge—autognosis—can be a valuable tool for organizing this data and naming specific problem areas (Messner, 1979).

Autognosis involves a process of introspection identifying perceptions, intuitive processes, feelings, emotions, thoughts, values, mores, fantasies, attitudes, motivations, and judgments. The nurse uses this awareness to understand the client's plight. Thus, an empathetic response comes directly from the nurse's own self-knowledge. For example, the nurse who has personally experienced the chaos of an alcoholic family and has resolved surrounding issues of conflict, ambivalence, separation, and individuation can more effectively guide the client who is experiencing these issues.

TRANSFERENCE AND COUNTERTRANSFERENCE

At times, the therapeutic relationship may be blocked by the nurse's unconscious projections toward the client. Since the term *transference* has been used to describe the client's feelings and attitudes toward the therapist, the term *countertransference* brings the nurse's feelings and attitudes into the therapeutic picture. Clients may experience the therapeutic relationship in much the same way as they did in a past relationship with a friend or loved one; nurses need to be aware of their own potential reactions to this situation. For example, a nurse could be led to feel increased self-importance by a client who sees and reacts to the nurse as he would to an authoritarian figure like a parent. In a similar way, the nurse may approach the client as a parent does a child. The nurse who has not completely resolved a relationship with a parent may experience many feelings in such a situation, including attraction, warmth, guilt, boredom, discouragement, or anger. These feelings, although unconscious initially, may eventually guide the nurse into unproductive behaviors. For instance, a nurse who feels compelled to "rescue" a client because of the client's striking physical or behavioral resemblance to the nurse's father may overcompensate by providing inappropriate nurturing or establishing unrealistic expectations. On the other hand, nurses who have struggled through the separation-individuation process with their own parents may be more empathetic and realistic when setting goals for the client.

Certain nurse reactions to psychiatric client behaviors are common (see Table 1.1). Most clinicians experience these feelings at one time or another; unusually intense reactions, however, require quick attention by the nurse and the clinical supervisor in order to facilitate further understanding of self and avoid interference with the therapeutic relationship. When the nurse becomes aware of inappropriate responses to a client in treatment, autognosis, peer consultation, and clinical supervision are often helpful in correcting the situation.

CLINICAL COLLABORATION

Many of the intense emotional reactions experienced by nurses in their day-to-day interactions with clients are displayed by others in the field of psychiatric–mental health care. Nevertheless, these reactions can make the nurse feel quite alone. Such questions as "Am I crazy?" or "Why is this client so hard to treat?" are common. Clinical supervisors can help nurses to explore their feelings and develop strategies for overcoming negative, stressful reactions to clients. Nurses themselves are best-suited for this supervisory task. Although psychiatrists, social workers, and psychologists may be quite adept at helping nurses foster theoretical understanding and clinical psychotherapeutic expertise, clinical nurse specialists best understand the problems and perspectives of other nurses.

SUMMARY

The psychiatric nurse's most valuable tool is the ability to initiate, foster, and maintain a therapeutic relationship with the client. Just as the client brings much "baggage" (an individual history and effective and ineffective ways of coping) to the therapeutic relationship, so too does the nurse

Continued on page 12

COMMON COUNTERTRANSFERENCE REACTIONS TO PSYCHIATRIC CLIENT BEHAVIORS

Table 1.1

Nurses commonly experience countertransference feelings. Once these become conscious, the nurse can use them for self-analysis, resulting in understanding those feelings that may inhibit nurse-client communication.

Feeling in Nurse	Characteristic Nurse Behaviors
Boredom Sleepiness	—Inattention —Frequently asking the client to repeat statements —Cryptic responses
Rescue	—Reaching for unattainable goals —Resisting peer feedback and supervisory recommendations
Overinvolvement	—Coming to work early, leaving late —Ignoring peer suggestions, resisting assistance —Buying client clothes, gifts —Behaving judgmentally at family interventions —Keeping secrets —Calling client when off-duty
Overidentification	—Special agendas, secrets —Increased self-disclosure —Feelings of omnipotence —Physical attraction

Self-Analysis	Solution
—Is the *content* of what the client presents uninteresting? Or is it the style of communication? Does the client exhibit an obnoxious style of communication? —Have you anything else on your mind that may be distracting you from the client's needs? —Is the client discussing an issue that makes you anxious?	—Redirect client if he provides more information than you need or goes "off the track." —Clarify information with client. —Confront ineffective modes of communication.
—What behavior stimulates your perceived need to rescue the client? —Has anyone evoked such feelings in you in the past? Who? —What are your fears or fantasies about failing to meet the client's needs?	—Avoid secret alliances. —Develop realistic goals. —Do not alter meeting schedule. —Let the client guide the interaction.
—What particular client characteristics are attractive? —Does client remind you of someone? Who? —Does your current behavior differ from your treatment of similar clients in the past?	—Establish firm treatment boundaries, goals, and nursing expectations. —Avoid self-disclosure. —Avoid calling the client when off-duty.
—With which of the client's physical, emotional, cognitive, or situational characteristics do you identify? —Recall similar circumstances in your own life. How did you deal with the issues now being recreated by the client?	—Allow the client to direct the issues. —Encourage a problem-solving approach from the client's perspective. —Avoid self-disclosure.

Continued

Common Countertransference Reactions to Psychiatric Client Behaviors
continued

Feeling in Nurse	Characteristic Nurse Behaviors
Misuse of honesty	—Withholding information —Lying
Anger	—Withdrawal —Speaking loudly —Using profanity —Asking to be taken off case
Helplessness or hopelessness	—Sadness

bring a past filled with various beliefs, feelings, and behaviors associated with relationships. This past affects the way in which the nurse formulates a nursing care plan for a particular client. Thus, the nurse's own self-awareness and introspection are essential to understanding the client's plight.

A good teacher imparts knowledge that has been mastered. In the same light, the nurse who has "worked through" and mastered difficult aspects of interpersonal relations (specifically intimacy, separation, individuation) can then impart knowledge and experiential data to the client. The psychiatric nurse thusly becomes the master of introspection—one who is mindful of reactions to client behaviors, has an awareness of where such reactions originate, and can deliver psychiatric nursing care in a thoughtful, purposeful manner.

REFERENCES

Messner, E. "Autognosis: Diagnosis by the Use of Self," in *Outpatient Psychiatry*. Baltimore: Williams & Wilkins Co., 1979.

Self-Analysis	Solution
—Why are you protecting the client? —What are your fears about the client's learning the truth?	—Be clear in your responses and aware of your hesitation; do not "hedge." —If you cannot provide information, tell the client and give your rationale. —Avoid keeping secrets. —Reinform the client about the interdisciplinary nature of treatment.
—What client behaviors are offensive to you? —What dynamic from your past may this client be recreating?	—Determine the origin of anger (nurse, client, or both). —Explore roots of client anger. —Avoid contact with client if anger is not understood.
—Which client behaviors evoke these feelings in you? —Has anyone evoked similar feelings in the past? Who? —What expectations were placed on you (verbally and nonverbally) by this person?	—Maintain therapeutic involvement. —Explore and focus on the client's experience rather than on your own.

Peplau, H. *Interpersonal Relations in Nursing*. New York: G.P. Putnam's Sons, 1952.

SELECTED BIBLIOGRAPHY

Ackerhalt, J. "Nurse-Client Relationship," in *Comprehensive Psychiatric Nursing,* 3rd ed. Edited by Haber, J., et al. New York: McGraw-Hill Book Co., 1987.

Bettelheim, B. "The Love That Is Enough: Countertransference and the Ego Processes of Staff Members in a Therapeutic Milieu," in *Countertransference*. Edited by Giovacchini, P. New York: Basic Books, 1967.

Blumenfield, M. *Applied Supervision in Psychotherapy*. New York: Grune & Stratton, 1982.

Burgess, A., and Lazare, A. *Psychiatric Nursing in the Hospital and the Community*. Englewood Cliffs, N.J.: Prentice-Hall, 1973.

Stein, M. *Jungian Analysis*. London: Open Court Publishing Co., 1982.

The Process of Nursing Diagnosis

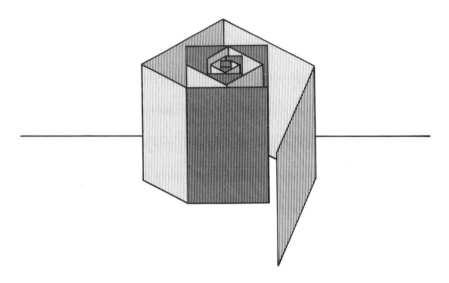

Luc R. Pelletier

Although some people believe that changes in client behavior are regulated by fate or some cosmic force, most academicians and clinicians believe that change is the result of purposeful, thoughtfully developed plans of treatment. Whether or not the nursing care plan is accorded a specific place in the medical record, the professional nurse must ensure that the issues addressed by nursing are clearly identified. Over the past few years, the nursing community has implemented a means by which diagnosis has been formally added to the nursing process. Nursing diagnosis, then, has become the process of collecting, interpreting, clustering, and naming information in preparation for later treatment by nurses (Gordon, 1987).

This book has been written to highlight the process of nursing diagnosis and to develop nursing care plans in the psychiatric setting (see Figure 2.1). Care plans developed by experts in the field are presented in Sections I and II. Section III presents the advanced work of clinical nurse specialists in treating clients with common mental illnesses. Case studies provide the background information from which the reader can evaluate functional health patterns and determine nursing diagnoses (see Figures 2.2, 2.3, and 2.4). The following steps will guide the reader through this experiential process:

Continued on page 22

THE PROCESS OF COLLECTING, CLUSTERING, AND LABELING DATA TO PLAN, IMPLEMENT, AND EVALUATE NURSING CARE

Figure 2.1

This diagram illustrates the series of steps a nurse follows in planning, implementing, and evaluating nursing care.

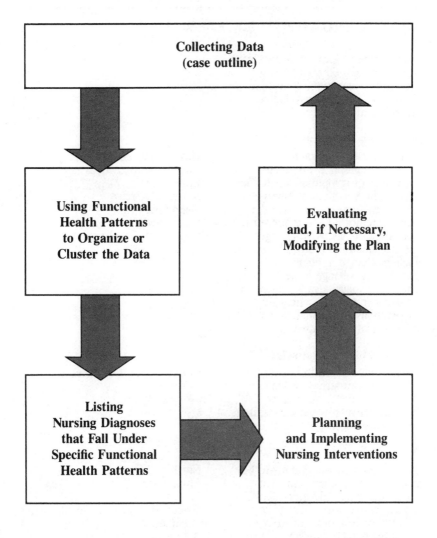

POSSIBLE FUNCTIONAL PATTERNS REPRESENTED IN CASE OUTLINE

Figure 2.2

This figure points to the various functional health patterns that may be represented under specific psychiatric history headings.

CASE OUTLINE (Banchik, 1983)	FUNCTIONAL PATTERN (Gordon, 1987a)
Identifying Information	
Age, sex, religion, ethnicity, marital status, general location of residence (urban, rural), others in living situation, occupation, education, number of previous psychiatric hospitalizations.	Health Management/Perception Value/Belief
Presenting Problems	
Date of onset, precipitants to seeking attention at this time, formation of symptoms, conditions under which symptoms emerge and abate, reactions of others to the client (premorbid and at present), losses, neurovegetative changes (sleep, appetite, libido), change in feeling, change in cognitive functioning, change in perception, change in consciousness, change in adjustment patterns, client's expectations of hospitalization, client's goals of treatment.	Health Management/Perception Nutritional/Metabolic Elimination Activity/Exercise Sleep/Rest Cognitive/Perceptual Coping/Stress Tolerance
Past Psychiatric Contacts	
Length, type of institution, treatment approaches utilized, diagnoses, client's account of benefit, between contacts: stability, progress, or decompensation.	Coping/Stress Tolerance
Medical History	
Any medical illness that could be contributory to client's present emotional state, allergies, alcohol consumption, drug abuse history, current medications, for women: age at menarche, menstrual cycle, contraceptive use.	Nutrition/Metabolic Elimination Sleep/Rest Health Management/Health Perception Activity/Exercise Cognitive/Perceptual

CASE OUTLINE	FUNCTIONAL PATTERN

Medical History
continued
Self-Perception/Self-Concept
Role Relationship
Sexuality/Reproductive
Coping/Stress Tolerance
Value/Belief

Social/Developmental History

Recollections of childhood, symptoms of behavioral problems, interactions with others, earliest and recurrent dreams and memories, friendships, school history, psychological and physical trauma (family problems, abuse, incest, geographical moves, deaths and other losses), puberty and adolescence, sexuality and sexual activity, occupational history.	Self-Perception/Self-Concept Role Relationship Sexuality/Reproductive Cognitive/Perceptual

Family History

Demographic descriptions of family members, ethnicity, education, occupation, medical and psychiatric histories, relationships between client and each family member.	Health Management/Perception Self-Perception/Self-Concept Role Relationship Sexuality/Reproductive Coping/Stress Tolerance Value/Belief

Mental Status

General appearance, emotional state, speech, nonverbal communication, state of consciousness, content of thought, perceptual state, coping strategies, cognitive functioning (orientation, memory, general fund of knowledge, attention, concentration, abstraction capacity, judgment), perception and coordination, attitude toward the interviewer.	Cognitive/Perceptual Coping/Stress Tolerance Self-Perception/Self-Concept

LIST OF NURSING DIAGNOSES

Figure 2.3

The accepted list from the North American Nursing Diagnosis Association (NANDA) (McLane, 1987).

Activity Intolerance
Activity Intolerance, Potential
Adjustment, Impaired
Airway Clearance, Ineffective
Anxiety
Body Image Disturbance
Body Temperature, Potential
   Alteration in
Bowel Elimination, Altered:
   Constipation
Bowel Elimination, Altered:
   Diarrhea
Bowel Elimination, Altered:
   Incontinence
Breathing Pattern, Ineffective
Cardiac Output, Altered:
   Decreased
Comfort, Altered: Pain
Comfort, Altered: Chronic Pain
Communication, Impaired Verbal
Coping, Ineffective Individual
Coping, Ineffective Family:
   Compromised
Coping, Ineffective Family:
   Disabling
Coping, Family: Potential for
   Growth
†Developmental Delay:
   —Bowel/Bladder Control
   —Communications Skills
   —Mobility
   —Physical Growth and
      Development
   —Self-Care Skills
   —Social Skills
   —Specify Cognitive Area
   —Specify Coping/Stress
      Tolerance Area
   —Specify Self-Perceptual/Self-
      Concept Area
Diversional Activity Deficit
Family Processes, Altered

Fear
Fluid Volume, Altered: Excess *or*
   Excess Fluid Volume
Fluid Volume Deficit, Actual
Fluid Volume Deficit, Potential
Gas Exchange, Impaired
Grieving, Anticipatory
Grieving, Dysfunctional
Growth and Development, Altered
Health Maintenance, Altered
Home Maintenance Management,
   Impaired (Mild, Moderate,
   Severe, Potential, Chronic)
Hopelessness
Hyperthermia
Hypothermia
Incontinence:
   —Functional
   —Reflex
   —Stress
   —Total
   —Urge
Infection, Potential for
Injury (Trauma): Potential for
   —Poisoning: Potential for
   —Suffocation: Potential for
Knowledge Deficit (Specify)
Mobility, Impaired Physical
Noncompliance (Specify)
Nutrition, Altered: Less Than Body
   Requirements *or Nutritional*
   Deficit (Specify)
Nutrition, Altered: More Than
   Body Requirements *or*
   Exogenous Obesity
Nutrition, Altered: Potential for
   More Than Body Requirements
   or Potential for Obesity
Oral Mucous Membrane, Altered
Parenting, Altered: Actual or
   Potential
Personal Identity Confusion

Post-Trauma Response
Powerlessness (Severe, Low, Moderate)
Rape-Trauma Syndrome
—Compounded
—Silent Reaction
Role Performance, Disturbance in
Self-Care Deficit:
—Feeding
—Bathing/Hygiene
—Dressing/Grooming
—Toileting
—Total
Self-Esteem Disturbance
Sensory-Perceptual Alterations: Input Excess
Sensory-Perceptual Alterations: Input Deficit
Sexual Dysfunction
Sexuality Patterns, Altered
Skin Integrity, Impaired, Actual *or Skin Breakdown*
Skin Integrity, Impaired, Potential *or Potential Skin Breakdown*

Sleep Pattern Disturbance
Social Interaction, Impaired
Social Isolation (Rejection)
Spiritual Distress (Distress of the Human Spirit)
Swallowing, Impaired *or Uncompensated Swallowing Impairment*
Thermoregulation, Ineffective
Thought Processes, Altered
Tissue Integrity, Impaired
Tissue Perfusion, Altered:
—Cerebral
—Cardiopulmonary
—Renal
—Gastrointestinal
—Peripheral
Unilateral Neglect
Urinary Elimination, Altered Patterns of
Urinary Retention
Violence, Potential for (Self-Directed or Directed at Others)

---

†Clinically useful diagnoses developed by the editor within the accepted NANDA diagnosis: Altered Growth and Development
Italics indicate suggested changes in wording by Gordon (1987b).
The term "alteration in" has been changed to "altered" by the editor.

NURSING DIAGNOSES CATEGORIZED UNDER FUNCTIONAL HEALTH PATTERNS*

Figure 2.4

The accepted NANDA list of nursing diagnoses categorized under Gordon's Functional Health Patterns.

Health perception/health management

**Growth and Development, Altered (see Developmental Delay)
Health Maintenance, Altered
Infection, Potential for
Injury (Trauma): Potential for
—Poisoning: Potential for
—Suffocation: Potential for
Noncompliance (Specify)

Nutritional/metabolic

Body Temperature, Potential Alteration in
Developmental Delay: Physical Growth and Development
†Fluid Volume, Altered: Excess *or Excess Fluid Volume*
Fluid Volume Deficit, Actual
Fluid Volume Deficit, Potential
†Nutrition, Altered: Less Than Body Requirements *or Nutritional Deficit (Specify)*
†Nutrition, Altered: More Than Body Requirements *or Exogenous Obesity*
†Nutrition, Altered: Potential for More Than Body Requirements or *Potential for Obesity*
Oral Mucous Membrane, Altered
†Skin Integrity, Impaired *or Skin Breakdown*
†Skin Integrity, Impaired, Potential *or Potential Skin Breakdown*
†Swallowing, Impaired *or Uncompensated Swallowing Impairment*
Tissue Integrity, Impaired

Elimination

Bowel Elimination, Altered:
—Constipation
—Diarrhea
—Incontinence
Developmental Delay: Bowel/ Bladder Control
Incontinence:
—Functional
—Reflex
—Stress
—Total
—Urge
Urinary Elimination, Altered Patterns of
Urinary Retention

Activity/exercise

Activity Intolerance
Activity Intolerance, Potential
Airway Clearance, Ineffective
Breathing Pattern, Ineffective
Cardiac Output, Altered: Decreased
Developmental Delay: Mobility
Developmental Delay: Self-Care Skills
Diversional Activity Deficit
Gas Exchange, Impaired
Home Maintenance Management, Impaired (Mild, Moderate, Severe, Potential, Chronic)
Mobility, Impaired Physical
Self-Care Deficit:
—Feeding
—Bathing/Hygiene
—Dressing/Grooming
—Toileting
—Total
Tissue Perfusion, Altered:
—Cerebral
—Cardiopulmonary
—Renal
—Gastrointestinal
—Peripheral

Sleep/rest

Sleep Pattern Disturbance

Cognitive/perceptual

Comfort, Altered: Pain
Comfort, Altered: Chronic Pain
Developmental Delay: (Specify
  Cognitive Area; attention,
  decision making, etc.)
Hyperthermia
Hypothermia
Knowledge Deficit (Specify)
Sensory-Perceptual Alterations:
  Input Excess
Sensory-Perceptual Alterations:
  Input Deficit
Thermoregulation, Ineffective
Thought Processes, Altered
Unilateral Neglect

Self-perception/self-concept

Anxiety
Body Image Disturbance
Fear
Hopelessness
Personal Identity Confusion
Powerlessness (Severe, Low,
  Moderate)
Self-Esteem Disturbance

Role relationship

Communication, Impaired Verbal
Developmental Delay:
  Communication Skills
Developmental Delay: Social
  Skills

Family Processes, Altered
Grieving, Anticipatory
Grieving, Dysfunctional
Parenting, Altered: Actual or
  Potential
Role Performance, Disturbance in
Social Interactions, Impaired
Social Isolation (Rejection)

Sexuality/reproductive

Rape-Trauma Syndrome
  —Compound Reaction
  —Silent Reaction
Sexual Dysfunction
Sexuality Patterns, Altered

Coping/stress tolerance

Adjustment, Impaired
Coping, Ineffective Individual
Coping, Ineffective Family:
  Compromised
Coping, Ineffective Family:
  Disabling
Coping, Family: Potential for
  Growth
Developmental Delay (Specify
  area)
Post-Trauma Response
Violence, Potential for (Self-
  Directed or Directed at Others)

Value/belief

Spiritual Distress (Distress of
  Human Spirit)

---

*According to Gordon (1987a) with some changes made by editor.

**For purpose of clarity, Altered Growth and Development has been broken down into treatable
  "Developmental Delays."

†Italics represent suggested changes in wording by Gordon (1987b).

Reprinted with permission from Gordon, M., *Nursing Diagnosis: Process and Application*, 2nd
ed. New York: McGraw-Hill Book Co., 1987.

1. Read the case carefully, keeping in mind the 11 functional patterns identified by Gordon (1987):
• Health management/health perception: Describes the client's perceived pattern of health and well-being and how health is managed
• Nutritional/metabolic: Describes the pattern of food and fluid consumption relative to metabolic need and the pattern indicators of local nutrient supply
• Elimination: Describes patterns of excretory function (bowel, bladder, and skin)
• Activity/exercise: Describes patterns of exercise, activity, leisure, and recreation
• Cognitive/perceptual: Describes sensory-perceptual and cognitive patterns
• Sleep/rest: Describes patterns of sleep, rest, and relaxation
• Self-perception/self-concept: Describes the self-concept pattern and perceptions of self (e.g., body comfort, body image, feeling state)
• Role relationship: Describes patterns of role engagements and relationships
• Sexuality/reproductive: Describes the client's satisfaction and dissatisfaction with sexuality patterns; describes reproductive patterns
• Coping/stress tolerance: Describes the client's general coping pattern and effectiveness of the pattern in terms of stress tolerance
• Value/belief: Describes the client's patterns of values, beliefs (including spiritual), or goals that guide choices or decisions

2. After each case, record the data under functional health patterns and review the list of nursing diagnoses. Check the box next to the nursing diagnosis that represents the data presented.

3. From these diagnoses, consider strategies for nursing interventions and identify goals and outcome criteria for the problems addressed.

4. After the exercises, read how experts in the field formulated the case and treated the client (Formulation, Diagnostic Summary, Nursing Care Plan, and Summary).

REFERENCES

Banchik, D. "Psychiatric Assessment and Case Formulation," in *Handbook of Psychiatric–Mental Health Nursing*. Edited by Adams, C., and Macione, A. New York: John Wiley & Sons, 1983.

Gordon, M. *Manual of Nursing Diagnoses (1986-1987)*. New York: McGraw-Hill Book Co., 1987a.

Gordon, M. *Nursing Diagnosis: Process and Application*, 2nd ed. New York: McGraw-Hill Book Co., 1987b.

McLane, A. *Classification of Nursing Diagnoses: Proceedings of the Seventh Conference (1986)*. St. Louis: C.V. Mosby Co., 1987.

SELECTED BIBLIOGRAPHY

Carpenito, L.J. *Nursing Diagnosis Application to Clinical Practice*. Philadelphia: J.B. Lippincott Co., 1983.

Gebbie, K. *Summary of the Second National Conference—Classification of Nursing Diagnoses*. St. Louis: The Clearinghouse, St. Louis University, 1976.

Hurley, M. *Classification of Nursing Diagnoses: Proceedings of the Sixth Conference*. St. Louis: C.V. Mosby Co., 1986.

Kim, M., and Moritz, D. *Classification of Nursing Diagnoses: Proceedings of the Third and Fourth National Conferences*. New York: McGraw-Hill Book Co., 1981.

Kim, M., et al. *Classification of Nursing Diagnoses: Proceedings of the Fifth National Conference*. St. Louis: C.V. Mosby Co., 1984.

McFarland, G., and Wasli, E. *Nursing Diagnoses and Process in Psychiatric Mental Health Nursing*. Philadelphia: J.B. Lippincott Co., 1986.

Nursing of Clients in Inpatient Psychiatric Settings

Hal:
Acute Mania

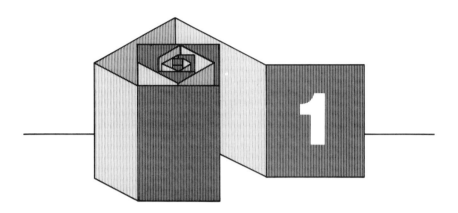

Stephen William Foster, PhD, MSN, RN

The treatment of acute mania is a recurrent and formidable "crisis" on inpatient units with a forensic focus. The nursing management of such episodes must go forward on a number of fronts—behavioral, emotional, social, pharmacologic—and must be attentive to clinical data encompassing diverse domains—past psychiatric history, family dynamics and difficulties, drug and alcohol use, and ongoing assessment of self-care and coping skills. Initial interventions include close supervision of the acutely manic client in order to maintain safety, to obtain clinical data for continuous reassessment, and to control symptoms of agitation, delusions, and poor impulse control by limiting stimulus input. Plans for nursing care must be revised continuously as the client's acuity decreases.

The following case study, which is based on a composite derived from a number of clients treated at a metropolitan general hospital over a 2-year period, not only covers the essential problems often encountered in managing acutely manic clients, but also takes note of possible medical and legal issues secondary to manic behavior. When providing nursing care for such a client on a security unit, the main tasks during the acute phase involve providing meticulous surveillance and intervention in order to maintain safety, promote recompensation, and limit or otherwise control stimulus input. The particular characteristics of the security unit (including the presence of numerous security guards around the clock and added physical barriers for security) facilitate these objectives in some ways but complicate them in others. In the less-acute phases of the illness, the nurse must initiate client education when possible, both as a means of encouraging medication compliance and as a way of preventing subsequent acute crises.

CASE STUDY

Hal was a 37-year-old, unmarried white male who had been chronically unemployed (currently on Social Security Disability) and had multiple inpatient psychiatric hospitalizations since his return from Viet Nam in the late 1960s. He had lived on the city streets, in several single-room occupancy hotels in the Tenderloin district of downtown San Francisco, and in a number of psychiatric extended-care facilities after his mother found that she could no longer manage him at home.

Hal's latest admission was precipitated by a visit to his mother's home. During the visit, he began screaming, shouting, and threatening his mother, and finally chased her from the apartment. She called the police, who soon arrived on the scene and transported Hal to the psychiatric emergency clinic of a local general hospital.

On admission, Hal was delusional, labile, hostile, and acutely disorganized, and his speech was pressured and incoherent. He was placed on a 72-hour mental health hold for psychiatric evaluation and treatment as a danger to himself and others. In the clinic, he initially appeared somewhat calmer and was allowed to smoke. But when he quickly brought a lit cigarette up to his eyes (as if to burn himself), it was taken away. When asked, "Why are you here?" he stated, "I'm Christ and this freckle proves it. I'm going to grab your prick and save the world. You're Dracula and you want to suck my blood." He was unable to state treatment goals for himself or to express his expectations for treatment.

According to Hal's mother, Hal had been living in the streets for a number of weeks prior to admission. He had been drinking heavily during this period and hadn't slept in 4 days. After Hal's admission to the emergency clinic, the police charged him with disorderly conduct and possession of stolen property. He was then admitted to the hospital's security unit, pending court proceedings.

Hal had been hospitalized many times during his adult life, both as an inpatient at general hospital psychiatric units for periods ranging from a week to several months and on a long-term basis at a nearby state mental hospital. Diagnoses during these past hospitalizations included schizophrenia, schizoaffective disorder, and bipolar affective disorder, with concurrent diagnoses of alcohol dependence and antisocial personality disorder. He had been treated with several different drugs, including chlorpromazine (Thorazine), haloperidol (Haldol), fluphenazine hydrochloride (Prolixin), and lithium carbonate (Lithane, Eskolith, Lithonate) with good results although he was prone to extrapyramidal side effects from these drugs, particularly Haldol. However, he was extremely non-compliant with his medication regimen when not in a closely supervised setting; without medication, he rapidly would become delusional and disorganized.

According to Hal's mother, Hal had a history of violent "acting out" behavior and had become more difficult to maintain in the community since his return from Vietnam. He frequently complained of poor sleep (restlessness and middle-of-the-night awakenings) since his return. His numerous hospital admissions were generally precipitated by disruptive, delusional, or sexually inappropriate behavior in public. His hospitalizations were characterized by hostility, disorganization, or sexual inappropriateness. In various records, he was described as a disruptive and manipulative character with poor impulse control and as a client who "really knows how to use the mental health system." In 1982, he was hospitalized at a local psychiatric hospital after being found lying on the ground at an airport and talking bizarrely. About 2 years previously, he was arrested for possession of marijuana; after attempting to hang himself in jail, he was hospitalized on a hospital security unit. On that admission, he was hostile, belligerent, and provocative. He was placed on Thorazine (up to 1200 mg per day) for agitation, as well as lithium carbonate 600 mg twice daily and 900 mg at hour of sleep, which resulted in lithium levels of 1.06 to 1.30. After 10 days, he became more manageable and his agitation decreased. He was first placed on a 14-day mental health hold as gravely impaired, and then on a temporary conservatorship. During this time, he was cooperative and pleasant, and readily agreed that he needed a more structured setting. Since he had outstanding legal charges at that time, however, he was discharged to jail. In jail, he refused to take his medications, subsequently decompensated, and then was returned to the hospital for another course of treatment. His presentation at that time was similar to that observed on his latest admission.

Approximately 1 year after this hospitalization, he had again been incarcerated for misdemeanor charges. While in jail, he became intrusive, bizarre, and sexually preoccupied, with rambling speech and tangential thought processes. He had superficially lacerated his forearm with a razor blade and was again admitted to the hospital for stabilization on medication.

Hal had no known medication allergies. He did have a history of long-term alcohol abuse and extensive use of marijuana and LSD. His medical history was difficult to assess, since he was an unreliable historian in this and other areas. Physical examination revealed no surgical scars or other abnormalities, except for several scars on one arm from the self-inflicted razor blade lacerations. His personal hygiene was grossly inadequate; but although disheveled and unkempt, he appeared adequately nourished. He was treated for lice and scabies, which had produced multiple lesions on his trunk and extremities. He was also treated for cellulitis of the left leg with oral dicloxacillin.

According to Hal's self-report, he was the product of an unremarkable pregnancy and delivery and met developmental milestones age-appropriately. His childhood was unremarkable for medical problems (except for the usual childhood illnesses), and he was ostensibly free of psychiatric disorders. His problems began to evidence themselves at age 14, when he started to withdraw from social activities and wrote several bizarre, elaborate letters to his teachers. At age 19, he made his first suicide attempt. At age 21, he was in Vietnam, working for a construction company contracted by the U.S. government. He began using marijuana and cocaine during this period, and it was at this time that his many psychiatric hospitalizations began.

The details of Hal's family history were difficult to assemble, since he did not respond productively to questions in this area. Hence, the exact role of family themes in Hal's development and problems was unclear. His mother had obtained a restraining order on him, claiming that he had pulled a knife on her and threatened to kill her. She was not helpful in corroborating the details of the family history that Hal provided.

Hal had two younger, adult sisters (one married and one single), both in good health and free of any history of mental illness. His parents divorced when Hal was age 10. His father, who changed his legal name to "Father Christmas" after the divorce, exhibited hypersocial, hyperactive behavior suggestive of mania during his intermittent phone calls to Hal at the hospital. Although he exhibited objective signs of psychopathology, a formal psychiatric history was unknown.

For his formal mental status examination, Hal was brought to the unit dressed in hospital clothing—standard procedure on the security unit. He presented as a 37-year-old white, unmarried male who appeared his stated age. His hair and beard were unkempt, and his personal hygiene had been neglected. He was unable to respond to questioning regarding orientation. His affect was labile, fluctuating from angry and hostile to pleasant and cooperative. His speech was pressured and consisted of "word salad." His thought processes were characterized by marked looseness of association and grandiose delusions; he appeared to be responding to auditory hallucinations of a punitive nature. His attention span and concentration were nonexistent, and he was altogether lacking in insight and judgment. He was also sexually preoccupied; he tried to masturbate

Continued on page 36

RECORDING THE DATA

After you have read the case, cluster significant data into functional health patterns.

Health management/health perception _____

_____

_____

_____

_____

Nutritional/metabolic _____

_____

_____

_____

Elimination _____

_____

_____

_____

Activity/exercise _____

_____

_____

_____

Cognitive/perceptual _____

_____

_____

_____

Sleep/rest _____

_____

_____

_____

Self-perception/self-concept _____

_____

_____

_____

Role relationship _____

_____

_____

_____

Sexuality/reproductive _____

_____

_____

_____

Coping/stress tolerance _____

_____

_____

_____

Value/belief _____

_____

_____

_____

ASSIGNING NURSING DIAGNOSES

Use your clustered data to select appropriate nursing diagnoses.

Health perception/health management

- [ ] Growth and Development, Altered (see Developmental Delay)
- [ ] Health Maintenance, Altered
- [ ] Infection, Potential for
- [ ] Injury (Trauma): Potential for
- [ ] Noncompliance (Specify)
- [ ] Poisoning: Potential for
- [ ] Suffocation: Potential for

Nutritional/metabolic

- [ ] Body Temperature, Potential Alteration in
- [ ] Developmental Delay: Physical Growth and Development
- [ ] Fluid Volume, Altered: Excess or Excess Fluid Volume
- [ ] Fluid Volume Deficit, Actual
- [ ] Fluid Volume Deficit, Potential
- [ ] Nutrition, Altered: Less Than Body Requirements or Nutritional Deficit (Specify)
- [ ] Nutrition, Altered: More Than Body Requirements or Exogenous Obesity
- [ ] Nutrition, Altered: Potential for More Than Body Requirements or Potential for Obesity
- [ ] Oral Mucous Membrane, Altered
- [ ] Skin Integrity, Impaired or Skin Breakdown
- [ ] Skin Integrity, Impaired or Potential Skin Breakdown
- [ ] Swallowing, Impaired or Uncompensated Swallowing Impairment
- [ ] Tissue Integrity, Impaired

Elimination

- [ ] Bowel Elimination, Altered: Constipation
- [ ] Bowel Elimination, Altered: Diarrhea
- [ ] Bowel Elimination, Altered: Incontinence

- [ ] Developmental Delay: Bowel/Bladder Control
- [ ] Incontinence: Functional
- [ ] Incontinence: Reflex
- [ ] Incontinence: Stress
- [ ] Incontinence: Total
- [ ] Incontinence: Urge
- [ ] Urinary Elimination, Altered Patterns of
- [ ] Urinary Retention

Activity/exercise

- [ ] Activity Intolerance
- [ ] Activity Intolerance, Potential
- [ ] Airway Clearance, Ineffective
- [ ] Breathing Pattern, Ineffective
- [ ] Cardiac Output, Altered: Decreased
- [ ] Developmental Delay: Mobility
- [ ] Developmental Delay: Self-Care Skills
- [ ] Diversional Activity Deficit
- [ ] Gas Exchange, Impaired
- [ ] Home Maintenance Management, Impaired (Mild, Moderate, Severe, Potential, Chronic)
- [ ] Mobility, Impaired Physical
- [ ] Self-Care Deficit: Feeding
- [ ] Self-Care Deficit: Bathing/Hygiene
- [ ] Self-Care Deficit: Dressing/Grooming
- [ ] Self-Care Deficit: Toileting
- [ ] Self-Care Deficit: Total
- [ ] Tissue Perfusion, Altered: (Specify)

Sleep/rest

- [ ] Sleep Pattern Disturbance

Cognitive/perceptual

- [ ] Comfort, Altered: Pain
- [ ] Comfort, Altered: Chronic Pain

☐ Developmental Delay: (Specify Cognitive Area; attention, decision making, etc.)
☐ Hypothermia
☐ Hyperthermia
☐ Knowledge Deficit (Specify)
☐ Sensory-Perceptual Alteration: Input Excess or Sensory Overload
☐ Sensory-Perceptual Alteration: Input Deficit or Sensory Deprivation
☐ Thermoregulation, Ineffective
☐ Thought Processes, Altered
☐ Unilateral Neglect

Self-perception/self-concept

☐ Anxiety
☐ Body Image Disturbance
☐ Fear
☐ Hopelessness
☐ Personal Identity Confusion
☐ Powerlessness (Severe, Low, Moderate)
☐ Self-Esteem Disturbance

Role relationship

☐ Communication, Impaired Verbal
☐ Developmental Delay: Communication Skills
☐ Developmental Delay: Social Skills
☐ Family Processes, Altered
☐ Grieving, Anticipatory
☐ Grieving, Dysfunctional
☐ Parenting, Altered: Actual or Potential

☐ Role Performance, Disturbance in
☐ Social Interactions, Impaired
☐ Social Isolation (Rejection)

Sexuality/reproductive

☐ Rape-Trauma Syndrome: Compounded
☐ Rape-Trauma Syndrome: Silent Reaction
☐ Sexual Dysfunction
☐ Sexuality Patterns, Altered

Coping/stress tolerance

☐ Adjustment, Impaired
☐ Coping, Ineffective Individual
☐ Coping, Ineffective Family: Compromised
☐ Coping, Ineffective Family: Disabling
☐ Coping, Family: Potential for Growth
☐ Developmental Delay (Specify area)
☐ Post-Trauma Response
☐ Violence, Potential for (Self-Directed or Directed at Others)

Value/belief

☐ Spiritual Distress (Distress of Human Spirit)

You are now ready to develop a nursing care plan for this client. Use the following blank pages to do so. Then refer to the author's formulation, diagnostic summary, care plan, and summary.

NURSING CARE PLAN

Complete the chart below to develop a nursing care plan for this client.

Discharge outcomes/long-term goals	

Nursing diagnosis	Nursing intervention	

	Predicted outcomes/short-term goals (include time frame)	**Date/signature**

Return to Formulation, page 36

whenever possible, and his speech exhibited much sexual content. He exhibited no coherent suicidal or homicidal ideation, perhaps because he was too disorganized to be volitional around these actions. But because of disinhibition, poor judgment and impulse control, and a history of suicide attempts, he was placed on assault, A.W.O.L., and suicide precautions.

Reader may now complete Recording the Data, Assigning Nursing Diagnoses, and Nursing Care Plan.

FORMULATION

Hal was a chronic psychiatric client who was noncompliant with his medication regimen and typically presented as acutely disorganized, delusional, internally preoccupied, and hyperactive. The details of his psychosocial and familial history were unclear, so exact family and social stressors could not be identified. But obviously, Hal's relationship with his mother had become strained as a result of his illness, a situation which may have in turn acted as a stressor that synergistically exacerbated his symptoms. Given his father's possible manic behavior, Hal's problems may have had genetic roots. If his father had become ill at intervals while with the family, this would have added to familial stressors and even provided "role modeling" for Hal.

Again speculatively, other important precipitants may have included Hal's experience in Vietnam and particularly his extensive use of "hard drugs" during that period. His alcoholism, while appearing to him subjectively as a means of self-treatment, falls into a similar category.

Finally, Hal's current presentation needed to be understood in the context of his status as an "institutionalized" mental health "patient". He had successfully learned to play this role to facilitate social "adaptation" and to create a context for "acting out" his emotions and feelings. After numerous hospitalizations, he had extensive contact with the mental health system; his dependency upon the system served as an "institutional transference" which provided him, at least intermittently, with basic needs. The mental health system provided a backdrop for the unfolding of his illness, accepting or permitting it while at the same time intervening to resolve it.

The ironic duality of Hal's neediness and his skill in getting those needs met indicated a regressive, childlike element. This element also was suggested by his sexual preoccupations and public masturbation (as though he was a little boy showing his parents what he has). This scenario also may have been in part a dramatization of his powerful institutional transference.

Continued on page 43

DIAGNOSTIC SUMMARY FOR HAL

Data	Functional health pattern	Nursing diagnosis
—Exhibits acutely disorganized thought processes (e.g., word salad) —Expresses delusions of grandeur; hallucinations of punitive nature —Brought lit cigarette to eyes during evaluation —Has a history of "acting-out" behavior —Has been drinking heavily during past 2 weeks —In 1984, attempted to hang self in jail; in 1985, superficially lacerated left arm with razor blade during previous hospitalization	Health management/ Health perception	Potential for violence to self and others related to manic dyscontrol secondary to agitation and suicidality
—Stated "I'm Christ and this freckle proves it. I'm going to grab your—and save the world. You're Dracula and you want to suck my blood." —Has been drinking heavily the past 2 weeks —Exhibits pressured, incoherent speech —Is unable to respond to questioning regarding orientation —On formal mental status examination, demonstrated: labile affect; speech consisting of word salad; marked looseness of association and grandiose delusions; response to hallucinations of a punitive nature; nonexistent attention span and concentration; frequent attempts at much sexual content in speech	Cognitive/Perceptual	Altered thought processes related to mania, as manifested by auditory hallucinations, delusions, and sexual preoccupations Potential altered comfort related to recent 2-week alcohol binge
—Has been living in the streets for a number of weeks —Currently charged with disorderly conduct and possession of stolen property —Experiences periodic drinking binges that often herald decompensation —Presents with unkempt hair and beard, neglected personal hygiene	Activity/Exercise	Self-care Deficit: Total related to acute disorganization and hyperactivity secondary to mania Potential altered comfort related to recent 2-week alcohol binge

Continued

Diagnostic Summary for Hal *continued*

Data	Functional health pattern	Nursing diagnosis
—Has been living in the streets for a number of weeks and drinking heavily the past 2 weeks	Nutrition/Metabolic	Potential Altered Nutrition: Less Than Body Requirements related to recently living in streets and increased alcohol consumption
—Demonstrates labile affect fluctuating from angry and hostile to pleasant and cooperative —On formal mental status examination, appeared to be responding to auditory hallucinations of a punitive nature	Self-Perception/Self-Concept	Fear related to decreased sense of security as manifested by punitive auditory hallucinations
—Has been sleep-deprived the past 4 days —Reports frequent restlessness and middle-of-the-night awakenings	Sleep/Rest	Sleep pattern disturbance related to hypervigilance and hyperactivity secondary to mania, as manifested by frequent awakenings
—Has a long history of noncompliance with medications and outpatient follow-up	Cognitive/Perceptual	Knowledge Deficit: medications and legal status related to unknown etiology

NURSING CARE PLAN

Complete the chart below to develop a nursing care plan for this client.

Discharge outcome/long-term goals			
1. HAL WILL BE FREE OF MANIC EPISODES. 2. HE WILL COMPLY WITH HIS MEDICA- TION REGIMEN (LITHIUM). 3. HIS LEGAL CHARGES WILL BE CLARIFIED OR RESOLVED.		4. LONG-TERM RESIDENTIAL OR TREAT- MENT PLACEMENT WILL BE ARRANGED. 5. HAL WILL IMPROVE HIS LEVEL OF SELF-CARE.	

Nursing diagnosis	Nursing intervention	Predicted outcome/short-term goals (include time frame)	Date/signature
POTENTIAL FOR VIOLENCE TO SELF AND OTHERS RELATED TO MANIC DYS- CONTROL SEC- ONDARY TO AGI- TATION AND SUICIDALITY	—PHYSICAL INTERVENTIONS: ·MAINTAIN SECLUSION AND RESTRAINTS P.R.N. ·TAKE SUICIDE PRECAUTIONS —CHEMICAL INTERVENTIONS: ·PROVIDE RAPID TRAN- QUILIZATION ·ADMINISTER P.R.N. MED- ICATIONS ·MONITOR VITAL SIGNS ·OBSERVE FOR EPS AND ADMINISTER MEDICATION AS ORDERED	—HAL WILL NOT HURT HIMSELF WHILE IN THE HOSPITAL —ACUTE AGITATION WILL DECREASE WITHIN 24 HOURS OF ADMISSION	6/8 DWF
	—LITHIUM THERAPY: ·COMPLETE LITHIUM WORKUP ·BEGIN LITHIUM ADMIN- ISTRATION ·ASSESS FOR POSSIBLE TOXIC EFFECTS AND DRUG INTERACTIONS (LITHIUM- PSYCHOTROPICS) ·MONITOR LITHIUM LEVELS EACH MONDAY, WEDNES- DAY AND FRIDAY ·REPORT ADVERSE EFFECTS TO PHYSICIAN PROMPTLY AND DOCUMENT	—WITHIN 1 WEEK, HAL WILL BE COMPLIANT WITH HIS MEDICA- TION REGIMEN —HAL WILL VERBALIZE KNOW- LEDGE OF LITHIUM'S PURPOSE, ACTION, AND SIDE EFFECTS WITHIN 2 WEEKS —HAL WILL NOT EXPERIENCE LITHIUM TOXICITY WHILE IN THE HOSPITAL	
	—DECREASE SENSORY STIMULI: ·MAINTAIN SECLUSION (AS ABOVE) ·PROVIDE TIME-OUT IN ROOM ·PROVIDE A QUIET ROOM FOR ONE-TO-ONE SES- SION AT LEAST EVERY SHIFT	—HAL WILL NOT HURT HIMSELF WHILE IN THE HOSPITAL —HAL WILL REQUIRE NO TIME- OUTS WITHIN 7 DAYS POST- ADMISSION	
ALTERED THOUGHT PROCESSES RE- LATED TO MANIA AS MANIFESTED BY AUDITORY HALLUCINATIONS, DELUSIONS, AND SEXUAL PRE- OCCUPATIONS	—CHEMICAL INTERVENTIONS (SEE INTERVENTIONS UNDER "POTENTIAL FOR VIOLENCE") —VERBAL INTERVENTIONS: ·SET FIRM, CLEAR LIMITS ·MAKE DECISIONS FOR HAL, BUT ALLOW HIM SOME CHOICES ·IDENTIFY UNACCEPTABLE BEHAVIOR AND CONFRONT	—SEE "OUTCOMES/SHORT-TERM GOALS" ABOVE —HAL WILL EXHIBIT NO SEXUALLY INAPPROPRIATE BEHAVIOR WITHIN 1 WEEK —HAL WILL RESPOND TO LIMIT- SETTING WITHIN 2 WEEKS —HAL WILL BE ABLE TO COMPLETE SIMPLE ASSIGNED TASKS	6/8 DWF

Continued

Nursing Care Plan *continued*

Nursing diagnosis	Nursing intervention	Predicted outcome/short-term goals (include time frame)	Date/signature
	HAL WITH SAME, GENTLY STATE CONSEQUENCES OF ACTIONS · ASSIGN SHORT, ATTAINABLE TASKS · ORIENT HAL TO REALITY EVERY SHIFT · REINFORCE AND PRAISE ACCEPTABLE BEHAVIOR		
SELF-CARE DEFICITS: TOTAL RELATED TO ACUTE DISORGANIZATION AND HYPERACTIVITY SECONDARY TO MANIA	—SET UP ROUTINE FOR BATHING, SHAVING, ORAL CARE, BOWEL HABITS, AND DRESSING —SUPERVISE HAL UNTIL THIS PATTERN IS ESTABLISHED —ROUTINIZE MEAL SCHEDULE AND ONE-TO-ONE AT MEALTIMES IN QUIET AREA. INTEGRATE HAL SLOWLY WITH OTHER CLIENTS FOR MEALS	—HAL WILL PERFORM ADLs ROUTINELY WITH SUPERVISION BY THE END OF THE FIRST WEEK OF HOSPITALIZATION; WITHOUT SUPERVISION, BY THE END OF THE SECOND WEEK —HAL WILL MAINTAIN NUTRITIONAL INTAKE AT 80 PERCENT OF REGULAR DIET WITHIN 5 DAYS OF HOSPITALIZATION	6/8 JWF
POTENTIAL ALTERED NUTRITION: LESS THAN BODY REQUIREMENTS RELATED TO RECENTLY LIVING IN STREETS AND INCREASED ALCOHOL CONSUMPTION	—OBTAIN DIET HISTORY —MONITOR FOOD AND FLUID CONSUMPTION DURING MEALS —ASSIST HAL WITH CHOOSING FOODS FROM ALL FOUR FOOD GROUPS	—HAL WILL MAINTAIN AN ADEQUATE FOOD AND FLUID INTAKE DURING HOSPITALIZATION	6/8 JWF
POTENTIAL ALTERED COMFORT RELATED TO RECENT 2-WEEK ALCOHOL BINGE	—DOCUMENT SIGNS AND SYMPTOMS OF WITHDRAWAL. NOTIFY PHYSICIAN IF PRESENT —MONITOR VITAL SIGNS EVERY SHIFT —TEACH HAL TO CONTROL DISCOMFORT THROUGH RELAXATION EXERCISES	—WITHIN 3 DAYS, HAL WILL REPORT DISCOMFORT TO NURSE AND IMPLEMENT RELAXATION TECHNIQUES	6/5 JWF
FEAR RELATED TO DECREASED SENSE OF SECURITY AS MANIFESTED BY PUNITIVE AUDITORY HALLUCINATIONS	—IF HAL IS ABLE TO VERBALIZE, TALK ABOUT HIS FEELINGS, GIVING PERMISSION AND EXPLORING PRECIPITANTS —IMPLEMENT RELAXATION TECHNIQUES —PROVIDE PROTECTION FROM PEERS: · SET LIMITS · PROVIDE INFORMATION · CALIBRATE RELATIONS	—HAL WILL EXHIBIT DECREASED NEEDINESS, AS INDICATED BY DECREASED FREQUENCY OF QUESTIONS AND REQUESTS —HAL WILL WORK THROUGH CONFLICTS WITH PEERS WITH ASSISTANCE FROM STAFF WITHIN 1 WEEK AND UNSUPERVISED WITHIN 2 WEEKS	6/8 JWF

Nursing diagnosis	Nursing intervention	Predicted outcome/short-term goals (include time frame)	Date/signature
	WITH PEERS		
	—PROVIDE HAL WITH FRE-		
	QUENT REASSURANCES		
	THAT HE IS IN A SAFE		
	ENVIRONMENT AND MAK-		
	ING POSITIVE MOVES		
	TOWARD HEALTH		
	—WHEN HAL IS LUCID, EX-		
	PLORE THE RELATIONSHIP		
	BETWEEN HIS FEARS AND		
	THE OCCURENCE OF AUDI-		
	TORY HALLUCINATIONS		
SLEEP PATTERN DISTURBANCE RELATED TO HYPER-VIGILANCE AND HYPERACTIVITY SECONDARY TO MANIA, AS MANIFESTED BY FREQUENT AWAKENINGS	—CHEMICAL INTERVEN-TIONS, PRNs AS ORDERED (SEE ABOVE UNDER "POTENTIAL FOR VIOLENCE") —SCHEDULE HOUR-OF-SLEEP INTERVENTIONS ·IMPLEMENT RELAXATION EXERCISES ·ORIENT HAL TO TIME ·REASSURE HAL THAT RELAXATION AND/OR MEDICATIONS WILL BE EFFECTIVE ·SET GENTLE, FIRM LIMITS FOR "LIGHTS OUT" ·REINFORCE HAL'S AWARENESS OF STAFF AVAILABILITY THROUGHOUT NIGHT ·MONITOR HAL'S ACTUAL HOURS OF SLEEP THROUGH ½-HOUR ROUNDS	—HAL WILL SLEEP 6 HOURS PER NIGHT AFTER 5 DAYS	6/8 DWF
	·APPROACH TREATMENT TEAM REGARDING REFERRING HAL TO A SLEEP DISORDER CLINIC FOR TREATMENT OF LONG-TERM SLEEP PATTERN DISTURBANCE	—IF ORDERED BY THE TREATMENT TEAM, HAL WILL AGREE TO AN EVALUATION BY A SLEEP DISORDER CLINIC	
KNOWLEDGE DEFICIT: MEDICATIONS AND LEGAL STATUS RELATED TO UNKNOWN ETIOLOGY	—GENERAL INTERVENTIONS: ·EXPLORE COPING MECH-ANISMS ·TEACH PROBLEM-SOLVING TECHNIQUES ·IDENTIFY SPECIFIC PROBLEMS ·HELP ARRANGE PRIORITIES —PROVIDE INFORMATION ON LITHIUM: ·RATIONALE FOR USE ·DOSAGE AND SCHEDULE ·SIGNS OF TOXICITY AND SIDE EFFECTS	—WITHIN 2 WEEKS, HAL WILL BE ABLE TO CONTRACT TO COMPLY WITH MEDICATION AND ABLE TO VERBALIZE RATIONALE, SCHEDULE AND ADVERSE EFFECTS, AND TOXICITY OF MEDICATION	6/8 DWF

Continued

Nursing Care Plan *continued*

Nursing diagnosis	Nursing intervention	Predicted outcome/short-term goals (include time frame)	Date/signature
	·ROUTINE LITHIUM LEVELS		
	—ENCOURAGE HAL TO COME TO STAFF WHEN MEDICATION IS SCHEDULED		
	—CLARIFY HAL'S LEGAL STATUS:	—WITHIN 1 WEEK HAL WILL BE ABLE TO REPEAT RATIONALE FOR CONSERVATORSHIP AND DISCHARGE PLANS	
	·EXPLAIN MENTAL HEALTH HOLD AND CONSERVATORSHIP		
	·EXPLAIN LEGAL CHARGES AND COURT DATES		
	—REPEAT TEACHING EVERY DAY AND EVALUATE RESULTS	—HAL WILL EXHIBIT A DECREASE IN THE NUMBER OF QUESTIONS ABOUT LEGAL ISSUES WITHIN 2 WEEKS	
	—WHEN HAL IS LUCID, LINK HIS NONCOMPLIANCE WITH TREATMENT TO FREQUENT EXACERBATIONS		

In summary, Hal's problem involved florid behavioral distortions and tempestuous emotional disturbances, which were registered in delusions and symbolized in aspects of his overt actions. Once his neediness and regression were addressed, he resolved, and his potential for self-care improved. His ability to draw staff into alliances with him, and the positive countertransferences that resulted, provided the bridge for his recompensation.

SUMMARY

Nursing care for Hal on admission focused on his acute mania and targeted the following problem areas: disorganized behavior, impaired personal safety and hygiene, altered sleep patterns, perceptual distortions, delusions and hallucinations, and possible suicidal impulses. It also included the management of his physical comfort and nutritional status.

The immediate management of Hal's acute symptoms included suicide precautions with one-to-one attention from nursing staff, seclusion (to limit stimuli), supportive social intervention, and an aggressive yet carefully titrated use of medication. During the first 3 days of his hospitalization, Hal remained in his room and continued to be labile and irritable. He repeatedly disrobed and pulled the linen from his bed to the floor. He masturbated frequently, and occasionally attempted to submerge his head in the toilet bowl. (However, it is not clear whether this gesture was suicidal in nature or merely a result of his disorganization and poor impulse control.) Attempts to verbally redirect him produced control for only a period of 1 day. He did not sleep for 3 days, in spite of repeated doses of Haldol. Thus he was briefly placed on lorazepam (Ativan) in order to decrease his agitation.

Hal's psychosocial presentation or style during hospitalization proved highly important in his relations with staff and peers and critical to his eventual integration into the milieu. While he appeared needy and sometimes demanding in spite of his symptoms, he nevertheless was skillful in forging attachments and alliances with staff and became a favorite client of the nursing staff. As he recompensated, he displayed considerable wit and appeared earnest and well-intentioned. These traits were important strengths. As a result, the nursing staff became well-invested in his care, although the negative side of his style caused them to label him as "manipulative" and "a user of the system."

On admission and for 10 days afterwards Hal remained separate or partially separate from the milieu, but became a participant in unit activities in carefully graded steps after his lithium level reached 1.23 and he more easily tolerated the company of others. As his sleep patterns improved and his delusions and hallucinations resolved, he became sociable and easily manageable on the unit.

For Hal's long-term care and discharge planning, the nursing staff needed to address residential placement, social support services, medication compliance, and the problems associated with his legal status. Because of Hal's repeated failures to maintain himself in the community, outpatient treatment was deemed unrealistic. The likelihood that he could complete his jail term (if sentenced) without decompensating seemed slim, since he could not be constrained to take medications in that setting. Hence, the staff determined that continued hospitalization was indicated, pending placement in a long-term care facility. Medication compliance would continue to be a major treatment objective. Although this plan may be seen as colluding with Hal's "institutional transference" and potential dependence on the mental health delivery system, it seemed the best option. He was therefore placed on a permanent conservatorship.

The particular context of treatment constituted by the realities of an inpatient security unit had ambiguous implications for Hal's hospitalization. The added "structure" afforded by architectural barriers not found on regular inpatient units, the added restrictions, and the uninterrupted presence of security staff might be considered helpful in "containing" Hal's initial agitation and disorganization. While there may be some truth in this perception, this same "regime of power" along with that of the psychiatric setting actually added to Hal's anxieties during treatment. In particular, the guards' uniforms roused in him fears of being hurt. Therefore, social interventions in the form of frequent reassurances were a necessary component of his management on the unit. Hal's legal involvements and court proceedings, which were also stressors, were handled in a reality-based fashion with ongoing teaching and discussion of legal matters.

Following the acute stage of Hal's disorder, treatment focused on encouraging graded activities. At this point, continued supportive interventions helped facilitate Hal's gradual entry into the milieu as he became able to tolerate increasing social contact. Planning for Hal's discharge and long-term care had already begun soon after his admission and was finalized as his functional baseline was assessed. In general, this planning was based on this assessment, together with information from Hal's psychiatric history.

SELECTED BIBLIOGRAPHY

Harris, E. "Lithium," *American Journal of Nursing* 81(7):1310-15, 1981.

Jampala, V.C. "Mania with Emotional Blunting: Affective Disorder or Schizophrenia," *American Journal of Psychiatry* 142(5):608-12, 1985.

Kraepalin, E. *Manic Depressive Insanity and Paranoia*. New York: Arno, 1976.

Lazar, A. "Manic Behavior," in *Outpatient Psychiatry*. Edited by Lazare, A. Baltimore: Williams & Wilkins Co., 1979.

Modell, J.G. "Inpatient Clinical Trial of Lorazepam for the Management of Manic Agitation," *Journal of Clinical Psychopharmacology* 5(2):109-13, 1985.

U.S. National Institutes of Health, Clinical Center, Nursing Department. *Nursing Care of the Manic Depressive Patient*. Washington, D.C.: U.S. Government Printing Office, 1973.

Wadeson, H.S., and Bunney, W.E., Jr. "Manic Depressive Art," *Journal of Nervous and Mental Disease* 150:215-31, 1970.

Wittenborn, J.R., and Weiss, W. "Patients Diagnosed as Manic-Depressive Psychosis—Manic State," *Journal of Consulting Psychology* 16:193-98, 1952.

Wolpert, E.A. *Manic Depressive Illness*. New York: International University Press, 1977.

Mrs. Moore:
Bipolar, Depressed

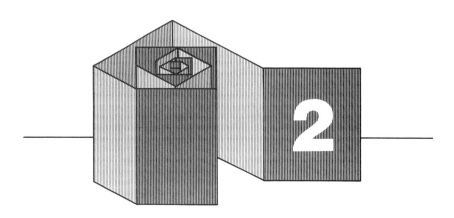

Billie Dixon Barringer, MA, RN

A client with manic-depressive illness (bipolar disorder) experiences recurrent mood swings that affect functioning in interpersonal and occupational relations. Severe exacerbations usually require hospitalization to stabilize the client in order to facilitate a return to the community. Frequently, exacerbations result from stresses of everyday life that interrupt the client's equilibrium. In this case, the loss of her job caused the client to reexperience previously experienced depressive symptoms. Her tenuous self-concept was damaged, as manifested by isolation and suicidal ideation.

The nurse's major role in this case involved an assessment of the client's previous coping and a thorough evaluation of her self-concept. Once this was determined, the nurse was able to plan interventions aimed at boosting the client's self-concept and teaching her effective communication and problem-solving skills to use in the future.

CASE STUDY

Mrs. Moore, a 45-year-old white female, was brought by a neighbor to the psychiatric hospital for treatment of bipolar disorder, depressed type.

While being escorted to her room, Mrs. Moore became resistive and loudly accused her neighbor of tricking her. She then began to cry and said she wished she were dead. Once Mrs. Moore was settled in her room, the nurse was able to conduct an admission interview.

Mrs. Moore felt her present problem began following her husband's death 2 years previously. She had been a homemaker for the previous 18 years, but her husband's death brought the prospect of financial insecurity, and she took a job as a typist for an automobile dealership. Mrs. Moore reported insecurity and lack of confidence in this return to the work force. Her emphasis during this time was on job success; she lost interest in gardening and sewing, two of her previously favorite pastimes. When a co-worker resigned, Mrs. Moore was faced with double work. To catch up, she went to work at 5:00 a.m., worked overtime, and did not stop for coffee breaks or lunch. She stayed awake nights worrying about getting the work done. She began suspecting her employer of talking about her behind her back and of thinking ill of her. After a confrontation, Mrs. Moore was fired.

But her nervousness and agitation continued at home. She was unable to stop thinking about her failure, even at night, which caused her to sleep poorly. She was fearful and usually isolated herself in the house. She refused to talk to anyone and would not take care of herself. Her friend, Mrs. Thomas, reported that sometimes when in the company of others, Mrs. Moore would become angry with seemingly no provocation and flee from the room. Finally, Mrs. Thomas talked Mrs. Moore into seeking treatment at the psychiatric hospital.

Along with feelings of failure, Mrs. Moore expressed her conviction that hospitalization proves her inadequacy. ("I can't even take care of myself—I have to have you take care of me. I'm ashamed....I don't have a say in my life anymore.") When questioned about her expectations of this hospitalization, Mrs. Moore replied that she wanted to learn to live at an "even pace," to cope with pressures of her present life, and to do something productive with herself.

Mrs. Moore's history includes a 6-week hospitalization in the state psychiatric facility at age 21. This admission followed her resignation from college, when she became despondent and threatened to kill herself with a knife. At the state facility she was diagnosed as having an adjustment reaction, treated with imipramine (Tofranil), and then released. She described herself as having "ups and downs" since then. She stated that she has always had difficulty getting along with others as a result of her erratic behavior. She felt this was because she is basically a "bad" person.

Mrs. Moore was admitted to a psychiatric hospital once again at age 37, following a hysterectomy. Upon this admission, she was aggressive, elated, and hyperactive. During the previous month, she had spent $2,000, an amount her family could not afford, on office equipment because she was writing three novels and needed a place to work.

Throughout this period, she survived on 4 hours of sleep a night. Finally, after threatening to burn down the house, she again entered the state hospital, where she received a diagnosis of manic-depressive reaction, manic type. Following treatment with Lithane and Thorazine and extensive individual psychotherapy, she returned home with plans for follow-up at the mental health center. She felt so well that she decided she needed neither the medication nor the clinical visits and stopped going. Her mood swings continued, but in manageable amounts.

No obvious medical problems contributed to Mrs. Moore's illness. She admitted to the occasional use of excessive amounts of alcohol during those times when she felt "high." She also described a weight loss of 20 pounds over the past month, which she attributed to "loss of appetite." She had not slept at all for 4 consecutive nights, and had been sleeping poorly for the previous 2 weeks.

Mrs. Moore's family history revealed multiple stress related to the responsibilities she was burdened with as a child. Both of Mrs. Moore's parents worked in order to support and advance the family in its middle-class community. As the oldest of five children, Mrs. Moore took care of her siblings and was performing many domestic chores by age 6. ("I can remember standing on a chair to do the dishes.") She described her parents as strict disciplinarians. Both of her parents shared similar lower-middle class, Protestant backgrounds. Her father worked for an insurance company, her mother taught elementary school. According to Mrs. Moore, her mother was the stronger of the two parents, although both shared in disciplining the children. Her parents had high aspirations for their family, worked hard, and managed money cautiously. Although Mrs. Moore never felt unloved, she never felt close to her parents. She held a great deal of respect for them and yearned for their approval. She expressed feeling closer to her brothers and sisters but refused to give information about them during the interview, saying that she "didn't want them involved."

Because of this and the family's modest financial circumstances, the children's basic needs were met only marginally. ("I never had the things other children had, like new clothes.") Her school years were unhappy; she felt others were making fun of her. She experienced alternating spurts of productivity and nonproductivity in the student role, and was seen several times by the school counselor for her inconsistent behavior. She had a few friends and occasional dates. After graduating from high school, she completed 1 year of college, then resigned during her sophomore year, before her first hospitalization. She worked for 1 year as a typist before marrying Mr. Moore. She described the marriage as happy. ("He was a good provider, and I had no worries.") Her life evolved around her husband and her home, to the exclusion of most other interests.

Mrs. Moore's family history also revealed that her maternal grandmother suffered from a "curious nerve problem" that caused her to have "complete mood swings." Mrs. Moore felt that she was "much like" this grandmother.

Mrs. Moore's mental status examination revealed a person oriented in four spheres with intact remote, recent, and immediate memory. The nurse who greeted Mrs. Moore found a tall, thin woman with dark circles under her eyes who was clearly agitated and irritable, unable to sit or stand still, and easily distracted. At one point, she yelled at the nurse, "Stop asking me all these stupid questions." She was clad in wrinkled, baggy slacks and a coffee-stained blouse, wore no make-up, and looked unhappy. Her personal hygiene was poor, with a foul body odor, oily hair, and dirty fingernails. Her thought processes appeared undisturbed, except for excessive worrying and negative thinking, which caused her to evaluate her present situation from the gloomy side. Abstracting ability was evident, but problem-solving was impaired. Mrs. Moore was resistive and suspicious during the beginning of the interview, but relaxed as the interview progressed. The nurse found her somewhat difficult to talk to because of her guardedness, especially around issues of siblings.

Reader may now complete Recording the Data, Assigning Nursing Diagnoses, and Nursing Care Plan.

FORMULATION

Mrs. Moore's major problem seemed to be one of ineffective individual coping that began following her husband's death. The pathology evidenced in her history indicated a disturbance in the affective sphere. According to Wolpert (1980), an affective reaction refers to "genetically controlled disorders in which spontaneous shifts of activity cycles cause typical symptoms of the disorder. Alternately, specific psychogenic factors meaning 'loss' act as triggers and can precipitate an episode, either manic or depressed." Mrs. Moore's disorder consistently had been set off by losses: an early symbolic loss of her parents due to their demands on her as the oldest child, a loss of self-esteem from her college failure, a hysterectomy, and her husband's death.

Essential features of the depressed type include a history of a previous manic episode; a depressed mood; loss of interest in usual activities; the inability to experience pleasure; sleep, appetite, and other somatic disturbances; weight change; psychomotor agitation or retardation; diminished energy level, feelings of guilt or worthlessness; and suicidal ideation. Associated features include depressed facies, tearfulness, anx-

Continued on page 56

RECORDING THE DATA

After you have read the case, cluster significant data into functional health patterns.

Health management/health perception ─────────────────────

───

───

───

───

Nutritional/metabolic ───────────────────────────

───

───

───

Elimination ──────────────────────────────

───

───

───

Activity/exercise ─────────────────────────────

───

───

───

Cognitive/perceptual ────────────────────────────

───

───

───

Sleep/rest _____

_____

_____

_____

Self-perception/self-concept _____

_____

_____

_____

Role relationship _____

_____

_____

_____

Sexuality/reproductive _____

_____

_____

_____

Coping/stress tolerance _____

_____

_____

_____

Value/belief _____

_____

_____

_____

ASSIGNING NURSING DIAGNOSES

Use your clustered data to select appropriate nursing diagnoses.

Health perception/health management

- [ ] Growth and Development, Altered (see Developmental Delay)
- [ ] Health Maintenance, Altered
- [ ] Infection, Potential for
- [ ] Injury (Trauma): Potential for
- [ ] Noncompliance (Specify)
- [ ] Poisoning: Potential for
- [ ] Suffocation: Potential for

Nutritional/metabolic

- [ ] Body Temperature, Potential Alteration in
- [ ] Developmental Delay: Physical Growth and Development
- [ ] Fluid Volume, Altered: Excess or Excess Fluid Volume
- [ ] Fluid Volume Deficit, Actual
- [ ] Fluid Volume Deficit, Potential
- [ ] Nutrition, Altered: Less Than Body Requirements or Nutritional Deficit (Specify)
- [ ] Nutrition, Altered: More Than Body Requirements or Exogenous Obesity
- [ ] Nutrition, Altered: Potential for More Than Body Requirements or Potential for Obesity
- [ ] Oral Mucous Membrane, Altered
- [ ] Skin Integrity, Impaired or Skin Breakdown
- [ ] Skin Integrity, Impaired or Potential Skin Breakdown
- [ ] Swallowing, Impaired or Uncompensated Swallowing Impairment
- [ ] Tissue Integrity, Impaired

Elimination

- [ ] Bowel Elimination, Altered: Constipation
- [ ] Bowel Elimination, Altered: Diarrhea
- [ ] Bowel Elimination, Altered: Incontinence
- [ ] Developmental Delay: Bowel/Bladder Control
- [ ] Incontinence: Functional
- [ ] Incontinence: Reflex
- [ ] Incontinence: Stress
- [ ] Incontinence: Total
- [ ] Incontinence: Urge
- [ ] Urinary Elimination, Altered Patterns of
- [ ] Urinary Retention

Activity/exercise

- [ ] Activity Intolerance
- [ ] Activity Intolerance, Potential
- [ ] Airway Clearance, Ineffective
- [ ] Breathing Pattern, Ineffective
- [ ] Cardiac Output, Altered: Decreased
- [ ] Developmental Delay: Mobility
- [ ] Developmental Delay: Self-Care Skills
- [ ] Diversional Activity Deficit
- [ ] Gas Exchange, Impaired
- [ ] Home Maintenance Management, Impaired (Mild, Moderate, Severe, Potential, Chronic)
- [ ] Mobility, Impaired Physical
- [ ] Self-Care Deficit: Feeding
- [ ] Self-Care Deficit: Bathing/Hygiene
- [ ] Self-Care Deficit: Dressing/Grooming
- [ ] Self-Care Deficit: Toileting
- [ ] Self-Care Deficit: Total
- [ ] Tissue Perfusion, Altered: (Specify)

Sleep/rest

- [ ] Sleep Pattern Disturbance

Cognitive/perceptual

- [ ] Comfort, Altered: Pain
- [ ] Comfort, Altered: Chronic Pain

☐ Developmental Delay: (Specify Cognitive Area; attention, decision making, etc.)
☐ Hypothermia
☐ Hyperthermia
☐ Knowledge Deficit (Specify)
☐ Sensory-Perceptual Alteration: Input Excess or Sensory Overload
☐ Sensory-Perceptual Alteration: Input Deficit or Sensory Deprivation
☐ Thermoregulation, Ineffective
☐ Thought Processes, Altered
☐ Unilateral Neglect

Self-perception/self-concept

☐ Anxiety
☐ Body Image Disturbance
☐ Fear
☐ Hopelessness
☐ Personal Identity Confusion
☐ Powerlessness (Severe, Low, Moderate)
☐ Self-Esteem Disturbance

Role relationship

☐ Communication, Impaired Verbal
☐ Developmental Delay: Communication Skills
☐ Developmental Delay: Social Skills
☐ Family Processes, Altered
☐ Grieving, Anticipatory
☐ Grieving, Dysfunctional
☐ Parenting, Altered: Actual or Potential

☐ Role Performance, Disturbance in
☐ Social Interactions, Impaired
☐ Social Isolation (Rejection)

Sexuality/reproductive

☐ Rape-Trauma Syndrome: Compounded
☐ Rape-Trauma Syndrome: Silent Reaction
☐ Sexual Dysfunction
☐ Sexuality Patterns, Altered

Coping/stress tolerance

☐ Adjustment, Impaired
☐ Coping, Ineffective Individual
☐ Coping, Ineffective Family: Compromised
☐ Coping, Ineffective Family: Disabling
☐ Coping, Family: Potential for Growth
☐ Developmental Delay (Specify area)
☐ Post-Trauma Response
☐ Violence, Potential for (Self-Directed or Directed at Others)

Value/belief

☐ Spiritual Distress (Distress of Human Spirit)

You are now ready to develop a nursing care plan for this client. Use the following blank pages to do so. Then refer to the author's formulation, diagnostic summary, care plan, and summary.

NURSING CARE PLAN

Complete the chart below to develop a nursing care plan for this client.

Discharge outcomes/long-term goals	

Nursing diagnosis	Nursing intervention	

	Predicted outcomes/short-term goals (include time frame)	**Date/signature**

Return to Formulation, page 49

iety, irritability, fearfulness, brooding, phobic attacks, paranoid symptoms, and delusions of poverty (Wolpert, 1980). Mrs. Moore exhibited all of the essential features and most of the associated features of the depressed type.

Mrs. Moore's overall mood was characterized by sadness and anger, with no evidence of pleasurable pursuits that might have served to counteract it. Her suspiciousness and accusations seemed to represent her internal anger, which interfered with her degree of insight. Her level of self-esteem was low; she described herself as a failure and characterized her situation as hopeless. Her persistent verbalization of the wish to die, plus her agitation, placed her at risk for potential self-injury.

Mrs. Moore's general appearance, sleep disturbance, and excessive weight loss indicated a decreased capacity for self-care, possibly due to her distractibility and agitation. She was unable to carry out responsible self-management (i.e., activities of daily living and work functions).

Mrs. Moore demonstrated a limited degree of insight into the basic facts about her illness; rather, she thought of herself as being "bad." She also demonstrated the overuse of the psychological defense mechanisms of projection and reaction formation, which contributed to her lack of insight. Largely, she did not seem to understand how her own nonassertive behavior contributed to the overall problem.

Mrs. Moore lived a lonely life with limited interpersonal contacts. Her negative way of thinking and her aggressiveness when hypomanic further diminished her social attractiveness. She neither had nor desired sexual contact although her capacity to trust and to love were evident in her history.

Mrs. Moore's only interaction with the community included occasionally attending church. She was dependent in her previous work setting, seeking approval by taking on additional projects and being unable to say no to excessive demands. This lack of autonomy may have served as a contributing factor to her isolation within the community. At a time when she needed to be productive and creative, a lack of confidence in her problem-solving skills prevented her from accomplishing many of the normal tasks associated with middle age.

In spite of Mrs. Moore's pessimism, she did have several strengths. She gardened and sewed for diversion. Mrs. Thomas, her neighbor and only friend, provided needed support. Although pessimistic, she had no serious cognitive disturbances. Finally, she possessed work skills.

Several factors may have accounted for Mrs. Moore's problem. Since one of her grandmothers suffered from mood swings, one basic factor could be heredity. Some evidence exists that bipolar affective disorder is transmitted by an X-linked dominant gene (Wetzel, 1984).

Likewise, the possible chemical basis of her problem should not be overlooked. Low levels of serotonin and norepinephrine have been implicated in bipolar disorder. A low serotonin level may be a predisposing factor to the development of the problem, and an imbalance of norepinephrine determines its direction. Depressive clients seem to have reduced norepinephrine levels; manics, increased norepinephrine levels (Dixson, 1981). Mrs. Moore did not understand the relationship of this chemical imbalance to her illness; rather, she blamed herself for being a "bad" person. While identifying her problem as a chemical imbalance would not negate her need to work on other relevant problems, knowing the facts would help relieve her self-critical tendency and promote the understanding necessary to help her recognize and prevent relapse.

Another reason for Mrs. Moore's problem is related to early object loss. According to Stuart and Sundeen (1983), two events apply: loss during childhood, which predisposes to adult depression; and separation in adult life, which results in sufficient stress to precipitate a depression. In Mrs. Moore's case, high parental expectations, harsh discipline, and the assumption of excess responsibility at an inappropriate maturational level may have caused her to perceive her parents as withdrawing from her. Love and hate, along with conformity to gain approval, are normal responses under these conditions. According to Dixson (1981), people who conform to such a complete degree tend to develop problems: they fail to learn to rely on themselves for problem solving, fail to develop sufficient trust in themselves, and experience anxiety from living in fear of further disapproval or loss. Mrs. Moore, having grown to adulthood with these characteristics, found herself vulnerable when Mr. Moore died. Therefore, Mrs. Moore's nursing treatment should be directed toward improving her problem-solving skills, improving her self-concept in the areas of confidence and self-esteem, and promoting self-understanding.

Of equal importance is the relationship of anger to Mrs. Moore's symptoms. The inability to deal effectively with anger can be explained from a psychodynamic point of view. Aggressive feelings result from object loss; however, direct expression of this anger is unsafe and forbidden by societal mores. Therefore, the aggression, which must be released in some way, becomes turned inward upon the self. Although initial theories considered inverted rage as a predisposing factor of depression (Freud, 1924), rage turned inward is now considered at times to be related to cognitive changes caused by the illness (Akiskal and McKinney, 1975). If the client never learns appropriate methods of expressing anger, therapy must be directed toward finding socially acceptable ways to release such anger. Suicide prevention receives high priority if the client presents suicidal ideation or intent as a coping strategy.

Mrs. Moore also exhibited a marked lack of autonomy. In becoming autonomous, a person learns to act independently, to make decisions, and to manipulate the environment in ways that bring positive rewards rather than the negative outcomes of shame and doubt. A lack of autonomy produces feelings of being unable to control events, helplessness, and powerlessness. Intervention for Mrs. Moore therefore needed to encourage autonomy and responsible assertive behaviors.

Failure to master an early conflict affects subsequent stages of development. Upon admission, Mrs. Moore was in the generativity versus stagnation stage (Erikson, 1963). Although this should be a productive phase, involving such tasks as developing satisfying social relationships, taking on civic and social responsibilities, and finding ways of utilizing leisure time, she was in fact suffering a crisis of stagnation, probably because of her dependent life-style. Thus, nursing interventions needed to be directed toward maximizing her potentials and encouraging her to take on the tasks of middle life.

Another etiology involves Mrs. Moore's family system. Within any family, roles are developed and played out by members. Harmony exists in a family as long as members live up to each other's expectations. Mrs. Moore's parents had high expectations of her at a very early age. She conformed to these expectations in order to survive and to gain approval, thus keeping the family in equilibrium at the expense of her own wishes, feelings, and desires.

Throughout her marriage, Mrs. Moore seemed to cope well. A closer look suggests that her dependency was allowed in that situation and that her own coping was enhanced by her husband's strength. In this manner, her family actually may have served her adversely, leaving her defenseless when her husband died. His death, following years of role complementarity, left quite a void in her life. Additional pressures and responsibilities caused by her need to take on additional roles are clearly evident. Stuart and Sundeen (1983) confirm the relevancy of role strain to affective states. Therefore the nursing staff needed to aim their interventions at assisting Mrs. Moore in her assumption of the work role and other social roles.

A final explanation for Mrs. Moore's depression draws from her sociocultural orientation. Wolpert (1980) describes the family of origin as upwardly mobile, both socially and economically, yet isolated in its community. Children are expected to conform to high standards of conduct and success to validate the family. Mrs. Moore's childhood recollections indicated the existence of this variable in her life. In addition, her reports of feeling inferior to other children in the community confirm

Continued on page 64

DIAGNOSTIC SUMMARY FOR MRS. MOORE

Data	Functional health pattern	Nursing diagnosis
—Reported being unable to stop thinking about her failure even at night; admits to not having slept well for 2 weeks —Has not slept for 4 consecutive nights —In the past, averaged 4 hours of sleep a night during "manic" episodes	Sleep/Rest	Sleep pattern disturbance related to hyperactivity and depression secondary to bipolar disorder
—Says she wishes she were dead —Feels problems began with husband's death 2 years ago —Has lost interest in favorite pastimes —Feels she is a "bad" person	Coping/Stress Tolerance	Potential for injury to self related to suicidal ideation secondary to feelings of hopelessness and worthlessness
—Worked overtime, did not stop for coffee breaks or lunch —Experienced a weight loss of 20 pounds over the past month; attributes this to "loss of appetite"	Nutritional/Metabolic	Altered nutrition; less than body requirements related to recent skipping of meals secondary to lack of interest in eating as part of depressed state
—Has become fearful and isolates herself in her house —Displays irritability; at one point yells at the nurse to "Stop asking me all of these stupid questions" —When in the company of others, often would become angry and flee from the room	Coping/Stress Tolerance	Ineffective individual coping, related to unknown etiology, as manifested by loss of control of anger and deficient problem-solving skills
—Expresses feelings of insecurity and lack of confidence in return to work —Believes the hospitalization proves her inadequacy: "I can't even take care of myself—I have to have you take care of me. I'm ashamed.... I don't have a say in my life anymore."	Self-Perception/Self-Concept	Self-esteem disturbance related to negative thinking secondary to feelings of hopelessness
—Has lost interest in gardening and sewing, two of her favorite pastimes —Was recently fired from her job	Activity/Exercise	Diversional activity deficit related to nonmotivation secondary to depression
—Has become fearful and usually isolates herself in her room —Refuses to talk to anyone —When in the company of others, often would become angry and flee from the room —Has only one friend, Mrs. Thomas	Role Relationship	Social isolation related to angry interpersonal style and lack of community supports

NURSING CARE PLAN

Complete the chart below to develop a nursing care plan for this client.

Discharge outcome/long-term goals	
I. MRS. MOORE WILL INCREASE HER COPING ABILITY AS EVIDENCED BY: — IDENTIFYING BEHAVIORS THAT INHIBIT SOCIALIZATION. — DEMONSTRATING IMPROVEMENT IN	SELF-CONCEPT THROUGH ALTERING NEGATIVE THINKING. — REINTEGRATING INTO THE COMMUNITY, AS EVIDENCED BY PARTICIPATION IN COMMUNITY AGENCY ACTIVITIES.

Nursing diagnosis	Nursing intervention	Predicted outcome/short-term goals (include time frame)	Date/signature
SLEEP PATTERN DISTURBANCE RELATED TO AGITATION AND DEPRESSION SECONDARY TO BIPOLAR DISORDER	— ASSIGN MRS. MOORE TO A PRIVATE ROOM — PROVIDE A QUIET AND NON-STIMULATING ENVIRONMENT — PROVIDE A WINDING-DOWN PERIOD PRIOR TO SLEEP — ENCOURAGE REDUCTION IN INTAKE OF COFFEE, COLA, TEA; RECORD INTAKE — PROVIDE HOT MILK AT HOUR OF SLEEP AS NEEDED — HAVE MRS. MOORE TAKE A BATH OR SHOWER AT HOUR OF SLEEP AS NEEDED — HAVE MRS. MOORE RETIRE AND ARISE AT SAME TIME EACH DAY — ENCOURAGE HER PARTICIPATION IN DAYTIME ACTIVITIES AND DISCOURAGE SLEEP DURING THE DAY — OBSERVE AND RECORD HER ACTUAL HOURS OF SLEEP	— MRS. MOORE WILL GET 8 HOURS OF UNDISTURBED SLEEP WITHIN 24 HOURS	1/21 BB
POTENTIAL FOR INJURY TO SELF RELATED TO SUICIDAL IDEATION SECONDARY TO FEELINGS OF HOPELESSNESS AND WORTHLESSNESS	— ALERT ALL PERSONNEL TO MRS. MOORE'S SUICIDE OBSERVATION STATUS — ASSIGN NURSING STAFF TO WATCH HER AT ALL TIMES — REDUCE ENVIRONMENTAL HAZARDS (REMOVE POTENTIALLY DANGEROUS OBJECTS FROM ENVIRONMENT) — AVOID PROVIDING MRS. MOORE WITH SECONDARY GAIN TO SUICIDAL THINKING — IF SELF-INJURY OCCURS, BE PREPARED TO DEAL WITH IT IN A MATTER-OF-FACT MANNER SO AS NOT TO REINFORCE THE SUICIDAL ACT	— MRS. MOORE WILL NOT HARM HERSELF DURING THE HOSPITAL STAY	1/21 BB

MRS. MOORE: BIPOLAR, DEPRESSED

Nursing diagnosis	Nursing intervention	Predicted outcome/short-term goals (include time frame)	Date/signature
ALTERED NUTRI- TION; LESS THAN BODY REQUIRE- MENTS RELATED TO RECENT SKIPPING OF MEALS SECOND- ARY TO LACK OF INTEREST IN EATING AS PART OF DEPRESSED STATE	—DETERMINE MRS. MOORE'S FOOD LIKES AND DISLIKES; HELP HER CHOOSE FOODS FROM ALL FOUR FOOD GROUPS —MONITOR AND RECORD HER FOOD INTAKE —WEIGH HER WEEKLY AND RECORD —WHILE MRS. MOORE IS AGITATED, HAVE HER EAT ALONE —ENCOURAGE EATING AND PROMOTE HER ATTENTION TO EATING —CONSULT WITH DIETICIAN REGARDING ADEQUATE (CALORIC) NUTRITIONAL INTAKE	—MRS. MOORE WILL EAT THREE MEALS A DAY AND BETWEEN- MEAL SNACKS THROUGHOUT HER HOSPITALIZATION —SHE WILL GAIN 2 POUNDS A WEEK, FOR A TOTAL WEIGHT GAIN OF UP TO 10 POUNDS BY 2/26	1/21 BB
INEFFECTIVE IN- DIVIDUAL COPING RELATED TO UN- KNOWN ETIOLOGY AS MANIFESTED BY LOSS OF CON- TROL OF ANGER AND DEFICIENT PROBLEM-SOLV- ING SKILLS	—FOR LOSS OF CONTROL OF ANGER: ·ENCOURAGE VERBAL EX- PRESSION OF ANGER ·HAVE PRIMARY NURSE DISCUSS JOURNAL NOTA- TIONS WEEKLY ·INVOLVE MRS. MOORE IN ASSERTIVENESS TRAINING ·REWARD ASSERTIVENESS; DIFFERENTIATE IT FROM AGGRESSION ·ENCOURAGE MRS. MOORE TO ATTEND OCCUPATIONAL THERAPY AS A WAY OF CHANNELING ANGER; RECREATION THERAPY FOR EXERCISE ·ENCOURAGE PARTICIPA- TION IN GROUP THERAPY —FOR DEFICIENT PROBLEM- SOLVING SKILLS: ·TEACH MRS. MOORE THE STEPS OF PROBLEM- SOLVING ·ROLE-PLAY PROBLEM- SOLVING WITH HER THREE TIMES A WEEK ·HAVE HER APPLY THE PROCESS TO PROBLEMS THAT ARISE WHILE SHE IS IN THE HOSPITAL (e.g., IN-MILIEU ACTIVITIES GROUP PSYCHOTHERAPY)	—MRS. MOORE WILL KEEP AN "ANGRY JOURNAL" BY 2/29 —MRS. MOORE WILL CONTROL HER ANGER AS EVIDENCED BY AN ABILITY TO VERBALIZE ANGER AND PROPOSE NEW COPING STRATEGIES; i.e., VENT WITH NURSE FIRST, VERBALIZE TO OBJECT OF ANGER LATER —MRS. MOORE WILL UTILIZE STEPS OF THE PROBLEM- SOLVING PROCESS BY 2/27	1/21 BB

Continued

Nursing Care Plan *continued*

Nursing diagnosis	Nursing intervention	Predicted outcome/short-term goals (include time frame)	Date/signature
SELF-ESTEEM DISTURBANCE RELATED TO NEGATIVE THINKING SECONDARY TO FEELINGS OF HOPELESSNESS	—SEEK MRS. MOORE OUT EACH DAY FOR BRIEF ½-HOUR ONE-TO-ONE SESSION —ENCOURAGE AND PRAISE HER INVOLVEMENT IN ACTIVITIES —TEACH HER THE PROCESS OF GOAL-SETTING —ASSIST HER IN SETTING HER REALISTIC, REACH-ABLE GOALS —CLARIFY AND TEACH HER GENETIC AND CHEMICAL COMPONENTS OF ILLNESS —DISCOURAGE SELF-DEP-RECATING REMARKS —INCLUDE HER IN ALL PHASES OF THE NURSING PROCESS —ALLOW HER TO MAKE SIMPLE DECISIONS, THEN GRADUATE HER TO MORE DIFFICULT ONES —ENCOURAGE RESPONSI-BILITY FOR SELF-CARE —LISTEN TO (BUT DO NOT AGREE WITH) HER EXPRES-SIONS OF HELPLESS-NESS —DIFFERENTIATE "I CAN'T" FROM "I WON'T" AND HELP HER SEE HER CHOICES IN LIFE EVENTS —PRAISE HER PROGRESS	—MRS. MOORE'S SELF-CONCEPT WILL IMPROVE BY 2/12, AS EVIDENCE BY POSITIVE COMMENTS ABOUT SELF AND VERBALIZING AN EXAMPLE OF REALISTIC GOAL-SETTING	1/21 BB
DIVERSIONAL ACTIVITY DEFICIT RELATED TO NONMOTIVATION SECONDARY TO DEPRESSION	—MONITOR PROGRESS IN OCCUPATIONAL THERAPY (OT); HELP MRS. MOORE WORK ON AN OT PROJECT ON THE UNIT —PROVIDE SEWING MAT-ERIALS AND ASSIST HER IN CHOOSING A PATTERN FOR A PATCHWORK PILLOW —PRAISE EFFORT AND PROGRESS —INVOLVE HER IN ASSIST-ING OT WITH A GAR-DENING PROJECT OR TEACHING ANOTHER CLIENT TO SEW	—MRS. MOORE WILL SHOW RE-NEWED INTEREST IN GARDEN-ING AND SEWING ACTIVITIES BY 2/7	1/21 BB

MRS. MOORE: BIPOLAR, DEPRESSED

Nursing diagnosis	Nursing intervention	Predicted outcome/short-term goals (include time frame)	Date/signature
SOCIAL ISOLATION RELATED TO ANGRY INTER-PERSONAL STYLE AND LACK OF COMMUNITY SUPPORTS	—FOR ANGRY INTERPERSONAL STYLE: · ESTABLISH A POSITIVE NURSE-PATIENT RELATIONSHIP · PROVIDE FEEDBACK WITH A NONCRITICAL STYLE · ENCOURAGE MRS. MOORE'S INVOLVEMENT IN GROUP THERAPY · PROVIDE ASSERTIVENESS TRAINING AS PREVIOUSLY MENTIONED	—MRS. MOORE WILL ASSOCIATE WITH OTHERS IN A MANNER WHICH IS NEITHER ABRASIVE OR PESSIMISTIC AND WILL ACCEPT CRITICISM WITHOUT ANGRY OUTBURSTS	1/21 BB
	—FOR LACK OF COMMUNITY SUPPORTS: · ENCOURAGE SOCIALIZATION WITH OTHERS; MONITOR INTERACTIONS	—MRS. MOORE WILL INITIATE SOCIAL CONTACT WITH THREE PEOPLE A DAY BY 2/5. SHE WILL CONTACT TWO COMMUNITY AGENCIES BY 2/14	
	· ENCOURAGE MRS. MOORE TO CALL MRS. THOMAS AND TO INVITE HER TO VISIT · INVESTIGATE EMPLOYMENT OPPORTUNITIES IN COLLABORATION WITH SOCIAL SERVICES STAFF · HAVE MRS. MOORE MAKE A STUDY OF AVAILABLE COMMUNITY RESOURCES SHE COULD UTILIZE FOR SUPPORT		

the connection of poverty to depression. A trend of inferiority as a result of economic deprivation could still serve as a motivating factor in Mrs. Moore's isolation from her community as an adult. Therapeutic interventions were thus directed toward improving her self-concept in the area of self-esteem.

SUMMARY

Mrs. Moore improved as the nursing care plan was implemented. By the end of the first week, she was sleeping, eating, caring for her own hygienic needs, and beginning to utilize her leisure time through diversional activities. (The nursing staff found it necessary to extend the time frames for the more intermediate goals of improved individual coping and self-concept, in order to allow sufficient time for these goals to be reached.) Gradually, Mrs. Moore became more confident (as evidenced by positive statements) and increased her socialization with others. Self-understanding (through the use of an "angry journal"), in terms of recognizing her anger and the way her interpersonal style influenced interactions with others, was resolved through individual nurse-client interaction and group therapy. These issues would need to be continuously addressed in further outpatient therapy.

By the time of discharge, Mrs. Moore understood the facts surrounding her illness. She expressed relief at knowing she was not totally responsible and confidence in her ability to care for herself. She was referred to the mental health center for follow-up. At the center, she was to continue individual counseling and attend an adult stabilization day hospital program in order to improve her social skills. Before discharge, she made contact with vocational rehabilitation for possible job placement and appeared committed to the idea of reintegrating herself into her community.

REFERENCES

Akiskal, H.S., and McKinney, W.T. "Overview of Recent Research on Depression: Integration of 10 Conceptual Models into a Comprehensive Clinical Frame," *Archives of General Psychiatry* 32:285-305, 1975.

Dixson, D. "Manic Depression: An Overview," *Journal of Psychiatric Nursing* 28-29, June 1981.

Erikson, E.H. *Childhood and Society*. New York: W.W. Norton & Co., 1963.

Freud, S. "Mourning and Melancholia," in *Complete Psychological Works of Sigmund Freud,* vol. XIV. London: Hogarth Press, 1924.

Stuart, G.W., and Sundeen, S.J. *Principles and Practice of Psychiatric Nursing*. St. Louis: C.V. Mosby Co., 1983.

Wetzel, J.W. *Clinical Handbook of Depression*. New York: Gardner Press, 1984.

Wolpert, E. "Major Affective Disorders," in *Comprehensive Textbook of Psychiatry,* vol. 2. Edited by Kaplan, H., et al. Baltimore: Williams & Wilkins Co., 1980.

SELECTED BIBLIOGRAPHY

Banchik, D. "Psychiatric Assessment and Case Formulation," in *Handbook of Psychiatric-Mental Health Nursing*. Edited by Adams, C., and Macione, A. New York: John Wiley & Sons, 1983.

Corker, E. "Manic Depression," *Nursing Mirror* 157(2):43-45, 1983.

Davis, J.M., and Mass, J.W. *The Affective Disorders*. Washington, D.C.: American Psychiatric Association, 1983.

Freden, L. *Psychosocial Aspects of Depression*. New York: John Wiley & Sons, 1982.

Gordon, M. *Manual of Nursing Diagnosis*. New York: McGraw-Hill Book Co., 1985.

Kim, M.J., et al. *Classification of Nursing Diagnoses: Proceedings of the Fifth National Conference (1982)*. St. Louis: C.V. Mosby Co., 1984.

Klerman, G. "Overview of Affective Disorders," in *Comprehensive Textbook of Psychiatry,* vol. 2. Edited by Kaplan, H., et al. Baltimore: Williams & Wilkins Co., 1980.

Pawlicki, R., and Heitkemper, T. Behavioral Management of Insomnia," *Journal of Psychosocial Nursing* 14-18, July 1985.

Pelletier, L. "Depression Update," *Journal of Emergency Nursing* 10(2):315-18, 1984.

Rowe, D. "Helping the Depressed Patient," *Nursing Times* 79(43):62-63, 1983.

Smith, L. "Problems Associated with Manic Depressive Patients," *Nursing81* 1:1307-90, 1981.

Richard:
Obsessive-Compulsive Disorder

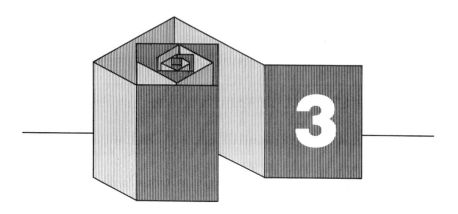

Geoffry W. McEnany, MS, RN

Everyone experiences anxiety, and most people are aware of its potentially paralyzing effects. In one way or another, people behave in ways that help stave off the discomforting experience inherent to an anxious state. Although an oversimplification of the process, obsessive-compulsive disorder (OCD) can be defined as a maladaptive means of dealing with the internal experience commonly labeled as anxiety.

Despite multiform theories on the etiology of OCD—including learning, cognitive, biological, and psychoanalytical theories (Emmelkamp, 1982)—OCD is not clearly understood from a biological perspective; hence, treatment is difficult and cure rare. In this case study, elements of behavioristic and psychobiological theories guide treatment, and nursing intervention is grounded in the conceptual framework of self-care.

The client with OCD presents nursing with an arduous task. Key elements to successful nursing care of such a client include patience, consistency of approach, and inclusion of the client in the planning of inpatient care. Additionally, ongoing evaluation of the effectiveness of nursing strategies help the staff and client monitor their progress in meeting goals for care and treatment.

CASE STUDY

Richard, a 40-year-old white, single, unemployed Protestant male of British ancestry, lived alone in a residence hotel in an eastern suburban town. Although his family maintained strong Christian ideals and actively participated in church events, Richard did not attend church due to his psychiatric disability. Rather, he remained at home, reading the Bible as his major source of spiritual enrichment.

Richard had functioned for 12 years with volunteer employment, disability payments, and pharmacological intervention, despite moderately incapacitating continuation of obsessive-compulsive symptoms. At age 40, upon the recommendation of his physician, Richard presented himself to a voluntary psychiatric inpatient unit for reevaluation of treatment. Richard's symptoms had become resistant to pharmacological treatment, as he spent up to 12 hours each day in ritualistic behavior. Other than the recalcitrant nature of the symptoms to psychopharmacological intervention, no other clear precipitant to this, his fourth hospitalization, was identifiable.

During the admission interview, Richard delved deeply into his psychiatric history. He marked the onset of his psychiatric difficulties at age 15. According to his report, "It was difficult to socialize with classmates, and I was very shy with girls; I never really fit in." Concurrent with his socializing difficulties, Richard remembered having "violent, defiling thoughts about God and His creations" that left him "feeling anxious and fearful." Despite concurrent, often severe anxiety in the early stages of his illness, Richard completed high school and, shortly after graduation, took a job as an office clerk. Within 6 months of his employment, Richard's anxiety and fearfulness increased as he began to experience an escalation of intrusive, negativistic thoughts about God. In an effort to counteract his "unacceptable thoughts," he developed an elaborate routine of ritualistic behaviors that, according to Richard, led to the "neutralization" of the hampering thoughts and subsequently decreased his level of anxiety. Examples of these "neutralizing" behaviors included walking a prescribed number of steps forward and backward, repeating certain words out loud while closing and opening his eyes, or repeatedly walking through a doorway. Richard reported having to reenact these rituals until the unwanted thoughts either abated or "converted to something more positive."

During the year following his employment as a clerk, Richard's symptoms worsened. In addition to intrusive thoughts about God, a variety of new behaviors began to precipitate severe anxiety and fearfulness: walking over thresholds, crossing town and city boundaries, removing clothing for hygiene or eliminative functions, or touching items such as soap or doorknobs. In an effort to counteract the anxiety produced by the aforementioned events, Richard developed a series of "clean thoughts" which he used while enacting the anxiety-producing behaviors. If an intrusive "bad thought" occurred during the time that he was engaged in a "cleansing or neutralizing" ritual, he often stopped the ritual and returned to the beginning steps of the purification scenario; Richard reported frequently having to repeat the ritual up to 20 times before it was acceptable to him.

As Richard's behavioral problems increased to age 19, so did his social isolation and deterioration in functional abilities at work. By the time Richard reached age 19½, he had started to use alcohol to cope with his ritualistic behavior. He reportedly drank up to 6 ounces of hard liquor each day to get through his activities of daily living. Because of an escalation in his rituals and an inability to cope, he quit his job and remained totally isolated in his apartment for weeks at a time. One month before his twentieth birthday, Richard entered a psychiatric hospital for a 12-month inpatient treatment course for his obsessive-compulsive behaviors.

Following his first hospitalization, Richard returned to work and functioned marginally for the next 3 years. He reported that during those 3 years he had periods of severe social and occupational dysfunction, forcing him at times to take up to 2 weeks of leave from work to regain control of the symptoms. Additionally, Richard reported shifts in the patterns of his thoughts. Whereas in the past he was able to connect stressful periods with increasing obsessive thoughts and compulsive rituals, he now was no longer able to maintain insight into his behavior. Severe dysfunction and inability to care for self precipitated his second hospitalization, which occurred over a 6-week period, on a voluntary inpatient unit.

Upon his second discharge, Richard returned to work as a part-time dishwasher in a restaurant. Since he could no longer afford his apartment, he moved into a single-room occupancy hotel. These changes in his job and living situation, coupled with a deteriorating psychiatric condition, caused increased feelings of low self-esteem and waning confidence. He consequently withdrew socially, thus weakening his social support network. His only contacts with people were at his place of employment. Richard believed that he was a "social leper" whose presence in society was "disgusting and disgraceful." He believed that others viewed him as a "freak" as he progressively lost control over his symptoms and began to enact ritualistic behaviors in public places. Richard offered the following illustration of how his symptoms interfered with his functioning. While at work one day, he became fearful of touching the doorknob to the men's restroom. He took several clean cloths and wiped the knob for 10 minutes at a time. Despite the knob-cleaning ritual, Richard was convinced that the doorknob was dirty and that by touching it, he would become prey to some transmittable disease. After an hour of attempting to get into the bathroom, he was incontinent of urine, a situation which he viewed as thoroughly humiliating.

Richard's behavioral difficulties waxed and waned for the next 4 years, and he returned to using alcohol as a self-medication to cope with his ritualistic behavior. When the alcohol failed to diminish the severity of his symptoms, Richard was voluntarily rehospitalized at age 28 for 6 weeks. At the time of this third admission, Richard had become so fearful of soap and hygiene rituals that he had not bathed in 3 months.

Following his third hospitalization, Richard did not return to work; instead, he was placed on permanent disability. He did take a part-time volunteer position with a charitable organization doing light clerical duties. Since he refused psychiatric follow-up treatment, he was cared for by a general practitioner, who prescribed psychotropic medications to control obsessive-compulsive behaviors.

Richard's history of hospital admissions for treatment of his symptoms offered significant data to this case. His first hospitalization occurred over a 12-month period in a state hospital. He received the diagnosis of OCD as in all other hospital stays, but treatment during the first admission consisted mainly of electroconvulsive therapy and psychotherapy, with reported transient benefit. The latter two hospitalizations were brief (6 weeks each) in comparison to the first hospital admission. During these two hospitalizations, he received psychopharmacological intervention with tricyclic antidepressant, benzodiazepine, and neuroleptic medications. While these medications were of some help, Richard's intermittent non-compliance with drug therapy made the long-term assessment of medication effectiveness difficult.

Richard's third hospital stay included a comprehensive program of classic behavioral interventions (e.g., desensitization and conditioning), in addition to medication for control of behavioral difficulties while learning new patterns of coping. Decompensation between hospital contacts resulted mainly from Richard's unwillingness to comply with psychiatric follow-up treatment, compounded by his impoverished social support network.

Looking at possible psychobiological contributants to Richard's illness, some data was readily available. When Richard was age 38, his physician noted mild hypertension on physical exam; this condition was well controlled with a sodium-restricted diet. Contributing to his hypertension and anxiety states was his excessive intake of caffeine (up to ten cups of coffee or cola per day), tobacco (two packs of cigarettes per day), and alcohol as previously noted.

From birth to early adolescence, Richard's developmental history was unremarkable. His birth was of normal vaginal delivery after an uneventful gestation period of 9 months. He met normal developmental milestones in infancy and early childhood. He attended public schools and was happily active in church activities and the Boy Scouts. Although never very popular, he always had a few friends.

Richard rarely dated; he was "always shy of girls," despite the fact that he "liked several girls a lot." He never married and recounted only one sexual experience, at age 26, that culminated in intercourse. According to Richard, in order for him to engage in sexual activity he had to be "very drunk." He admitted that his consequent feelings of guilt, remorse, and dissatisfaction were "overwhelming." As he moved into his late 20s, he "gave up on the idea of being married" because the "intimate emotional contact was just too painful to bear."

At the time of admission, Richard had only one person in his life whom he considered a friend—a local minister who visited him once a week to bring groceries and to provide some social contact. Outside of this social contact, Richard suffered gross social isolation secondary to his own social withdrawal.

Richard's family history provided few insights into his persistent difficulties. Richard was the second eldest and the only male in a family of four children. All of his sisters were happily married and lived in a neighboring state; they maintained telephone contacts with Richard, and he viewed them as "distantly supportive." His mother and father lived with one of his sisters. Richard noted that despite their age, both his mother and father were healthy and "considerably active." The family history was negative for psychiatric disorders, including alcohol or drug abuse.

Richard recounted his family history with warmth and pride for the varied accomplishments of his family members. His father was a retired surgeon, and his mother a retired nurse; both parents retired more than 10 years previously. Two of Richard's sisters were practicing physicians, and one a university professor. Richard left his family at age 17 "to strike out on my own" and to prove his ability to care for himself, "being the only son in my family." When he developed behavioral difficulties after leaving his family, he felt "being too ashamed to return home," despite many offers from his family to help in his times of need. He believed that over the years, his family "became discouraged" with his chronic difficulties and refusals of help; he felt that they were now "less invested" in aiding him in his efforts toward wellness.

On his latest admission, Richard presented as a generally cooperative male who appeared older than his stated age. His affect was anxious, his mood, mildly depressed. His thought content focused on themes of incapacitation related to his symptoms, which he viewed as "unbearable." He denied suicidal and homicidal ideation and any visual, auditory, or tactile hallucinations. His speech was slow and hyphenated with pauses, and he engaged in repetitive gestures such as seesawing movements of his arms. He occasionally stood up, took two steps forward and one backward, and then returned to his chair; he explained that this behavior "neutralized bad thoughts." Richard's thought process demonstrated marked obsessiveness and hesitation, despite his stated need to "get all sentences out in the most precise way." Objectively, however, his thought process was circumstantial, maintaining a fragmented storytelling quality. The interviewer noted no loosening of associations. Cognitively, Richard was alert and oriented to person, time, place, and situation. He calculated serial sevens without difficulty or error. His immediate memory was impaired, evidenced by the ability to recall only one object out of four after 5 minutes. His long-term memory was intact; he remembered all the presidents back to Truman. His fund of knowledge was average. His insight was poor and judgment fair. Richard was aware of his deteriorating condition and noted several behaviorally dysfunctional changes. He stated that his sleep was generally of poor quality and duration, although he usually felt better in the morning. He believed that his compulsive behavior exacerbated with fatigue and feelings of helplessness or anger.

Reader may now complete Recording the Data, Assigning Nursing Diagnoses, and Nursing Care Plan.

FORMULATION

According to the *Diagnostic and Statistical Manual of Mental Disorders-III (DSM-III)*, the most prominent features of OCD are "recurrent, persistent ideas, thoughts, images, or impulses that are ego dystonic...that invade consciousness and are experienced as senseless or repugnant [obsessions]; and repetitive and seemingly purposeful behaviors that are performed according to certain rules or in a stereotyped fashion [compulsions]" (APA, 1980). Compulsive behavior in OCD is an attempt to mitigate the subjective discomfort of the obsession and to relieve the concurrent anxiety that occurs with the intrusive obsessive thought.

In Richard's case, obsessions were evident, inasmuch as he had repetitive, intrusive thoughts about God, contaminations, and sexuality which he found totally unacceptable and a major source of distress. His obsessions gave way to compulsions such as modulated behaviors in gait, repetitive behaviors while passing through doorways or across town, county, or state lines, and significant difficulty in maintaining adequate hygiene. Richard maintained a series of cleansing rituals, especially concerning touching doorknobs or people (e.g., handshaking). Usually, he

Continued on page 78

RECORDING THE DATA

After you have read the case, cluster significant data into functional health patterns.

Health management/health perception _____

_____

_____

_____

_____

Nutritional/metabolic _____

_____

_____

_____

Elimination _____

_____

_____

_____

Activity/exercise _____

_____

_____

_____

Cognitive/perceptual _____

_____

_____

_____

Sleep/rest _____

_____

_____

_____

Self-perception/self-concept _____

_____

_____

_____

Role relationship _____

_____

_____

_____

Sexuality/reproductive _____

_____

_____

_____

Coping/stress tolerance _____

_____

_____

_____

Value/belief _____

_____

_____

_____

ASSIGNING NURSING DIAGNOSES

Use your clustered data to select appropriate nursing diagnoses.

Health perception/health management

- ☐ Growth and Development, Altered (see Developmental Delay)
- ☐ Health Maintenance, Altered
- ☐ Infection, Potential for
- ☐ Injury (Trauma): Potential for
- ☐ Noncompliance (Specify)
- ☐ Poisoning: Potential for
- ☐ Suffocation: Potential for

Nutritional/metabolic

- ☐ Body Temperature, Potential Alteration in
- ☐ Developmental Delay: Physical Growth and Development
- ☐ Fluid Volume, Altered: Excess or Excess Fluid Volume
- ☐ Fluid Volume Deficit, Actual
- ☐ Fluid Volume Deficit, Potential
- ☐ Nutrition, Altered: Less Than Body Requirements or Nutritional Deficit (Specify)
- ☐ Nutrition, Altered: More Than Body Requirements or Exogenous Obesity
- ☐ Nutrition, Altered: Potential for More Than Body Requirements or Potential for Obesity
- ☐ Oral Mucous Membrane, Altered
- ☐ Skin Integrity, Impaired or Skin Breakdown
- ☐ Skin Integrity, Impaired or Potential Skin Breakdown
- ☐ Swallowing, Impaired or Uncompensated Swallowing Impairment
- ☐ Tissue Integrity, Impaired

Elimination

- ☐ Bowel Elimination, Altered: Constipation
- ☐ Bowel Elimination, Altered: Diarrhea
- ☐ Bowel Elimination, Altered: Incontinence
- ☐ Developmental Delay: Bowel/Bladder Control
- ☐ Incontinence: Functional
- ☐ Incontinence: Reflex
- ☐ Incontinence: Stress
- ☐ Incontinence: Total
- ☐ Incontinence: Urge
- ☐ Urinary Elimination, Altered Patterns of
- ☐ Urinary Retention

Activity/exercise

- ☐ Activity Intolerance
- ☐ Activity Intolerance, Potential
- ☐ Airway Clearance, Ineffective
- ☐ Breathing Pattern, Ineffective
- ☐ Cardiac Output, Altered: Decreased
- ☐ Developmental Delay: Mobility
- ☐ Developmental Delay: Self-Care Skills
- ☐ Diversional Activity Deficit
- ☐ Gas Exchange, Impaired
- ☐ Home Maintenance Management, Impaired (Mild, Moderate, Severe, Potential, Chronic)
- ☐ Mobility, Impaired Physical
- ☐ Self-Care Deficit: Feeding
- ☐ Self-Care Deficit: Bathing/Hygiene
- ☐ Self-Care Deficit: Dressing/Grooming
- ☐ Self-Care Deficit: Toileting
- ☐ Self-Care Deficit: Total
- ☐ Tissue Perfusion, Altered: (Specify)

Sleep/rest

- ☐ Sleep Pattern Disturbance

Cognitive/perceptual

- ☐ Comfort, Altered: Pain
- ☐ Comfort, Altered: Chronic Pain

☐ Developmental Delay: (Specify Cognitive Area; attention, decision making, etc.)
☐ Hypothermia
☐ Hyperthermia
☐ Knowledge Deficit (Specify)
☐ Sensory-Perceptual Alteration: Input Excess or Sensory Overload
☐ Sensory-Perceptual Alteration: Input Deficit or Sensory Deprivation
☐ Thermoregulation, Ineffective
☐ Thought Processes, Altered
☐ Unilateral Neglect

Self-perception/self-concept

☐ Anxiety
☐ Body Image Disturbance
☐ Fear
☐ Hopelessness
☐ Personal Identity Confusion
☐ Powerlessness (Severe, Low, Moderate)
☐ Self-Esteem Disturbance

Role relationship

☐ Communication, Impaired Verbal
☐ Developmental Delay: Communication Skills
☐ Developmental Delay: Social Skills
☐ Family Processes, Altered
☐ Grieving, Anticipatory
☐ Grieving, Dysfunctional
☐ Parenting, Altered: Actual or Potential

☐ Role Performance, Disturbance in
☐ Social Interactions, Impaired
☐ Social Isolation (Rejection)

Sexuality/reproductive

☐ Rape-Trauma Syndrome: Compounded
☐ Rape-Trauma Syndrome: Silent Reaction
☐ Sexual Dysfunction
☐ Sexuality Patterns, Altered

Coping/stress tolerance

☐ Adjustment, Impaired
☐ Coping, Ineffective Individual
☐ Coping, Ineffective Family: Compromised
☐ Coping, Ineffective Family: Disabling
☐ Coping, Family: Potential for Growth
☐ Developmental Delay (Specify area)
☐ Post-Trauma Response
☐ Violence, Potential for (Self-Directed or Directed at Others)

Value/belief

☐ Spiritual Distress (Distress of Human Spirit)

You are now ready to develop a nursing care plan for this client. Use the following blank pages to do so. Then refer to the author's formulation, diagnostic summary, care plan, and summary.

NURSING CARE PLAN

Complete the chart below to develop a nursing care plan for this client.

Discharge outcomes/long-term goals	

Nursing diagnosis	Nursing intervention	

	Predicted outcomes/short-term goals (include time frame)	Date/signature

Return to Formulation, page 71

found some relief of anxiety by executing his compulsions. However, these compulsive behaviors gradually lost their power to abate his high level of anxiety, and he increasingly needed to resort to substances such as alcohol to cope with his secondary dysphoria.

DSM-III addresses several classical associated features of OCD exhibited in Richard's clinical behavior. We reported depression and anxiety as the most prominently related symptoms of his condition. His anxiety increased with actual or anticipated events that he perceived as threatening. *DSM-III* points out that the age of onset for OCD is usually sometime in adolescence, and the course of the disorder includes exacerbations and remissions but generally follows a chronic routine. Impairment, such as Richard experienced, is usual for clients with OCD; loss of social and occupational functioning is not uncommon. Complications of the disorder are similar to those that Richard suffered, namely alcohol and/or drug abuse to control associated symptoms of OCD, especially anxiety and depression.

Kaplan and Sadock (1982) discuss the causes of OCD from the perspectives of psychodynamic and learning theories. From the psychodynamic focus, three major defenses are in cooperation with each other: isolation, undoing, and reaction formation. Richard clearly demonstrated these defenses in his behavior. In the early stages of his illness, and during periods of remission, Richard was able to separate affect and anxiety-provoking impulses, keeping them unconsciously repressed. However, as his defenses deteriorated, his symptoms reappeared in a frighteningly strong fashion, leading to the emergence of compulsive behavior. In undoing, Richard attempted to counteract an obsessive thought with a particular behavior, as was the case with his rituals surrounding hygiene activities, crossing through doorways, and other actions. Reaction formation—a defense in which a person behaves overtly in an opposing fashion to the intent of an impulse—was manifested in Richard's frequent attention to the detail of scriptures and his interpretation of the Bible, when in essence his thoughts often included the defilement of God.

The learning theorists, according to Kaplan and Sadock (1982), view obsessive-compulsive behavior as a conditioned relief-seeking response to anxiety. Because the intrusion of an unwanted thought yields anxiety, and the person is able to control the anxiety through a specific act or series of modulated behaviors, the latter serves to reinforce the former.

Insel (1982) believes that OCD is not a homogeneous syndrome of behaviors; rather, people with OCD may "fit" into several subcategories of behavior, including those who show affective symptoms versus those with neuroendocrine and/or sleep EEG abnormalities. Such data points to possibly a more psychobiologically oriented model in discovering the etiology of OCD. Insel and colleagues (1983) discuss the fact that until recently, OCD was fairly refractory to intervention. However, with the development of such behavior techniques as "response prevention, exposure in vivo...and the use of antidepressant medications," treatment outcomes have greatly improved.

In addition to medications to treat OCD and its associated features, well-planned, theoretically based, prescriptive nursing interventions are essential to the comprehensive inpatient care of persons suffering from this debilitating and often demoralizing condition. Nurses working with clients carrying the diagnosis of OCD need to be aware of several facts relating to the behavioral manifestations of the disorder: the maladaptive patterns of OCD clients are not within direct, conscious control; at the time of hospitalization, OCD clients are often under extreme stress and distress and must be approached with a keen sensitivity and awareness of their specialized, albeit complex, needs; hospitalization often heightens the OCD client's sense of vulnerability and loss of control, often exacerbating their behavioral symptoms; and the client needs to be actively involved in the development of the nursing care plan and treatment plan for the outcome of care to be successful.

The following nursing care plan delineates one approach to treating clients with OCD. It has the potential for success in a wide range of clients, providing that nurses mold the plan to the contours of their client's specific presenting difficulties. Interdisciplinary collaboration is essential; the nursing care plan for the client with OCD must dovetail with the plans of other disciplines. Providing that the client is sufficiently motivated and capable of engaging in a collaborative approach to care, the outcome of inpatient treatment is likely to yield positive behavioral changes and greater autonomy.

SUMMARY

Richard's clinical care plan provides an excellent example of interdisciplinary teamwork that required input and cooperation from psychiatry, psychology, nursing, social work, and rehabilitation therapy.

While this case study focuses mainly on the nursing care of the client, other interventions merit strong consideration in evaluating the behavioral outcomes of this hospitalization. While consistent behavioral intervention is essential for the treatment of OCD, the nurse must also consider the influence of psychoactive medications on the client's psychobiological states and subsequent behavior. In their discussion of the pharmacological treatment of OCD, Insel and Murphy (1981) point to

Continued on page 89

DIAGNOSTIC SUMMARY FOR RICHARD

Data	Functional health pattern	Nursing diagnosis
—Spends up to 12 hours a day engaged in ritualistic behavior —Must reenact rituals until unwanted thoughts either abate or "convert to something more positive" —Finds his symptoms unbearable	Activity/Exercise	Self-Care Deficit: Feeding, related to rituals in getting to dining room secondary to obsessive-compulsive disorder
—In the past, eliminative functions precipitated severe anxiety and fearfulness —In the past, was fearful of touching the doorknob to the men's restroom; resultant knob-cleaning ritual caused incontinence of urine	Activity/Exercise	Self-Care Deficit: Toileting, related to obsessions of touching the bathroom doorknob secondary to obsessive-compulsive disorder
—Spends up to 12 hours a day engaged in ritualistic behavior —Has "overwhelming" feelings of guilt, remorse, and dissatisfaction regarding sexual activity —Before his third admission, was so fearful of soap and hygiene rituals that he had not bathed in 3 months	Activity/Exercise	Self-Care Deficit: Bathing/Hygiene, related to religious obsessions and fears of undressing secondary to obsessive-compulsive disorder
—Engaged in "neutralizing behaviors," including repeatedly walking through a doorway —Walking over thresholds precipitated severe anxiety and fearfulness	Activity/Exercise	Activity Intolerance related to obsessive-compulsive rituals as manifested by fear of walking through doorways
—Refused psychiatric follow-up treatment after his last hospitalization —In the past, was noncompliant with drug therapy —Has demonstrated unwillingness to comply with psychiatric follow-up treatment	Health Management/Health Perception	Noncompliance related to lack of knowledge, poor impulse control, and poor concentration secondary to obsessive-compulsive disorder, as manifested by lack of follow-up with medications and outpatient therapy
—Uses excessive amounts of caffeine: up to 10 cups of coffee or cola per day	Self-Perception/Self-Concept	Anxiety related to unknown etiology, as manifested by ritualistic behavior
—In the past, experienced increased feelings of low self-esteem and waning confidence that led to social withdrawal, thus weakening his social support network —Has only one friend, a minister; suffers gross social isolation secondary to his own social withdrawal	Role Relationship	Social isolation related to embarrassment with regard to ritualistic behavior

NURSING CARE PLAN

Complete the chart below to develop a nursing care plan for this client.

Discharge outcome/long-term goals		
1. RICHARD WILL LIVE IN A STRUCTURED LIVING SETTING FOR 3 MONTHS AFTER DISCHARGE AS A TRANSITIONAL AID TO INDEPENDENT LIVING. 2. BY HIS DISCHARGE DATE, RICHARD WILL	HAVE, WITH STAFF ASSISTANCE, STARTED WORK WITH A VOLUNTEER AGENCY. 3. RICHARD WILL FOLLOW THROUGH WITH POST-DISCHARGE CARE BY ACCEPTING OUTPATIENT PSYCHOTHERAPY. 4. RICHARD WILL CONTINUE TO WORK WITH	

Nursing diagnosis	Nursing intervention	Predicted outcome/short-term goals (include time frame)	Date/signature
SELF-CARE DEFICIT: FEEDING RELATED TO RITUALS IN GETTING TO THE DINING ROOM SECONDARY TO OBSESSIVE-COMPULSIVE DISORDER	—ADMINISTER BENZODIAZEPINE ½-HOUR BEFORE MEALS, PER MEDICAL ORDER AND AT RICHARD'S REQUEST, TO DECREASE ANXIETY AROUND RITUALISTIC BEHAVIOR AT MEALS —BETWEEN 10/1 AND 10/14, NOTIFY RICHARD ½-HOUR BEFORE MEALS THAT MEALS WILL BE ARRIVING IN 30 MINUTES. AT THIS TIME, HE MAY REQUEST BENZODIAZEPINE FOR ANXIETY —DESCRIBE THE RITUAL REDUCTION SCHEDULE LISTED IN THE "PREDICTED OUTCOMES". USING A PARADOXICAL APPROACH, TELL RICHARD THAT HE MUST REMAIN ENGAGED IN THE RITUALS FOR THE TIMES SPECIFIED —DO NOT INTERVENE IN THE RITUALIZED BEHAVIORS DURING THE TIMES SPECIFIED —REMIND HIM THAT HIS TIME IS UP IF RICHARD PERSEVERATES IN HIS RITUALS BEYOND THE ALOTTED TIME —OFFER VERBAL ASSISTANCE TO GET HIM TO THE DINING ROOM; RESPECT HIS RESPONSE —EVALUATE RESPONSE TO THIS PLAN ON A DAILY BASIS	—RICHARD WILL ATTEND MEALS AND MAINTAIN AN ADEQUATE NUTRITIONAL INTAKE TO PREVENT PHYSIOLOGICAL IMBALANCE: ·BETWEEN 10/1-10/7, RICHARD WILL TAKE NO LONGER THAN 15 MINUTES INVOLVED IN RITUALS TO GET TO THE DINING ROOM ·BETWEEN 10/8-10/14, RICHARD WILL TAKE NO LONGER THAN 10 MINUTES TO GET TO THE DINING ROOM ·BETWEEN 10/15-10/28, RICHARD WILL TAKE RESPONSIBILITY FOR KNOWING WHEN MEALS ARRIVE AND WILL REQUEST PRE-MEAL MEDICATIONS INDEPENDENTLY ·BETWEEN 10/15-10/21, RICHARD WILL TAKE NO LONGER THAN 5 MINUTES TO GET TO THE DINING ROOM ·RICHARD WILL ENTER THE DINING ROOM SPONTANEOUSLY, WITHOUT RITUAL	10/1 DM
SELF-CARE DEFICIT: TOILETING RELATED TO OBSESSIONS OF TOUCHING THE BATHROOM DOORKNOB SECONDARY TO OBSESSIVE-	—AS PER "PREDICTED OUTCOMES" —DO NOT ASK RICHARD ABOUT HIS NEED FOR ASSISTANCE —DO NOT VARY FROM OUTCOME SCHEDULE; REMIND RICHARD THAT IT IS	—RICHARD WILL ASK FOR STAFF ASSISTANCE AS NEEDED, PER OUTCOME GUIDELINES —BETWEEN 10/1-10/7, RICHARD WILL REQUEST THAT STAFF OPEN THE BATHROOM DOOR AS HE EXITS THE BATHROOM; DURING THIS TIME PERIOD, RICHARD	10/1 DM

Continued

Nursing Care Plan *continued*

Discharge outcome/long-term goals			
PROFESSIONAL CAREGIVERS IN THE DEVELOPMENT OF STRATEGIES FOR HIS CARE.			

Nursing diagnosis	Nursing intervention	Predicted outcome/short-term goals (include time frame)	Date/signature
COMPULSIVE DISORDER	ESSENTIAL TO FOLLOW GUIDELINES —DOCUMENT RICHARD'S RESPONSE IN THE PROGRESS NOTES	WILL OPEN THE DOOR ENTERING THE BATHROOM —RICHARD WILL OPEN THE BATH-ROOM DOOR, PLACE A DOORSTOP, AND REMOVE THE DOORSTOP UPON EXITING —RICHARD WILL ENTER/EXIT THE BATHROOM WITH VERBAL ASSIST-ANCE ONLY FROM THE STAFF —BETWEEN 10/22-10/28, RICHARD WILL USE THE BATHROOM INDEPENDENTLY	
SELF-CARE DEFICIT: BATH-ING/HYGIENE, RELATED TO RELIGIOUS OB-SESSIONS AND FEARS OF UN-DRESSING SEC-ONDARY TO OB-SESSIVE-COM-PULSIVE DIS-ORDER	—IMPLEMENT PARADOXICAL INTENT PROGRAM (SEE "PREDICTED OUTCOMES") —DO NOT ATTEMPT TO PERSUADE RICHARD TO IN-CREASE SELF-CARE ABILITIES IN HYGIENE AT THIS TIME, AS DISCUSSION OF THIS ISSUE INCREASES HIS ANXIETY —FOR MORNING HYGIENE PROGRAM, CLOSELY MAIN-TAIN SCHEDULE —ENCOURAGE RICHARD TO FOLLOW THE HYGIENE PROGRAM —GUIDE AND DIRECT RICHARD THROUGH BE-HAVIORAL PROGRAM, GIV-ING VERBAL PROMPTS WHEN NEEDED —ADMINISTER ANTI-ANX-IETY MEDICATION FOR HYGIENE TASKS AS RE-QUESTED BY RICHARD —EVALUATE EFFECTIVE-NESS OF MEDICATION IN FACILITATING BEHAVIOR-AL PROGRAM —EVALUATE PROGRESS WITH THIS SCHEDULE ON A DAILY BASIS —REVIEW AND PRAISE RICHARD FOR PROGRESS —ALLOW HIM TO REQUEST ANTIANXIETY MEDICATION	—RICHARD WILL COMPLETE A PROGRESSIVE DESENSITIZA-TION PROGRAM BY 10/28 —RICHARD WILL ACCOMPLISH HYGIENE TASKS INDEPENDENTLY BY DISCHARGE —HE WILL SHOWER THREE TIMES PER WEEK AND LAUNDER CLOTHING WEEKLY BY DISCHARGE —10/1—RICHARD WILL SIT IN HIS ROOM FOR 1/2-HOUR WORRYING ABOUT GETTING TO THE SHOWER, THEN WALK TO THE SHOWER ROOM. HE IS NOT TO SHOWER 10/2—SAME AS ABOVE 10/3—10/4—RICHARD WILL SIT IN HIS ROOM, WORRY FOR 1/2-HOUR, THEN WALK WITH STAFF INTO THE SHOWER ROOM AND REMAIN THERE FOR 5 MINUTES, THEN LEAVE. NO SHOWER 10/5—10/6—WORRY IN ROOM FOR 1/2-HOUR, THEN WALK WITH STAFF TO SHOWER ROOM, REMAIN IN SHOWER ROOM FOR 5 MINUTES, THEN LEAVE. NO SHOWER 10/7—10/8—WORRY IN ROOM FOR 15 MINUTES. GO TO SHOWER ROOM FOR 5 MINUTES, WASH FACE, THEN LEAVE 10/9—10/11—WORRY IN ROOM FOR 15 MINUTES, GO TO SHOWER ROOM FOR 2 MINUTES, WASH FACE, THEN LEAVE 10/12—10/14—WORRY IN ROOM	10/1 M.B.

Nursing diagnosis	Nursing intervention	Predicted outcome/short-term goals (include time frame)	Date/signature
	FOR HYGIENE TASKS AS PER MEDICAL ORDERS — DOCUMENT HIS PROGRESS	FOR 15 MINUTES, GO TO SHOWER ROOM FOR 2 MINUTES, WASH FACE, THEN LEAVE	
		10/15 — WORRY IN ROOM FOR 5 MINUTES, GO TO SHOWER ROOM, WASH FACE, SHAVE AND LEAVE	
		10/16 – 10/18 — WORRY IN ROOM FOR 5 MINUTES, GO TO SHOWER ROOM, WASH FACE, SHAVE, TURN ON SHOWER (BUT DO NOT ENTER SHOWER), WHILE WASHING/SHAVING TURN OFF SHOWER AND LEAVE	
		10/19 — WORRY IN ROOM FOR 2 MINUTES, GO TO SHOWER ROOM, TURN ON SHOWER AND GET IN SHOWER TO WASH AND SHAVE FOR 5 MINUTES	
		10/20 — WORRY IN ROOM FOR 2 MINUTES, GO INTO LAUNDRY ROOM FOR 2 MINUTES EN ROUTE TO SHOWER (HE WILL NOT LAUNDER HIS CLOTHES). LEAVE LAUNDRY ROOM AND GO TO SHOWER ROOM TO WASH FACE, SHAVE, AND BRUSH TEETH	
		10/21 — SAME AS 10/20	
		10/22 — WITHOUT WORRY IN ROOM, REPEAT ROUTINE OF 10/20	
		10/23 — GO TO LAUNDRY ROOM FOR 2 MINUTES, PLACE CLOTHES IN WASHER, THEN GO TO SHOWER ROOM TO WASH FACE, SHAVE, AND BRUSH TEETH	
		10/24 — GO TO SHOWER ROOM, TURN ON SHOWER, GET INTO SHOWER FOR 10 MINUTES: WASH/SHAVE. TURN OFF SHOWER AND BRUSH TEETH	
		10/25 — GO TO SHOWER ROOM TO WASH, SHAVE, AND BRUSH TEETH	
		10/26 — GO TO LAUNDRY ROOM TO PLACE CLOTHES IN WASHER EN ROUTE TO SHOWER ROOM TO WASH, SHAVE, AND BRUSH TEETH	
		10/27 — GO TO SHOWER ROOM	

Continued

Nursing Care Plan *continued*

Nursing diagnosis	Nursing intervention	Predicted outcome/short-term goals (include time frame)	Date/signature
		TO WASH, SHAVE, AND BRUSH TEETH	
		10/28-40 TO LAUNDRY ROOM TO PLACE CLOTHES IN WASHER EN ROUTE TO SHOWER ROOM TO SHOWER FOR 10 MINUTES	
ACTIVITY INTOLERANCE RELATED TO OBSESSIVE-COMPULSIVE RITUALS, AS MANIFESTED BY FEAR OF WALKING THROUGH DOORS	—FOR THE WEEK OF 10/1-10/8, REVIEW THE FOLLOWING SCHEDULED EVENTS FOR THE DAY —REVIEW SPECIFIC TASKS BEFORE RICHARD ATTEMPTS ACTIVITIES —EMPHASIZE CRITICAL POINTS WITH RICHARD, e.g., THAT HE IS NOT TO GO THROUGH DOOR ON 10/1 —GUIDE AND DIRECT RICHARD THROUGH ACTIVITY —ALLOW HIM TO EXPRESS HIS FEELINGS (e.g., FRUSTRATION) AFTER THE RITUALS —REINFORCE ADAPTIVE CLIENT BEHAVIORS BY PRAISING RICHARDS PROGRESS AND REVIEWING AREAS FOR GROWTH —ACCOMPANY RICHARD OFF THE UNIT DURING RITUALS AND EVALUATE HIS PROGRESS	—RICHARD WILL PARTICIPATE IN THE DEVELOPMENT OF A TOLERABLE ACTIVITY SCHEDULE —HE WILL MEET ESTABLISHED GOALS FOR EACH WEEKS ACTIVITIES —RICHARD WILL DEMONSTRATE IMPROVED TOLERANCE FOR ACTIVITY BY DISCHARGE, EVIDENCED BY COMPLETION OF AT LEAST ONE ACTIVITY PER DAY —RICHARD WILL SPEND 30 MINUTES BEFORE EACH ACTIVITY WORRYING ABOUT THE ANTICIPATED EVENT, INCREASED EXPECTATION OF SELF, AND TASKS RELATED TO LEAVING THE HOSPITAL: 10/1—WALK FROM HIS ROOM TO THE DOOR OF THE UNIT 10/2—SAME AS 10/1 10/3—WALK TO THE DOOR OF THE UNIT AND STAND ON THE THRESHOLD, BUT HE WILL NOT GO THROUGH THE DOOR 10/4—SAME AS 10/3 10/5—WALK TO THE FRONT DOOR OF THE UNIT, THROUGH THE DOOR AND INTO THE ADJOINING HALL, AND THEN IMMEDIATELY RETURN TO THE UNIT 10/6—SAME AS 10/5 10/7—WALK THROUGH THE FRONT DOOR AND HALFWAY DOWN THE ADJOINING HALL 10/8—SAME AS 10/7 —FOR THE WEEK OF 10/9— 10/16, RICHARD WILL FOLLOW THE SAME PREPARATORY ROUTINE, EXCEPT HAVE RICHARD ENACT THE FOLLOWING ACTIVITIES: 10/9 AND 10/10—WALK	10/1 DM

Nursing diagnosis	Nursing intervention	Predicted outcome/short-term goals (include time frame)	Date/signature
		THROUGH THE UNIT DOOR TO THE THERAPIST'S OFFICE, BUT WILL NOT GO THROUGH THE THERAPIST'S OFFICE DOOR	
		10/11 — WALK TO THE THERAPIST'S DOOR, REMAIN FOR 15 MINUTES, THEN RETURN TO THE UNIT	
		10/12 — WALK FROM THE UNIT, THROUGH TWO SETS OF DOORS TO THE ELEVATOR	
		10/13 — SAME AS 10/12	
		10/14 — WALK FROM THE UNIT THROUGH TWO SETS OF DOORS TO THE ELEVATOR, PRESS ELEVATOR CALL BUTTON, WAIT FOR THE ELEVATOR TO ARRIVE, BUT WILL NOT GET ON THE ELEVATOR	
		10/15 — SAME AS 10/14	
		— FOR THE FOLLOWING WEEK, RICHARD'S WORRY TIME WILL BE REDUCED TO 15 MINUTES EACH DAY, AND HE WILL ENACT THE FOLLOWING ACTIVITIES:	
		10/16 — GO TO THE ELEVATOR, PUSH THE CALL BUTTON, GET ON THE ELEVATOR, AND RIDE IT TO THE FIRST FLOOR. HE WILL NOT GET OFF THE ELEVATOR, BUT WILL RETURN TO THE UNIT	
		10/17 — SAME AS 10/16	
		10/18 — GO TO FIRST FLOOR ON ELEVATOR, GET OFF AND REMAIN ON FIRST FLOOR FOR 2 MINUTES (NO LONGER), THEN RETURN TO UNIT	
		10/19 — SAME AS 10/18	
		10/20 — GO TO FIRST FLOOR AND STAND AT FRONT DOOR OF HOSPITAL, BUT WILL NOT GO OUT DOORS!	
		10/21 — SAME AS 10/20	
		10/22 — GO TO THE FRONT STEPS OF THE HOSPITAL AND REMAIN OUT OF DOORS FOR 5 MINUTES	
		— FOR THE FOLLOWING WEEK, RICHARD WILL NOT TAKE ANY PREPARATORY WORRY TIME, AND ENACT THE FOLLOWING ACTIVITIES:	

Continued

Nursing Care Plan *continued*

Nursing diagnosis	Nursing intervention	Predicted outcome/short-term goals (include time frame)	Date/signature
		10/23 – (ACCOMPANIED) HE WILL GO TO THE SIDEWALK IN FRONT OF THE HOSPITAL, AND REMAIN THERE FOR 10 MINUTES	
		10/24 – SAME AS 10/23	
		10/25 – (ACCOMPANIED) HE WILL GO TO A NEARBY STORE AND PURCHASE SOME FRUIT	
		10/26 – (ACCOMPANIED) HE WILL TAKE A BUS FROM OUTSIDE THE HOSPITAL TO A NEARBY SHOPPING PLAZA TO EAT LUNCH	
		10/27 – SAME AS 10/26	
		10/28 – (UNACCOMPANIED BY STAFF) RICHARD WILL TAKE A BUS TO THE VOLUNTEER AGENCY TO INTERVIEW FOR A VOLUN- TEER JOB	
NONCOMPLIANCE RELATED TO LACK OF KNOWLEDGE, POOR IMPULSE CONTROL, AND POOR CONCEN- TRATION SEC- ONDARY TO OBSESSIVE- COMPULSIVE DISORDER, AS MANIFESTED BY LACK OF FOLLOW-UP WITH MEDI- CATIONS AND OUTPATIENT THERAPY	– PROVIDE MEDICATION TEACHING THREE TIMES WEEKLY TO REINFORCE THE FOLLOWING: ·DRUG NAME(S) ·DOSE(S) ·ADMINISTRATION SCHEDULE(S) ·SIDE EFFECT(S) ·SELF-CARE MEASURES TO COUNTERACT SIDE EFFECT(S) ·PURPOSE/TARGET SYMPTOM(S) – INFORM RICHARD TO CONTACT STAFF TO RECEIVE ALL MEDI- CATION AFTER FIRST ITEM ABOVE – AT TIME OF ADMIN- ISTRATION, ASK HIM TO REITERATE ALL POINTS OUTLINED IN FIRST ITEM ABOVE – EVALUATE WEEKLY PROGRESS IN PATIENT'S NOTES re: LEARNING ABILITY AND COOPER- ATION WITH TEACHING EFFORTS – INFORM RICHARD OF HOUSING OPTIONS FOR	– BY DISCHARGE, RICHARD WILL HAVE RECEIVED COMPLETE MEDICATION TEACHING, INCLUDING: ·DRUG NAME(S) ·DOSE(S) ·ADMINISTRATION SCHEDULE(S) ·SIDE EFFECT(S) ·SELF-CARE MEASURES TO COUNTERACT SIDE EFFECT(S) ·PURPOSE/TARGET SYMPTOM(S) – BY DISCHARGE, RICHARD WILL HAVE COLLABORATED WITH STAFF TO SECURE A STRUCTURED LIVING SITUA- TION AND OUTPATIENT THERAPIST	10/1 DM

Nursing diagnosis	Nursing intervention	Predicted outcome/short-term goals (include time frame)	Date/signature
	STRUCTURED SETTINGS; ASSIST WITH COMPLETION OF APPLICATIONS AND ARRANGING INTERVIEWS —INFORM RICHARD OF OPTIONS FOR FOLLOW-UP THERAPY AND ASSIST WITH ARRANGING THE SAME —REINFORCE IMPORTANCE OF COMPLIANCE WITH TREATMENT TO PREVENT RELAPSE		
ANXIETY RELATED TO UNKNOWN ETIOLOGY, AS MANIFESTED BY RITUALISTIC BEHAVIOR	—INSTRUCT RICHARD TO REPORT EARLY SYMPTOMS OF ANXIETY, e.g., TIGHTNESS IN BACK, UNCOMFORTABLE INTERNAL SENSATIONS —ALLOW HIM TO DISCUSS HIS ANXIETY-PROVOKING CONCERNS FOR 15 MINUTES —INTERVENE TO INTERRUPT PERSEVERATION OF ANXIOUS THEMES BY OFFERING ASSISTANCE WITH RELAXATION TECHNIQUES —AFTER HE COMPLETES RELAXATION EXERCISE, REDIRECT INTO DIVERSIONAL ACTIVITIES —SUGGEST THAT HE MAINTAIN A LOG OF EVENTS PRECEDING, DURING, AND AFTER BEING AWARE OF ANXIETY; USE THIS LOG TO CHECK FOR THEMES IN ANXIOUS PATTERNS AND TO TEACH PREVENTATIVE MEASURES —USE ABOVE MEASURES DURING DESENSITIZATION PROCEDURES —DOCUMENT EFFECTIVENESS OF ABOVE PLAN EVERY 3 DAYS —ADMINISTER ANXI-	—BY DISCHARGE, RICHARD WILL REPORT SUBJECTIVE IMPROVEMENT IN ANXIOUS SYMPTOMS —BY DISCHARGE, HE WILL LEARN AND DEMONSTRATE AT LEAST ONE NEW METHOD TO COPE WITH ANXIETY	10/1 D·M

Continued

Nursing Care Plan *continued*

Nursing diagnosis	Nursing intervention	Predicted outcome/short-term goals (include time frame)	Date/signature
	OLYTIC MEDICATIONS AS PER PHYSICIAN'S ORDERS; MONITOR AND EVALUATE EFFECTIVENESS OF MEDICATION —MEDICATION TEACHING, AS DESCRIBED UNDER "NONCOMPLIANCE"		
SOCIAL ISOLA-TION RELATED TO EMBARASS-MENT WITH REGARD TO RITUALISTIC BEHAVIOR	—STRESS THE IMPOR-TANCE OF COMPLIANCE WITH TREATMENT PLAN; THAT AS HE WORKS ON ANXIETY, EASE WITH OTHER INTERPERSONAL INTER-ACTIONS WILL FOLLOW —SUGGEST THAT RICHARD INTEGRATE ANXIETY WITH SOCIAL RELATIONS IN HIS DAILY LOG. REVIEW LOG ONCE A WEEK AND COMPLIMENT PROGRESS —INTEGRATE INTO MILIEU SLOWLY	—RICHARD WILL EAT WITH COMMUNITY MEMBERS BY 10/5 — HE WILL SOCIALIZE APPRO-PRIATELY FOR AT LEAST 2 HOURS EACH DAY START-ING 10/3	10/1 DM

the fact that while anxiolytic and neuroleptic medications yield inconsistent behavioral outcomes, antidepressant medications often produce encouraging results.

Richard's pharmacological treatment consisted of a trial of phenelzine (Nardil), a monoamine oxidase inhibitor, and alprazolam (Xanax), a benzodiazepine anxiolytic. The alprazolam served as an "as-needed" medication that helped modulate Richard's anxiety until the phenelzine began to reduce his obsessive-compulsive behaviors. As he experienced a therapeutic effect from the phenelzine, Richard was more able to participate in his behaviorally-oriented program of care. Noteworthy improvement occurred: he washed, bathed, laundered clothing, ate in a community setting, and socialized in a relatively appropriate fashion for the first time in months. He managed to secure a part-time volunteer job, doing clerical work for a charitable organization. Prior to his discharge from the hospital, Richard interviewed for and received acceptance at a halfway house; he was later referred to a program of graded steps to independent living.

Fortunately, Richard accepted follow-up treatment in psychotherapy for ongoing conflicts involving issues of interpersonal relationships and intimacy, as well as behavioral difficulties imposed by the OCD. During stressful periods, such as discharge from the hospital, Richard showed signs of regression to previous levels of maladaptive functioning. However, with behavioral and pharmacological assistance, he managed to avoid protracted periods of severe dysfunction. The staff at the halfway house where Richard resided after discharge agreed to continue carrying out the inpatient behavioral program of treatment.

REFERENCES

Diagnostic and Statistical Manual of Mental Disorders, 3rd ed. Washington, D.C.: American Psychiatric Association, 1980.

Emmelkamp, P. *Phobic and Obsessive-Compulsive Disorders.* New York: Plenum Press, 1982.

Insel, T. "Obsessive-Compulsive Disorder—Five Clinical Questions and a Suggested Approach," *Comprehensive Psychiatry* 3:241-51, 1982.

Insel, T., and Murphy, D. "The Psychopharmacological Treatment of Obsessive-Compulsive Disorder: A Review," *Journal of Clinical Psychopharmacology* 5:304-11, 1981.

Insel, T., et al. "Obsessive-Compulsive Disorder," *Archives of General Psychiatry* 40:605-12, 1983.

Kaplan, H., and Sadock, B. *Comprehensive Textbook of Psychiatry III.* Baltimore: Williams & Wilkins Co., 1982.

SELECTED BIBLIOGRAPHY

Anath, J. "Clomiprimine in Obsessive-Compulsive Disorder: A Review," *Psychosomatics* 24(8):723-27, 1983.

Cooper, J. "The Leyton Obsessive Inventory," *Psychological Medicine* 1:48-64, 1970.

Kneisl, C.R., and Wilson, H.S. *Handbook of Psychosocial Nursing Care.* Menlo Park, Calif.: Addison-Wesley Publishing Co., 1984.

Rebecca:
Generalized Anxiety Disorder

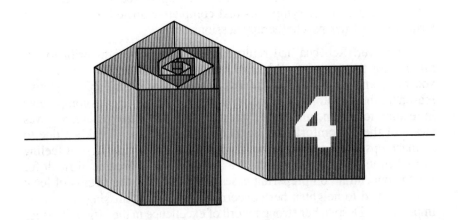

Geoffry W. McEnany, MS, RN

Nursing care of a client carrying the diagnosis of generalized anxiety disorder represents a major clinical challenge. Such a client suffers severe and often unyielding symptoms and requires adept, well-coordinated nursing care. Knowledge of the psychobiology of anxiety assists the nurse in understanding the physical manifestations of this condition. Additionally, the nurse working with such a client is well advised to become familiar with the different types of nursing interventions aimed at anxiety reduction, as well as the appropriate timing of these techniques to abate the client's anxious symptoms.

CASE STUDY

Rebecca was a 29-year-old, white, Catholic woman who worked as an associate in a small law firm in a large western city. Since her separation and subsequent divorce 2 years prior to admission, she had been living alone in a two-bedroom suburban apartment. Her former husband had custody of their only child, a 4-year-old girl; Rebecca saw the child for two weekends each month. Before her current hospitalization, Rebecca had never been hospitalized for psychiatric difficulties.

She had, however, been under the care of a psychiatric clinical nurse specialist at one time. At age 21, following the unexpected death of her older brother, she received treatment for symptoms of sleep disturbance and irritability. Rebecca characterized the 3-month course of outpatient psychotherapy as "brief therapy for the resolution of grief issues around my brother's death." She received no psychopharmacological intervention during the therapy, but reported that the experience was "extremely helpful," and that her symptoms had completely abated by the time of termination of her psychotherapy sessions.

However, Rebecca had returned to therapy 4 months prior to admission for treatment of subjective feelings of restlessness, unease, nervousness, and, at times, fearfulness without any identifiable objective reason for the symptoms. According to Rebecca, each day was comparable in relation to her uncomfortable internal state. Upon awakening, she was aware of the discomfort; she stopped eating her usual breakfast due to stomach upset and poor appetite. Once at work, she found herself feeling overwhelmed with the demands of a law practice. It became difficult for her to concentrate on preparing cases for court, and the details of legal briefs served to heighten her concern that she was "missing something important." Despite her strong record of excellence in the office, Rebecca became concerned that others were aware of her difficulties and afraid that she would be summoned by senior staff for reprimands about her performance. By noon of each day she had developed diarrhea, and as a consequence, began cancelling luncheon meetings with clients. She frequently spent her afternoons in court; during the week prior to contacting her psychotherapist, she encountered problems thinking clearly and difficulties in presenting her cases in a convincing fashion. At times in court, her mouth became dry, her hands shook, and she perspired excessively. She also noted her heart pounding and on at least two occasions became afraid that she was experiencing the initial symptoms of a myocardial infarction.

Her symptoms remissed in severity after court each day, but continued to persist into the evening. Because of the unpredictable complexity of her symptoms, Rebecca began to isolate herself, refusing invitations to professional and social events. Her evenings consisted of a series of events to curtail her anxiety; she often had a glass of wine before taking a warm bath, during which she listened to classical music or read. After her bath, she frequently prepared a light supper, had another glass of wine, and then went to bed. But despite her attempts at relaxation, Rebecca continued to feel tension and apprehension. In bed, she tossed and turned, often worrying about her child or thinking about the events of the day. Her sleep became riddled with bizarre, tortuous, often frightening dreams that kept her awake often for more than an hour at a time. The next morning, the onerous cycle would begin again.

Shortly after beginning psychotherapy, Rebecca received a prescription for lorazepam (Ativan), 1 mg every 3 hours as needed for symptom relief. Initially, she experienced some relief of somatic symptoms, but her internal sensations of fear and anxiety, although reduced, were never completely mollified. After 2 months of this medication regimen, most of the symptoms had recurred, despite increased daily doses. After discussing the medication's ineffectiveness and Rebecca's possible tolerance with her therapist, the psychiatrist discontinued the lorazepam and prescribed alprazolam (Xanax), 0.5 mg every 2 to 4 hours as needed for symptom relief. Again, the medication helped mitigate Rebecca's symptoms for a 3-week period, but by the end of the month, she was taking up to 4 mg of alprazolam daily without relief.

Throughout the course of her therapy, Rebecca experienced an actual decline in her ability to function professionally and socially. In her work, she developed major difficulties in her ability to concentrate and focus on the presentation of her cases to a judge and jury. Clients became impatient with her frequent inability to retain details and to keep facts in sequentially correct patterns. As clients demonstrated their disapproval of Rebecca's behavior, she became markedly more distressed. On several occasions, she was relieved of her duties on important cases and given more menial responsibilities. Eventually, her boss asked that she take a leave of absence and return to work only when her condition had significantly improved. This event precipitated her first psychiatric hospitalization.

No obvious biological/physical conditions contributed to Rebecca's psychiatric presentation. She was healthy and in excellent physical condition. She did not smoke or take illicit drugs; her intake of alcoholic beverages was moderate and often concurrent with an exacerbation of her psychological symptoms. Physical examination revealed no abnormalities. She had been hospitalized only once, for the birth of her daughter, and had no history of surgery, allergies, or medical conditions. Her only medication was the alprazolam prescribed by her physician.

Rebecca's developmental and family histories contributed some significant data to the understanding of this case. Rebecca was the middle child in a family of five children. She had an older brother and sister and a pair of younger twin brothers. Her mother was alive and well; her father died 5 years ago from the complications of alcoholism, specifically liver failure.

Rebecca remembered her childhood and adolescence as a painful and troublesome time in her life. Her father was an unsuccessful businessman who ran the family household "like a tight ship." She recounts her father's stern attitude "towards child-rearing as well as everything else...he always expected perfection from all of us all of the time." While Rebecca was in grade school, her father's alcoholism escalated to the

Continued on page 100

RECORDING THE DATA

After you have read the case, cluster significant data into functional health patterns.

Health management/health perception _____

_____

_____

_____

_____

Nutritional/metabolic _____

_____

_____

_____

Elimination _____

_____

_____

_____

Activity/exercise _____

_____

_____

_____

Cognitive/perceptual _____

_____

_____

_____

Sleep/rest _____

_____

_____

_____

Self-perception/self-concept _____

_____

_____

_____

Role relationship _____

_____

_____

_____

Sexuality/reproductive _____

_____

_____

_____

Coping/stress tolerance _____

_____

_____

_____

Value/belief _____

_____

_____

_____

ASSIGNING NURSING DIAGNOSES

Use your clustered data to select appropriate nursing diagnoses.

Health perception/health management

- ☐ Growth and Development, Altered (see Developmental Delay)
- ☐ Health Maintenance, Altered
- ☐ Infection, Potential for
- ☐ Injury (Trauma): Potential for
- ☐ Noncompliance (Specify)
- ☐ Poisoning: Potential for
- ☐ Suffocation: Potential for

Nutritional/metabolic

- ☐ Body Temperature, Potential Alteration in
- ☐ Developmental Delay: Physical Growth and Development
- ☐ Fluid Volume, Altered: Excess or Excess Fluid Volume
- ☐ Fluid Volume Deficit, Actual
- ☐ Fluid Volume Deficit, Potential
- ☐ Nutrition, Altered: Less Than Body Requirements or Nutritional Deficit (Specify)
- ☐ Nutrition, Altered: More Than Body Requirements or Exogenous Obesity
- ☐ Nutrition, Altered: Potential for More Than Body Requirements or Potential for Obesity
- ☐ Oral Mucous Membrane, Altered
- ☐ Skin Integrity, Impaired or Skin Breakdown
- ☐ Skin Integrity, Impaired or Potential Skin Breakdown
- ☐ Swallowing, Impaired or Uncompensated Swallowing Impairment
- ☐ Tissue Integrity, Impaired

Elimination

- ☐ Bowel Elimination, Altered: Constipation
- ☐ Bowel Elimination, Altered: Diarrhea
- ☐ Bowel Elimination, Altered: Incontinence

- ☐ Developmental Delay: Bowel/Bladder Control
- ☐ Incontinence: Functional
- ☐ Incontinence: Reflex
- ☐ Incontinence: Stress
- ☐ Incontinence: Total
- ☐ Incontinence: Urge
- ☐ Urinary Elimination, Altered Patterns of
- ☐ Urinary Retention

Activity/exercise

- ☐ Activity Intolerance
- ☐ Activity Intolerance, Potential
- ☐ Airway Clearance, Ineffective
- ☐ Breathing Pattern, Ineffective
- ☐ Cardiac Output, Altered: Decreased
- ☐ Developmental Delay: Mobility
- ☐ Developmental Delay: Self-Care Skills
- ☐ Diversional Activity Deficit
- ☐ Gas Exchange, Impaired
- ☐ Home Maintenance Management, Impaired (Mild, Moderate, Severe, Potential, Chronic)
- ☐ Mobility, Impaired Physical
- ☐ Self-Care Deficit: Feeding
- ☐ Self-Care Deficit: Bathing/Hygiene
- ☐ Self-Care Deficit: Dressing/Grooming
- ☐ Self-Care Deficit: Toileting
- ☐ Self-Care Deficit: Total
- ☐ Tissue Perfusion, Altered: (Specify)

Sleep/rest

- ☐ Sleep Pattern Disturbance

Cognitive/perceptual

- ☐ Comfort, Altered: Pain
- ☐ Comfort, Altered: Chronic Pain

☐ Developmental Delay: (Specify Cognitive Area; attention, decision making, etc.)

☐ Hypothermia

☐ Hyperthermia

☐ Knowledge Deficit (Specify)

☐ Sensory-Perceptual Alteration: Input Excess or Sensory Overload

☐ Sensory-Perceptual Alteration: Input Deficit or Sensory Deprivation

☐ Thermoregulation, Ineffective

☐ Thought Processes, Altered

☐ Unilateral Neglect

Self-perception/self-concept

☐ Anxiety

☐ Body Image Disturbance

☐ Fear

☐ Hopelessness

☐ Personal Identity Confusion

☐ Powerlessness (Severe, Low, Moderate)

☐ Self-Esteem Disturbance

Role relationship

☐ Communication, Impaired Verbal

☐ Developmental Delay: Communication Skills

☐ Developmental Delay: Social Skills

☐ Family Processes, Altered

☐ Grieving, Anticipatory

☐ Grieving, Dysfunctional

☐ Parenting, Altered: Actual or Potential

☐ Role Performance, Disturbance in

☐ Social Interactions, Impaired

☐ Social Isolation (Rejection)

Sexuality/reproductive

☐ Rape-Trauma Syndrome: Compounded

☐ Rape-Trauma Syndrome: Silent Reaction

☐ Sexual Dysfunction

☐ Sexuality Patterns, Altered

Coping/stress tolerance

☐ Adjustment, Impaired

☐ Coping, Ineffective Individual

☐ Coping, Ineffective Family: Compromised

☐ Coping, Ineffective Family: Disabling

☐ Coping, Family: Potential for Growth

☐ Developmental Delay (Specify area)

☐ Post-Trauma Response

☐ Violence, Potential for (Self-Directed or Directed at Others)

Value/belief

☐ Spiritual Distress (Distress of Human Spirit)

You are now ready to develop a nursing care plan for this client. Use the following blank pages to do so. Then refer to the author's formulation, diagnostic summary, care plan, and summary.

NURSING CARE PLAN

Complete the chart below to develop a nursing care plan for this client.

Discharge outcomes/long-term goals	

Nursing diagnosis	Nursing intervention	

	Predicted outcomes/short-term goals (include time frame)	**Date/signature**

Return to Formulation, page 101

point where he lost his job at the family-owned moving and storage company; this in turn further fueled his alcoholic behavior. Eventually, the family business went bankrupt, and the family lost their home to a foreclosure. The family moved to a small apartment, and Rebecca's mother was forced to go to work as a waitress in a local restaurant to support the household. Her father continued to drink heavily and was unable to hold a job for any extended period.

During high school, Rebecca dated and had many friends, although she was ashamed to bring friends home out of embarrassment of her alcoholic father. She and her siblings were actively involved in church and civic activities; they attended parochial schools until the family could no longer afford the costs of tuition. Rebecca characterizes her memories of childhood and adolescence as "a major life lesson in survival tactics." Her oldest brother drinks heavily; she describes him as "an alcoholic who has not yet hit bottom with his drinking."

After high school, Rebecca attended college, taking courses in preparation for law school; she graduated with honors from her undergraduate studies. During her college years she met John, and the couple dated for 2 years before marrying. Thirteen months after the wedding, Rebecca gave birth to a daughter. During her daughter's infancy, Rebecca attended law school while her daughter was in day care. Rebecca worked assiduously in school and again graduated with honors. Almost immediately after passing the state bar examination, she took a job with the law firm with which she is currently employed.

Rebecca viewed her family and social supports as warm and dependable. ("Outside of my alcoholic brother, I know that I can pick up the phone, call any one of them, and they will help me out with just about anything.") She reported a "close" relationship with her mother, stating that they talked on the telephone frequently and saw each other at least once a week.

On admission to the hospital, Rebecca presented as a casually dressed woman appearing older than her stated age. Her thought content was appropriate to the interviewer's questions; thought process was halting at times, but seemed mainly goal-directed. But, according to her report, concentration was poor. Her mood and affect were anxious, as evidenced by constant fidgeting and only fleeting eye contact. Her short-term memory was poor, as demonstrated by an inability to remember three objects after 5 minutes, while her short-term and remote memory capacities appeared intact. Her calculation abilities were mildly impaired; she stated irritably "I don't have the mind for that sort of thing right now." No evidence existed of hallucinations, delusions, or loosening of associations. Rebecca denied any past or present suicidal ideation, although she did state that, in her condition, "life isn't much fun." Her speech was mildly pressured, with normal tones and inflection. She seemed properly oriented to person, place, time, and situation. Her abstraction abilities were above average, as was her general knowledge, and her judgment and insight appeared fair.

Reader may now complete Recording the Data, Assigning Nursing Diagnoses, and Nursing Care Plan.

FORMULATION

Rebecca clearly meets the *DSM-III* diagnostic criteria for Generalized Anxiety Disorder. For such a diagnosis, *DSM-III* requires that an individual manifest persistent symptoms of anxiety continuously for at least 1 month, that the symptoms not be due to other mental disorders, and that the individual be at least 18 years of age. The behaviors that must be present include three of the following: "(1) Motor tension (shakiness, jitteriness, jumpiness...restlessness, etc.); (2) Autonomic hyperactivity (sweating, heart pounding or racing...dry mouth...upset stomach, etc.); (3) Apprehensive expectation (anxiety, worry, fear, rumination, anticipation of misfortune to self or others); (4) Vigilance and scanning (hyperattentiveness resulting in distractibility, difficulty in concentrating...irritability, etc.)" (APA, 1980).

Rebecca demonstrated behaviors in each of the four categories outlined in *DSM-III*. She complained of tremulous hands and restlessness, pounding heart, excessive perspiration, upset stomach, rumination, fears of harm to her daughter, and difficulty in concentration. Most of her symptoms had persisted for more than a month and were not markedly responsive to medication. She did not meet criteria for other mental disorders, even though she did report mild symptoms of intermittent depression.

Rebecca accepted voluntary hospitalization for the treatment of her symptoms. The following nursing care plan delineates the various nursing approaches utilized in the course of her 4-week hospital stay.

SUMMARY

The course of Rebecca's hospitalization provides an example of how multi-leveled intervention strategies can correct deficits and needs in the areas of biological, psychological, and social difficulties. In each of these categories, skillful nursing care and intervention yielded a positive influence on the client's successful outcome of treatment.

In the initial phase of hospitalization, Rebecca demonstrated severe

Continued on page 107

DIAGNOSTIC SUMMARY FOR REBECCA

Data	Functional health pattern	Nursing diagnosis
—Experiences subjective feelings of restlessness, unease, nervousness; fear without any identifiable objective reason for the symptoms —Symptoms made it difficult for her to concentrate on preparing cases for court —Symptoms worse in afternoon and evening	Self-Perception/Self-Concept	Anxiety related to unknown etiology as manifested by restlessness, heart pounding, and shakiness
—By noon of each day, had developed diarrhea and as a consequence, started cancelling luncheon meetings with clients	Elimination	Altered bowel elimination, diarrhea related to physiological effects of anxious state
—Despite the attempts at relaxation, continued to feel tension coupled with apprehension —Once in bed, tossed and turned, often worrying about her child or ruminating over the events of the day —Sleep riddled with bizarre dreams that keep her awake for often more than an hour at a time	Sleep/Rest	Sleep Pattern Disturbance related to anxiety as manifested by hyperattentiveness and interrupted sleep
—Because of the unpredictable complexity of symptoms, began to isolate herself, refusing invitations to professional and social events	Role Relationship	Social Isolation related to unpredictability of symptoms
—Has never taken clonazepam prior to this hospitalization	Cognitive/Perceptual	Knowledge Deficit related to lack of information re: new medication

NURSING CARE PLAN

Complete the chart below to develop a nursing care plan for this client.

Discharge outcome/long-term goals		
1. RETURN TO PREVIOUS LEVEL OF HIGH FUNCTIONING, AS EVIDENCED BY SAT-ISFACTORY FUNCTIONING AT WORK AND REINTEGRATION INTO SOCIAL SITUATIONS.	2. ABATEMENT OF TARGET SYMPTOMS SECONDARY TO GENERALIZED ANXIETY DISORDER	

Nursing diagnosis	Nursing intervention	Predicted outcome/short-term goals (include time frame)	Date/signature
ANXIETY RE-LATED TO UN-KNOWN ETIOL-OGY AS MAN-IFESTED BY RESTLESSNESS, HEART POUNDING AND SHAKINESS	—ASSIST REBECCA IN DEVELOPING A LIST OF BEHAVIORS THAT SHE IDENTIFIES AS SIGNS OF ESCALATING ANX-IETY; REBECCA IS TO SHARE THIS LIST WITH PRIMARY CARE NURSE ON A DAILY BASIS —ENCOURAGE REBECCA TO KEEP A RUNNING LOG OF: ·TIME WHEN SHE IS AWARE OF ANXIETY ·EVENTS SURROUNDING ANXIOUS FEELINGS ·HER OWN BEHAVIOR BEFORE, DURING, AND AFTER THE INCREASE IN ANXIETY —PRIMARY CARE NURSE IS TO REVIEW THE LOG WITH REBECCA ON A DAILY BASIS TO IDENT-IFY HER PATTERN OF ANXIETY AND RELIEF-SEEKING BEHAVIOR —INSTRUCT REBECCA TO REPORT EARLY SIGNS OF ANXIETY TO NURS-ING STAFF —FOLLOW THE PROCE-DURE BELOW FOR ANXIETY ABATEMENT: ·STAFF TO SIT WITH REBECCA FOR 5 MIN-UTES TO DISCUSS ANTE-CEDENTS TO HER ANXIOUS FEELINGS ·AFTER 5 MINUTES, REDIRECT REBECCA TO 30 MINUTES OF GUIDED IMAGERY RELAXATION —IF REBECCA DEMON-STRATES MODERATE TO SEVERE ANXIETY (e.g. POUNDING HEART, PERSPIRATION, RUM-INATION) FOLLOW THE PROCEDURE LISTED BE-	—REBECCA WILL DEMONSTRATE A DECREASE IN OBJECTIVE SIGNS OF ANXIETY, e.g. DIM-INISHED SHAKINESS, HEART POUNDING, INSOMNIA, AND HYPERATTENTIVENESS WITHIN 3 WEEKS —REBECCA WILL REPORT ANY SUBJECTIVE IMPROVEMENT IN HER ANXIOUS SYMPTOMS IMMEDIATELY —REBECCA WILL LEARN EARLY SIGNS AND SYMPTOMS OF ANXIETY AND LEARN AND EMPLOY METHODS OF EARLY INTERVENTIONS WITHIN 3 WEEKS	10/1 DM

Continued

Nursing Care Plan *continued*

Nursing diagnosis	Nursing intervention	Predicted outcome/short-term goals (include time frame)	Date/signature
	LOW: • REMAIN WITH REBECCA BUT DO NOT ENGAGE IN DISCUSSION OF ANXIETY-PROVOKING EVENT • BRING CLIENT TO A QUIET AREA • ASSESS FOR P.R.N. MEDICATION (ANXIOLYTIC) • ASSIST REBECCA WITH DEEP-BREATHING EXERCISES OR WHITE NOISE RELAXATION, e.g., RECORDED OCEAN WAVES, ETC • EVALUATE AND DOCUMENT EFFECTIVENESS OF INTERVENTION – INVOLVE REBECCA IN EXERCISE GROUP ON A DAILY BASIS		
ALTERED BOWEL ELIMINATION: DIARRHEA, RELATED TO PHYSIOLOGICAL EFFECTS OF ANXIOUS STATE	– REBECCA IS TO REPORT ANY INCIDENT OF DIARRHEA TO STAFF – WHEN DIARRHEA IS PRESENT, HAVE REBECCA INCORPORATE THE FOLLOWING FOODS INTO DIET: • RICE • APPLE JUICE • BANANAS – IF DIARRHEA PERSISTS NOTIFY PHYSICIAN – ASSESS THE EFFECTIVENESS OF ABOVE INTERVENTION	– REBECCA WILL REPORT DEVIATIONS FROM NORMAL AND EFFECTIVENESS OF INTERVENTIONS IMMEDIATELY – BY DISCHARGE, REBECCA WILL REPORT A RETURN TO NORMAL ELIMINATIVE FUNCTION	10/1 DM
SLEEP PATTERN DISTURBANCE RELATED TO ANXIETY AS MANIFESTED BY HYPERATTENTIVENESS AND INTERRUPTED SLEEP	– INSTRUCT REBECCA IN HIGH L-TRYPTOPHAN DIET – IF REBECCA AWAKENS DURING THE NIGHT, ADMINISTER A DOSE OF L-TRYPTOPHAN WITH A CARBOHYDRATE DRINK (FRUIT JUICE) AND ENCOURAGE HER TO LISTEN TO 30 MINUTES OF WHITE NOISE RELAXATION – EVALUATE EFFECTIVENESS OF PLAN	– BY DISCHARGE, REBECCA WILL FOLLOW THE FOLLOWING ROUTINE WITHOUT PROMPT: • LIMIT INTAKE OF CAFFEINATED BEVERAGES TO ONE CUP OF COFFEE OR ONE CAFFEINATED SODA PER DAY • NO CAFFEINATED BEVERAGES OR CHOCOLATE AFTER 5 PM • AT 7 PM, REBECCA WILL SPEND 30 MINUTES IN MODERATE EXERCISE, e.g., EXERCYCLE • AT 9 PM, REBECCA WILL TAKE A WARM BATH • AT 10 PM, REBECCA WILL DO	10/1 DM

Nursing diagnosis	Nursing intervention	Predicted outcome/short-term goals (include time frame)	Date/signature
		30 MINUTES OF PROGRES-SIVE RELAXATION EXERCISES	
		• AT 10:30 P.M., REBECCA WILL BE IN BED WITH LIGHTS OUT; SHE WILL LISTEN TO WHITE NOISE RE-LAXATION TAPE, e.g., TAPE OF OCEAN WAVES, ETC	
		— REBECCA WILL REPORT EFFECTIVENESS OF SLEEP PLAN TO NURSE AND PHY-SICIAN WITHIN 1 WEEK	
SOCIAL ISOLA-TION RELATED TO UNPREDICT-ABILITY OF SYMPTOMS	—EXPLORE SOURCES OF SOCIAL SUPPORT WITH REBECCA	— BY DISCHARGE, REBECCA WILL HAVE MADE CONTACT WITH AT LEAST TWO NEW SOURCES OR AGENCIES FOR SOCIAL SUPPORT	10/1 DM
	—OFFER REBECCA RECOMMENDATIONS FOR AGENCIES THAT ARE SENSITIVE TO THE NEEDS OF PROFESSIONAL WOMEN	— REBECCA, BY WEEK 2 OF HOSPITALIZATION, WILL AGREE TO SELECT ONE AGENCY AND ATTEND ONE FUNCTION OF THE AGENCY	
	—ENCOURAGE CONTACT WITH A SOCIAL AGENCY —ENCOURAGE REBECCA TO ATTEND A WOMAN'S GROUP ON THE UNIT TWICE WEEKLY	— REBECCA WILL KEEP AN ONGOING LOG OF HER LEVEL OF ANXIETY IN MAKING CONTACTS WITH NEW SOCIAL SITUATIONS	
	— PRIMARY CARE NURSE WILL REVIEW THE LOG WITH REBECCA TO EXPLORE BEHAVIORAL MEANS OF ANXIETY CONTROL		
KNOWLEDGE DEFICIT RE-LATED TO LACK OF INFORMA-TION RE: NEW MEDICATION	—REBECCA IS TO RECEIVE A WRITTEN COPY OF THE TEACHING PLAN FOR CLONAZEPAM WHEN SHE BEGINS THE MED-ICATION	—BY DISCHARGE, REBECCA WILL DEMONSTRATE AN ABILITY TO MEDICATE SELF	10/1 DM
	—REBECCA'S PRIMARY CARE NURSE WILL TEACH THE FOLLOWING ACCORDING TO THE MED-ICATION TEACHING GUIDE:	—BY DISCHARGE, REBECCA WILL VERBALIZE THE FOLLOW-ING CONCERNING HER MEDI-CATION:	
	•NAME OF MEDICATION •PURPOSE OF TAKING MEDICATION/TARGET SYMPTOMS •DOSAGE •SIDE EFFECTS •TIMES OF ADMINIS-TRATION	•NAME/PURPOSE/TARGET SYMPTOMS •DOSAGE •SIDE EFFECTS •TIMES OF ADMINISTRATION —DURING WEEK 2 OF HOSPI-TALIZATION, REBECCA WILL APPROACH STAFF AT MED-ICATION ADMINISTRATION TIMES TO REQUEST MEDICATION —WHEN REBECCA DEMON-	

Continued

Nursing Care Plan *continued*

Nursing diagnosis	Nursing intervention	Predicted outcome/short-term goals (include time frame)	Date/signature
	—THE PRIMARY CARE NURSE WILL REVIEW THE TEACHING FORM ON A WEEKLY BASIS —BEFORE ADMINISTER- ING THE MEDICATION, STAFF WILL DETERMINE REBECCA'S KNOWLEDGE OF THE FIVE POINTS OUTLINED ABOVE IN SECOND ITEM —ON MONDAY, WEDNES- DAY, AND FRIDAY OF EACH WEEK, THE PRIMARY CARE NURSE WILL DOCUMENT REBECCA'S PROGRESS IN HER UNDERSTAND- ING OF MEDICATION —SUPERVISE REBECCA AS APPROPRIATE —EVALUATE EFFECTIVE- NESS OF MEDICATION ON TARGET SYMPTOMS	STRATES MASTERY OF THE MEDICATION-RELATED INFORMATION, SHE WILL BE- GIN TO REQUEST AND POUR HER OWN MEDICATION WITH STAFF SUPERVISION	

anxiety, making behavioral intervention difficult without the use of psychopharmacological interventions. On admission, Rebecca was maintained on clonazepam (Clonopin). During the first 4 weeks of her hospitalization, she received 5 mg of clonazepam daily, in divided doses. This dose proved effective in relieving the paralytic effects of Rebecca's anxiety, enabling her to learn behavioral means of controlling her anxious feelings. During the course of her work in therapy and with the nursing staff, she reported a marked decrease in anxiety, as evidenced by a diminution of somatic manifestations as well as improved social and occupational functioning. With a series of day passes, Rebecca returned to work on a part-time basis before leaving the hospital. Additionally, she fostered her involvement in a local women's group while volunteering 8 hours of legal service per week to a women's resource center near her home.

Nursing assessment and intervention played an important role in Rebecca's recovery. Her primary care nurse worked with her to develop intervention strategies that effected changes on the psychobiological level of functioning. For example, on initial assessment, Rebecca demonstrated sleep patterns indicative of initial and middle insomnia. Such patterns of sleep pointed to the possibility of a disturbance of her circadian rhythms in sleep/wake cycles. Possible contributing factors to these disturbed sleep patterns included anxiety, caffeine intake, and the cumulative effects of poor sleep over an extended period of time (Moore-Ede et al., 1983). In an effort to assist Rebecca in "resetting" her circadian clock, while also managing her concurrent anxiety, the primary care nurse provided her with instructions on the use of a diet high in L-tryptophan, an amino acid abundant in many foods. Once ingested, these proteins selectively convert to neurotransmitters. Resulting changes include the establishment of a feedback mechanism that affects nutritional, metabolic, and neurochemical systems, resulting in possible behavioral changes (Wurtman, 1982). This high-L-tryptophan diet, along with supplemental tryptophan, anxiolytic medication, and the elimination of caffeine, resulted in abatement of the somatic manifestations of Rebecca's anxiety, which improved her sleep patterns.

Rebecca was discharged 4 weeks after her voluntary admission to the psychiatric inpatient unit. As evidenced by her subjective report and by the objective data, she made remarkable strides toward improvement during the course of her hospital stay.

Many variables influenced the outcome of Rebecca's treatment. In her case, factors such as a high level of motivation, a high level of premorbid functioning, and a multitude of personal strengths all worked in her favor towards a satisfactory recovery. Not all clients exhibit such strengths, however. Consequently, when planning care for a client with generalized anxiety disorder, the nursing staff must remember to gauge interventions and goals to levels that are achievable for the client. Such an approach not only aids the client toward recovery, but it also prevents any disappointment among staff in their capacity to provide effective care.

REFERENCES

Breier, A., et al. "The Diagnostic Validity of Anxiety Disorders and Their Relationship to Depressive Illness," *American Journal of Psychiatry* 142(7):787-97, 1985.

Diagnostic and Statistical Manual of Mental Disorders, 3rd ed. Washington, D.C.: American Psychiatric Association, 1980.

Hoehn-Saric, R. "Comparison of Generalized Anxiety Disorder with Panic Disorder Patients," *Psychopharmacology Bulletin* 14(4):104-08, 1982.

Moore-Ede, M.C., et al. "Circadian Time Keeping in Health and Disease: Basic Properties of Circadian Pacemakers," *New England Journal of Medicine* 309(8):469-76, 1983.

Raskin, M., et al. "Panic and Generalized Anxiety Disorders," *Archives of General Psychiatry* 39:687-89, 1982.

Wurtman, R.J. "Nutrients That Modify Brain Functions," *Scientific American* 246(50):59-60, 1982.

SELECTED BIBLIOGRAPHY

Alper, J. "Biology and Mental Illness," *The Atlantic Monthly* 70-76, December 1983.

Braestrup, C. "Neurotransmitters and CNS Disease," *The Lancet* 1030-34, November 1982.

Kneisl, C.R., and Wilson, H.S. *Handbook of Psychosocial Nursing Care.* Menlo Park, Calif.: Addison-Wesley Publishing Co., 1984.

Matthew, R.J., ed. *The Biology of Anxiety.* New York: Brunner-Mazel, 1982.

Pasnau, R.O., ed. *Diagnosis and Treatment of Anxiety.* Washington, D.C.: American Psychiatric Association, 1984.

Peter:
Chronic Schizophrenia

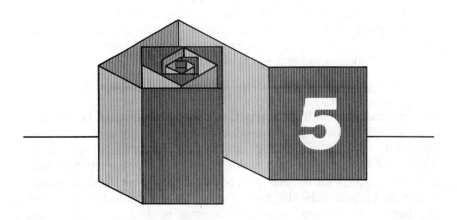

Barbara R. Garson, MSN, RN, CS

One of the most common disorders treated in a psychiatric inpatient setting is an exacerbation of chronic schizophrenia. The three major components of this disorder include disorganization of thought and emotion, deterioration of functioning, and a persistence of symptoms. A person experiencing acute symptoms of schizophrenia can benefit greatly from an environment that provides the structure, safety, reality testing, and judgment that the individual lacks. In addition, using the opportunity of hospitalization to assess and intervene in the individual's social system can do much to decrease the frequency of future hospitalization and other sequelae of the illness. The hospitalization is also an opportunity to promote the client's positive interpersonal interactions and to transfer this learning to situations encountered as an outpatient. Discharge plans based upon a thorough assessment of the individual and family's baseline dynamics, strengths, and weaknesses in communication can do much to maximize the client's functioning and enhance quality of life.

CASE STUDY

This was the first psychiatric admission and first psychiatric contact for Peter, a 19-year-old Catholic, unemployed, single white male living with his parents. Peter was admitted to the hospital with the chief complaint of "the FBI is out to get me."

Peter stated that he had been sick since he started college 7 months earlier. Shortly after arriving at college he began to feel suspicious of other people (particularly his roommate) and became convinced that the dormitory food was poisoned and worried that people were "out to get" him as well as his parents, who lived 3 hours away. He remained in college for the first semester, withdrawing socially and doing poorly academically. At the end of the semester, he returned home and did not return to school, stating that school was not a safe place for him.

On more specific questioning, Peter stated that since tenth grade he has been preoccupied with thoughts about religion and sin. He remembers speaking with the priest at his church about what he felt was his "calling" to God; he believed that God had spoken to him and instructed him to remain celibate. Peter also described receiving "messages" over the radio telling him that he was sinful and instructing him to avoid contact with females at school and to perform various rituals to cleanse himself if he did have contact. This happened at the same time that he had become attracted to a girl in his homeroom at school. He described running to the bathroom to wash his mouth out after talking with her and immediately washing his hands "to cleanse my soul" after holding hands in the hallway at school. Occasionally he would hear voices telling him he would be punished. At times he spent hours washing his hands and rinsing his mouth to try to make the voices go away. Peter believed his mother was the only woman with whom he was allowed to spend extended time without having to repent or cleanse himself.

Over the course of his sophomore and junior years, Peter felt increasingly anxious about his attraction to women at school. His grades suffered to some extent, and in his senior year he spent all of his free time alone at home or with his mother. During this time, Peter's father began to spend more time away from home. When home, he was generally quiet and isolated, spending his time watching television and drinking beer.

A few weeks after arriving at college, Peter went to a dance sponsored by his dormitory. There, he met a woman who asked him to dance. They danced and talked, and she asked him to walk her across campus to her dormitory. Peter stated that on his way back to his room he heard a woman's voice telling him that he was sinful and that he and his parents were in danger. He began to worry that the voice was a message from God and that some people wanted to hurt him. When he got back to his room, he repeatedly rinsed his mouth and washed his hands in the hope that this would cleanse him. The next morning, he went to church and stayed for the entire day, hoping that this would free him from the punishment he felt sure was ordered against him. Nevertheless, on the way back to his dormitory he felt convinced that God's messengers had taken the form of FBI agents and were out to harm or kill him. He became convinced that his roommate was a disguised FBI agent.

Over the next 2 months, Peter grew increasingly suspicious. He refused to eat the food in the dormitory, fearing it was poisoned. He was convinced that his roommate could read his mind and was trying to control his thoughts. He was also convinced that the Pope's planned visit to the U.S. President was arranged to oversee his persecution and ultimate execution. To Peter, each radio broadcast concerning the Pope's planned trip was a special personal message about the nature of his sins and his ultimate punishment. He found himself unable to concentrate on his schoolwork and failed four of his five courses. By the time he returned home at Christmas break he had lost 30 pounds and appeared quite distraught.

Peter told his mother how dangerous he felt things were at school and expressed concerns about his parents' safety. He refused to return to school; instead, he remained home and started working as a stock clerk in a local supermarket. But his fears continued. He avoided eating lunch and rarely spoke with other employees out of concern that the other clerks and cashiers were disguised FBI agents who might be trying to poison him. Unable to concentrate on stocking shelves because of his constant vigilance for disguised FBI agents, he voluntarily left his job after only 1 month.

Peter came to the hospital at his mother's insistence after she discovered that he was collecting knives and staying up all night to sharpen them for, as he put it, protection when the FBI descended upon the house. Before admission, he had not slept for 4 days. He did not want to come to the hospital and said he thought it could not help him. He said that he came because his mother had told him that a psychiatrist in the emergency room said that he may not have a choice about whether to be admitted.

Peter denied any drug or alcohol use, and his medical history was not remarkable. Peter is an only child, described by his mother as a quiet "loner type" during childhood. His mother and father reported that he never had many friends but always had done well in school. They stated that Peter's maternal aunt had a "nervous breakdown" while in her twenties and is now living with Peter's maternal grandmother. They reported no other family history of psychiatric illness or drug or alcohol abuse.

Peter's mother appeared to be very actively involved in her son's life but to have only a distant, intellectual relationship with her husband. She reported having no friends or activities of her own other than keeping house and taking care of her son, and admitted to having been lonely and distraught when he was away at college. Peter's father presented as a quiet, passive man. He reported that he kept busy with work and appeared disinterested in his wife's or son's life. He acknowledged the close relationship between his son and his wife.

At the time of admission, Peter was very suspicious of the staff and the other clients on the unit. During the initial interview with his primary nurse, he constantly shifted his eyes around the room, paced back and forth, and appeared to talk to someone next to him (although no one was there). When talking with his nurse, he would start a sentence and sometimes stop midway and become quiet. Frequently, he would jump from one subject to another even in the middle of a sentence. At other times when discussing his history, he would giggle or smile at inappropriate times. He told his nurse that he was sure the FBI was putting thoughts in his head and that the radio had sent him a message to be careful about putting any food in his mouth. He said this message was a warning that his food was poisoned.

Peter's primary nurse acknowledged and validated Peter's fears about being hurt, and reassured him in a simple and clear fashion that he was in a hospital and that the staff would not allow harm to come to him or to anyone else. She told Peter that the staff was concerned about how frightened he was feeling, and that a staff member would be outside his open door to assure his comfort and safety. She then asked him what he thought would help him feel safe. He stated that he wanted to be left alone in his room. She agreed that he should spend some quiet time alone, and suggested that he unpack his clothes and put them into the bureau drawers. She asked him if the voices he heard told him to harm himself or anyone else. Peter reiterated that the voices just repeated statements such as "you are sinful" and "don't trust her" (the nurse). The nurse asked Peter to let the staff know if the voices bothered him again. She also told him that she would like to help him feel more comfortable by giving him some medication that would make the voices bother him less. Peter refused, although he did agree to let the nurse speak with his mother regarding the medication's potential effects.

Peter's nurse met with Peter's mother, Mrs. K., who was waiting in the admission area outside the unit. She asked Mrs. K. if she would talk with Peter about taking his medication. The nurse answered Mrs. K.'s questions, acknowledging Peter's frightened state and outlining the initial plan of care to ensure his safety and decrease his anxiety.

Mrs. K. was able to help Peter agree to take the medication but was asked to leave shortly afterwards, when Peter became visibly more agitated as she began inspecting his bed linen and putting away his clothes. On her way out, Mrs. K. was encouraged to call the nurses' station at any time for a report on Peter's status.

On formal mental status examination, Peter presented as a 19-year-old who appeared his stated age. His hands were excoriated, and he was unshaven and disheveled. He appeared fatigued yet hypervigilant. He constantly shifted his gaze around the room and avoided eye contact with the examiner. Periodically, he fixed his gaze on the space next to him and appeared to be conversing with a nonexistent person. His speech was halting, with thought blocking. He was experiencing auditory and visual hallucinations with delusions of persecution, thought control, and thought insertion. His motor behavior was agitated, with constant pacing and a tense body posture. His affect was labile and generally fearful and anxious, with periodic inappropriate giggling and smiling. His primary coping strategies included withdrawal and hypervigilance. He was properly oriented to person, place, time, and situation. Memory and general fund of knowledge were not assessed due to lack of cooperation, but concentration, abstraction capacity, and judgment were poor. His visual perception was distorted, with visual hallucinations, but depth perception appeared normal, as did motor coordination. Peter reacted to the interviewer with suspiciousness.

Reader may now complete Recording the Data, Assigning Nursing Diagnoses, and Nursing Care Plan.

FORMULATION

This client, Peter, presented as disorganized in multiple spheres: cognitive and sensory perceptions, self care, and social and academic functioning. On a cognitive level, his ability to accurately perceive reality is grossly impaired. He experiences delusions of thought insertion and ideas of reference and shows evidence of blocking, ritualistic behavior associated with magical thinking, and delusions of persecution. Peter copes by presenting an aggressive stance as a response to the perception that others wish to hurt him. He refuses to eat or drink in an attempt to protect himself from the perceived danger of poisoning. His hypervigilance is a response to the perceived need to be on guard against attack. Because his delusions are not based upon reality, arguing or reasoning with him about his delusional content is not appropriate.

The following goals are based upon the assessment that Peter is responding to a perceived threat:
- remove any object of his concern, when possible
- encourage a more accurate perception of reality
- tell him that his perceptions are not shared by those around him
- help him feel in greater control and thus reduce his need for vigilant self-protection.

Continued on page 120

RECORDING THE DATA

After you have read the case, cluster significant data into functional health patterns.

Health management/health perception _____

_____

_____

_____

_____

Nutritional/metabolic _____

_____

_____

_____

Elimination _____

_____

_____

_____

Activity/exercise _____

_____

_____

_____

Cognitive/perceptual _____

_____

_____

_____

Sleep/rest _____

_____

_____

_____

Self-perception/self-concept _____

_____

_____

_____

Role relationship _____

_____

_____

_____

Sexuality/reproductive _____

_____

_____

_____

Coping/stress tolerance _____

_____

_____

_____

Value/belief _____

_____

_____

_____

ASSIGNING NURSING DIAGNOSES

Use your clustered data to select appropriate nursing diagnoses.

Health perception/health management

- [ ] Growth and Development, Altered (see Developmental Delay)
- [ ] Health Maintenance, Altered
- [ ] Infection, Potential for
- [ ] Injury (Trauma): Potential for
- [ ] Noncompliance (Specify)
- [ ] Poisoning: Potential for
- [ ] Suffocation: Potential for

Nutritional/metabolic

- [ ] Body Temperature, Potential Alteration in
- [ ] Developmental Delay: Physical Growth and Development
- [ ] Fluid Volume, Altered: Excess or Excess Fluid Volume
- [ ] Fluid Volume Deficit, Actual
- [ ] Fluid Volume Deficit, Potential
- [ ] Nutrition, Altered: Less Than Body Requirements or Nutritional Deficit (Specify)
- [ ] Nutrition, Altered: More Than Body Requirements or Exogenous Obesity
- [ ] Nutrition, Altered: Potential for More Than Body Requirements or Potential for Obesity
- [ ] Oral Mucous Membrane, Altered
- [ ] Skin Integrity, Impaired or Skin Breakdown
- [ ] Skin Integrity, Impaired or Potential Skin Breakdown
- [ ] Swallowing, Impaired or Uncompensated Swallowing Impairment
- [ ] Tissue Integrity, Impaired

Elimination

- [ ] Bowel Elimination, Altered: Constipation
- [ ] Bowel Elimination, Altered: Diarrhea
- [ ] Bowel Elimination, Altered: Incontinence
- [ ] Developmental Delay: Bowel/Bladder Control
- [ ] Incontinence: Functional
- [ ] Incontinence: Reflex
- [ ] Incontinence: Stress
- [ ] Incontinence: Total
- [ ] Incontinence: Urge
- [ ] Urinary Elimination, Altered Patterns of
- [ ] Urinary Retention

Activity/exercise

- [ ] Activity Intolerance
- [ ] Activity Intolerance, Potential
- [ ] Airway Clearance, Ineffective
- [ ] Breathing Pattern, Ineffective
- [ ] Cardiac Output, Altered: Decreased
- [ ] Developmental Delay: Mobility
- [ ] Developmental Delay: Self-Care Skills
- [ ] Diversional Activity Deficit
- [ ] Gas Exchange, Impaired
- [ ] Home Maintenance Management, Impaired (Mild, Moderate, Severe, Potential, Chronic)
- [ ] Mobility, Impaired Physical
- [ ] Self-Care Deficit: Feeding
- [ ] Self-Care Deficit: Bathing/Hygiene
- [ ] Self-Care Deficit: Dressing/Grooming
- [ ] Self-Care Deficit: Toileting
- [ ] Self-Care Deficit: Total
- [ ] Tissue Perfusion, Altered: (Specify)

Sleep/rest

- [ ] Sleep Pattern Disturbance

Cognitive/perceptual

- [ ] Comfort, Altered: Pain
- [ ] Comfort, Altered: Chronic Pain

☐ Developmental Delay: (Specify Cognitive Area; attention, decision making, etc.)
☐ Hypothermia
☐ Hyperthermia
☐ Knowledge Deficit (Specify)
☐ Sensory-Perceptual Alteration: Input Excess or Sensory Overload
☐ Sensory-Perceptual Alteration: Input Deficit or Sensory Deprivation
☐ Thermoregulation, Ineffective
☐ Thought Processes, Altered
☐ Unilateral Neglect

Self-perception/self-concept

☐ Anxiety
☐ Body Image Disturbance
☐ Fear
☐ Hopelessness
☐ Personal Identity Confusion
☐ Powerlessness (Severe, Low, Moderate)
☐ Self-Esteem Disturbance

Role relationship

☐ Communication, Impaired Verbal
☐ Developmental Delay: Communication Skills
☐ Developmental Delay: Social Skills
☐ Family Processes, Altered
☐ Grieving, Anticipatory
☐ Grieving, Dysfunctional
☐ Parenting, Altered: Actual or Potential

☐ Role Performance, Disturbance in
☐ Social Interactions, Impaired
☐ Social Isolation (Rejection)

Sexuality/reproductive

☐ Rape-Trauma Syndrome: Compounded
☐ Rape-Trauma Syndrome: Silent Reaction
☐ Sexual Dysfunction
☐ Sexuality Patterns, Altered

Coping/stress tolerance

☐ Adjustment, Impaired
☐ Coping, Ineffective Individual
☐ Coping, Ineffective Family: Compromised
☐ Coping, Ineffective Family: Disabling
☐ Coping, Family: Potential for Growth
☐ Developmental Delay (Specify area)
☐ Post-Trauma Response
☐ Violence, Potential for (Self-Directed or Directed at Others)

Value/belief

☐ Spiritual Distress (Distress of Human Spirit)

You are now ready to develop a nursing care plan for this client. Use the following blank pages to do so. Then refer to the author's formulation, diagnostic summary, care plan, and summary.

NURSING CARE PLAN

Complete the chart below to develop a nursing care plan for this client.

Discharge outcomes/long-term goals	

Nursing diagnosis	Nursing intervention	

	Predicted outcomes/short-term goals (include time frame)	Date/signature

Return to Formulation, page 113

Peter's sensory perceptions are also grossly impaired. He hears voices from internal stimulation but is unable to ascertain that the voices are not real. As is common, the voices are insulting ("You're a jerk"; "You're no good to the human race") as well as frightening in nature. Although Peter states that the voices are not commanding him to do anything harmful, this should be further assessed, given his delusions of persecution and his lack of trust in the staff.

Disorganization exists in the area of daily functioning. Peter has probably neglected his personal hygiene because of his inability to concentrate on anything other than the perceived threat to his life from the constant presence of delusions and hallucinations. His physical well-being is threatened by inadequate nutrition, lack of sleep, and poor hygiene. His general judgment regarding self-care is severely impaired.

Peter's coping skills—social isolation, an aggressive stance toward others, and avoidance of food—are attempts at self-protection. However, they are dysfunctional and render him at risk for harm to himself and others. Given Peter's poor judgment and his inability to perceive reality, the staff must provide protection. Although Peter communicated that he wished to be in control, he will be reassured when the staff takes over as needed.

Over the past 4 years, Peter's functioning has deteriorated significantly. Symptoms first appeared in the tenth grade with a noticeable decline in social functioning. Throughout high school, he was able to continue to function academically, but during his first college semester his academic performance declined markedly. Throughout this semester, Peter's ability to care for himself also deteriorated, as evidenced by a profound weight loss. The most recent significant decline in functioning occurred immediately prior to hospitalization, when Peter was unable to function in his job as a stock clerk, was unable to leave his home or eat, and for the 3 nights prior to hospitalization was unable to sleep.

Although this was Peter's first hospitalization and his first psychiatric contact, his history shows that his illness began in the tenth grade. His limited social contact and his family's tolerance of unusual behavior delayed the seeking of professional help. Given Peter's prolonged symptoms and lack of professional assistance, his family system probably supports his symptoms; i.e., his symptoms serve a purpose in the family. Rather than focusing on other issues in their structure, family members focus on Peter's psychopathology. Two questions are important in assessing the family system: Should Peter be dependent and live at home? Should he separate successfully from his family and achieve a life of his own? Significantly, Peter's first symptoms appeared around issues of sexual identity and puberty, hallmarks of impending adulthood and separation.

At the time of his hospitalization, Peter's most immediate need is safety. After Peter stabilizes, the staff must address and plan for his needs after discharge. In relation to discharge planning, three important components must be assessed: baseline functioning abilities, support systems, and family relationships. Based upon these assessments, a plan for follow-up care will be developed.

SUMMARY

After 10 days in the hospital, Peter appeared considerably less agitated. He no longer emphatically stated that the staff and other clients wanted to hurt him. He was sleeping and eating well. He continued to prefer to spend most of his time alone in his room; however, he began to spend more time in the community. The nursing staff had succeeded in helping him tolerate contact with other people so that he started to eat his food in the community dining room, although he sat alone. He also attended a community meeting, although he had not yet begun to attend other groups on the unit. Peter denied feeling the need to hurt anyone, and his status had been changed from constant observation to 15-minute check-ins after 2 days of hospitalization. After 7 days, he was able to approach the nurses' station himself to check in every 30 minutes and was able to make a contract with his primary nurse to let the staff know when he was feeling more upset or frightened, or if the voices were bothering him.

Peter consistently expressed suspicions about his medication and was given his antipsychotic medication in a liquid form to prevent "cheeking" of the pills. At least once a day, he would argue with his nurse about taking his medication but could eventually be convinced to take it.

Peter's mother first visited Peter the evening after his admission. During this visit, she was observed to be intrusive and inappropriately intimate with her son. For instance, she immediately opened his dresser drawers and criticized how he had placed his underwear inside. She commented on his every physical movement and began to give him a back rub when he said his back was sore. When she did this, Peter became much more agitated, pacing rapidly around his room, talking as though he was responding to voices and accusing a staff member of being a member of the FBI. At this point, the staff member explained to Peter and his mother the sensibleness of Peter's spending some time alone and suggested that he might benefit from time-limited visits. After this visit, Peter's primary nurse met with Mrs. K. and explained Peter's inability

Continued on page 130

DIAGNOSTIC SUMMARY FOR PETER

Data	Functional health pattern	Nursing diagnosis
—Is suspicious of other people he believes "are out to get him" —Experiences auditory hallucinations —Became delusional around the Pope's visit; special messages about the nature of his sins and ultimate punishment —Collected and sharpened knives to protect self	Coping/Stress Tolerance	Potential for violence to self and others related to poor impulse control secondary to psychosis
—Was convinced dormitory food was poisoned, and that people were out to get him —Believed God had spoken to him and instructed him to remain celibate in order to follow His calling —Heard voices telling him he'd be punished —Heard a woman's voice telling him that he was sinful and that his parents would be punished —Became delusional around FBI as "God's messengers" —Was convinced that his roommate could read his mind —Believed that the Pope's visit was to discuss him with the President, who would oversee his persecution and ultimate execution —Was unable to concentrate on schoolwork, failed four of five courses —Was giggling and smiling at inappropriate times during interview; appeared to be talking to someone next to him	Cognitive/Perceptual	Altered thought processes related to psychosis, as manifested by auditory hallucinations, paranoid ideation, and delusions
—Was convinced that dormitory food was poisoned —Lost 30 pounds in 3 months	Activity/Exercise	Self-Care Deficit: Feeding related to chronic thought disorder secondary to acute psychosis Self-Care Deficit: Bathing Hygiene related to chronic thought disorder secondary to psychosis Potential altered nutrition: less than body requirements related to inadequate food/fluid intake secondary to psychosis

Data	Functional health pattern	Nursing diagnosis
—Stayed up all night sharpening knives —Has not slept for 4 days	Coping/Stress Tolerance	Sleep pattern disturbance related to hypervigilance secondary to psychosis
—Peter's mother and father have a distant relationship —Peter's father is also distant from Peter —During a visit, Peter's mother was observed to be intrusive and inappropriately intimate with Peter	Coping/Stress Tolerance	Ineffective family coping related to conflictual parental relationship, as manifested by overintrusive mother and distant father

NURSING CARE PLAN

Complete the chart below to develop a nursing care plan for this client.

Discharge outcome/long-term goals	NURSE SPONTANEOUSLY AND COMPLYING WITH SPECIFIED REGIMENS.		
1. PETER WILL VERBALIZE FEELING INTERNAL CONTROL.			
2. PETER'S SUSPICIOUSNESS WILL DECREASE, AND HE WILL BEGIN TO TRUST PRIMARY NURSE, AS EVIDENCED BY SEEKING OUT THE			

Nursing diagnosis	Nursing intervention	Predicted outcome/short-term goals (include time frame)	Date/signature
POTENTIAL FOR VIOLENCE TO SELF AND OTHERS RE-LATED TO POOR IMPULSE CONTROL SECONDARY TO PSYCHOSIS	—PLACE PETER UNDER CON-STANT OBSERVATION IN A LOW-STIMULATION ENVIRON-MENT —ASSESS FOR PRESENCE OF COMMAND HALLUCINATIONS TO HURT SELF OR OTHERS EACH SHIFT	—PETER WILL NOT HURT HIMSELF OR OTHERS DURING HOSPITAL-IZATION, AS EVIDENCED BY: ABSENCE OF THREATS TO OTHERS AND DECREASED REPORTS THAT PETER PERCEIVES OTHERS AS THREATENING HIS SAFETY (10 DAYS)	2/4 B.R.
	—MEDICATE AS ORDERED AND EVALUATE EFFECTIVENESS OF MEDICATION —TEACH PETER DRUG NAME(S) DOSAGE(S), ADMINISTRATION SCHEDULE, SIDE EFFECT(S), AND PURPOSE OF MEDICA-TION(S)	—PETER WILL VERBALIZE NAME, DOSAGE, ADMINISTRATION SCHED-ULE, SIDE EFFECTS, AND PURPOSE OF ALL MEDICATIONS IN 2 WEEKS	
	—MONITOR PETER'S INTERACTIONS WITH OTHER PATIENTS AND TEST HIS REALITY ORIENTATION AS CONFLICTS ARISE —PROVIDE PETER WITH QUIET TIME IN HIS OWN ROOM OR A LESS-STIMULATING COMMUNITY AREA —ACKNOWLEDGE PETER'S FEARS; VERBALLY REINFORCE THAT HE WILL NOT BE PERMITTED TO LOSE CONTROL		

Discharge outcome/long-term goals	TION SOCIALLY AND VOCATIONALLY.		
1. PETER WILL ESTABLISH MAINTENANCE SCHEDULE.			
2. PETER WILL EXPERIENCE REDUCED DELU- SIONS, HALLUCINATIONS, AND PARANOID IDEATION, WHICH WILL ALLOW HIM TO FUNC-			

Nursing diagnosis	Nursing intervention	Predicted outcome/short-term goals (include time frame)	Date/signature
ALTERED THOUGHT PROCESSES RE- LATED TO PSY- CHOSIS, AS MAN- IFESTED BY AUDITORY HAL- LUCINATIONS, PARANOID IDEA- TION, AND DE- LUSIONS	—ADMINISTER PRESCRIBED ANTIPSYCHOTICS —MONITOR THERAPEUTIC RESPONSE (e.g., DECREASE IN PSYCHOTIC SYMPTOMS AND AGITATION) —MONITOR SIDE EFFECTS AND TEACH PETER TO IN- FORM STAFF OF SAME —ADMINISTER ANTI- PARKINSONIAN AGENTS PRN —TEACH PETER ABOUT MEDICATIONS AS UNDER DIAGNOSIS: VIOLENCE —PROVIDE A ROOM WITH LOW STIMULATION —INFORM PETER OF RATIO- NALE FOR CLOSE OBSERVATION —REASSURE PETER THAT HE WILL BE SAFE —SPEAK TO PETER IN SIMPLE, CLEAR TERMS; AVOID LENGTHY, COMPLEX CONVERSATIONS —DISCUSS PETER'S DELUSIONAL SYSTEM, BUT ONLY TO EXTENT NEEDED TO ASSESS SAFETY —PROVIDE REALITY TESTING EACH SHIFT AND MORE OFTEN IF NECESSARY	—PETER WILL EXPERIENCE A DE- CREASE IN AUDITORY HALLUCI- NATIONS, BLOCKING, DELUSIONS OF PERSECUTION, THOUGHT IN- SERTION AND IDEAS OF REFER- ENCE (1 WEEK) —PETER'S CONCENTRATION WILL INCREASE, ALLOWING HIM TO ATTEND TO MORE COMPLEX INFORMATION WITHIN 2 WEEKS —PETER WILL VERBALIZE A DE- CREASE IN AGITATION IN 1 WEEK —PETER WILL VERBALIZE NAME, DOSAGE, ADMINISTRATION SCHEDULE, SIDE EFFECTS, AND PURPOSE OF ALL MEDICATIONS IN 2 WEEKS	2/4 BM

Continued

Nursing Care Plan *continued*

Discharge outcome/long-term goals	
1. PETER WILL RE-ESTABLISH USUAL EATING PATTERN. 2. PETER WILL RE-ESTABLISH USUAL BATHING AND HYGIENE HABITS.	

Nursing diagnosis	Nursing intervention	Predicted outcome/short-term goals (include time frame)	Date/signature
SELF-CARE DEFICIT: FEEDING RELATED TO THOUGHT DIS- ORDER SECOND- ARY TO ACUTE PSYCHOSIS	— MONITOR INTAKE AND OUTPUT EACH SHIFT; WEIGHT EACH WEEK — PERFORM A COMPLETE PHYSICAL ASSESSMENT, CAREFULLY OBSERVING SKIN INTEGRITY, SKIN TURGOR, ETC.	— PETER WILL GAIN 1 LB. PER WEEK — PETER WILL FEEL ABSENCE OF PERMANENT INSULT TO PHYS- ICAL WELL-BEING DURING HOSPITALIZATION — PETER WILL PROVIDE FOR HIS PERSONAL HYGIENE NEEDS	2/4 BK
SELF-CARE DEFICIT: BATH- ING/HYGIENE RELATED TO THOUGHT DIS- ORDER SECOND- ARY TO ACUTE PSYCHOSIS	— DO NOT ATTEMPT TO FORCE FOOD OR FLUIDS — IF DEHYDRATION OR STARVATION EXISTS, AD- MINISTER NUTRIENTS VIA IV. PER ORDER. IF PETER RESISTS, HE MAY REQUIRE A MENTAL HEALTH HOLD FOR TREATMENT	WITHOUT STAFF ASSISTANCE WITHIN 3 WEEKS — PETER WILL ESTABLISH EAT- ING HABITS WITHOUT STAFF ASSISTANCE WITHIN 5 WEEKS	
POTENTIAL FOR ALTERED NUTRITION: LESS THAN BODY REQUIREMENTS RELATED TO IN- ADEQUATE FOOD AND FLUID INTAKE SECONDARY TO PSYCHOSIS	— PROVIDE PETER WITH UNOPENED, PREPACKAGED FOOD AND FLUIDS TO DECREASE HIS CONCERN ABOUT POISONING — OFFER PETER SMALL AMOUNTS OF FOOD AND FLUIDS AT FREQUENT INTERVALS IN A NON-STIMULATING ENVIRONMENT		
	— PROVIDE PETER WITH CHOICES BY ASKING WHAT HE PREFERS TO EAT AND DRINK — TEST PETER'S REALITY ORIENTATION WITH REGARD TO FEAR OF POISONING — ENCOURAGE PETER TO MAINTAIN PROPER HY- GIENE. ACCOMPANY HIM TO THE BATHROOM, PROVIDING HIM WITH SUPPLIES AND FACILITIES AT A QUIET, NON- THREATENING TIME — APPROACH PETER IN A GENTLE, NON-CONTROL- LING MANNER		

Discharge outcome/long-term goals		SLEEPING.	
1. PETER'S USUAL PATTERN OF SLEEP WILL BE RE-ESTABLISHED. 2. IN TIMES OF RESTLESS SLEEP PATTERN, PETER WILL SPONTANEOUSLY USE RELAXATION TECHNIQUES TO FACILITATE			
Nursing diagnosis	**Nursing intervention**	**Predicted outcome/short-term goals (include time frame)**	**Date/signature**
SLEEP PATTERN DISTURBANCE RELATED TO HYPERVIGILANCE SECONDARY TO PSYCHOSIS	- MONITOR PETER'S SLEEP-WAKE CYCLE - OFFER HIM RELAXATION TAPES, HOT MILK, TUB BATH BEFORE ADMINISTERING MEDICATIONS - ADMINISTER SLEEPING MEDICATION AS ORDERED EVALUATE ITS EFFECTIVENESS	- PETER WILL SLEEP 6 TO 8 HOURS UNINTERRUPTED EACH NIGHT (ONE WEEK)	2/4 BM

Continued

REVISED NURSING CARE PLAN

Complete the chart below to develop a nursing care plan for this client.

Discharge outcome/long-term goals	
1. PETER AND STAFF WILL BE FREE FROM HARM DURING HOSPITALIZATION.	

Nursing diagnosis	Nursing intervention	Predicted outcome/short-term goals (include time frame)	Date/signature
POTENTIAL FOR VIOLENCE TO OTHERS RELATED TO POOR IMPULSE CONTROL SECONDARY TO PSYCHOSIS AND FEAR	—ESTABLISH CONTRACT WITH PETER STATING THAT HE WILL LET STAFF KNOW WHEN HE'S FEELING MORE FRIGHTENED OR IF VOICES ARE BOTHERING HIM —CONTINUE TO ACKNOWLEDGE PETER'S FEARFUL FEELINGS, BUT PROVIDE REALITY TESTING —MONITOR FOR RESURGENCE OF ACUTE PARANOIA —ADMINISTER MEDICATION AS PREVIOUSLY DESCRIBED	—PETER WILL ESTABLISH PLANS TO DEAL WITH FEELING FRIGHTENED (e.g. LEAVING UPSETTING SITUATION, REALITY TESTING, PRN MEDICATION) WITHIN 1½ WEEKS	2/8 OR
ALTERED THOUGHT PROCESSES RELATED TO PSYCHOSIS	—CONTINUE TO ADMINISTER ANTIPSYCHOTIC MEDICATION EVALUATE ITS EFFECTIVENESS —REINFORCE MEDICATION TEACHING —PROVIDE PETER WITH A DAILY SCHEDULE TO HELP ORGANIZE HIS TIME. POST IT ON THE BULLETIN BOARD IN HIS BEDROOM —ASSESS PETER'S TOLERANCE FOR INCREASED STIMULATION IN GRADUAL STEPS —INCORPORATE PETER INITIALLY IN GROUP ACTIVITIES THAT DON'T DEMAND GOOD COMMUNICATION OR INTERPERSONAL SKILLS	—PETER WILL VERBALIZE POSITIVE FEELINGS ABOUT MEDICATION AND PLANS TO COMPLY WITH MEDICATION REGIMEN AFTER DISCHARGE WITHIN 2 WEEKS —PETER WILL DETERMINE LEVEL OF STIMULATION HE CAN TOLERATE WITHIN 1 WEEK	2/8 OR

Discharge outcome/long-term goals			
1. PETER'S FEEDING AND BATHING/HYGIENE PATTERNS WILL BE RE-ESTABLISHED. 2. PETER AND FAMILY WILL IDENTIFY THE ROLE EACH PLAYS IN THE FAMILY: DISTANT VERSUS INTRUSIVE RELATIONS.			
Nursing diagnosis	Nursing intervention	Predicted outcome/short-term goals (include time frame)	Date/signature
SELF-CARE DEFICIT: FEEDING, BATHING/ HYGIENE, RELATED TO PSYCHOSIS	—OBSERVE FOR ANY INCREASE IN SYMPTOMS SURROUNDING SUSPICIONS OF POISONED FOOD -ASSIGN A MALE STAFF MEMBER TO ASSIST PETER IN PERSONAL HYGIENE AND STRUCTURING OF HYGIENE SCHEDULE	—PETER WILL RECEIVE ADEQUATE DIETARY INTAKE IMMEDIATELY —PETER WILL MAINTAIN PERSONAL HYGIENE SCHEDULE WITHOUT PROMPTS FROM STAFF IN 1 WEEK	2/8 BR
INEFFECTIVE FAMILY COPING RELATED TO CONFLICTUAL PARENTAL RELATIONSHIP, OVERINTRUSIVE MOTHER AND DISTANT FATHER	—MONITOR FAMILY VISITS —WITH PETER'S PERMISSION, LIMIT VISITS TO 30 MINUTES AT FIRST AND INCREASE THEM GRADUALLY —WHEN PSYCHOSIS LIFTS, BEGIN TO DISCUSS PETER'S RELATIONSHIP WITH HIS MOTHER (INTRUSIVE) AND BEGIN TO TEACH HIM LIMIT-SETTING BEHAVIORS —EXPLORE HIS RELATIONSHIP WITH HIS FATHER AND PLAN ACTIVITIES ON UNIT FOR PETER AND HIS FATHER —COMMUNICATE OBSERVATIONS AND EVALUATIONS OF FAMILY INTERACTIONS TO SOCIAL WORKER AND CONTINUE COLLABORATIVE WORK —CONTINUE TO SPEAK TO PETER IN CLEAR, SIMPLE TERMS —CONTINUE TO PROVIDE REALITY TESTING EACH SHIFT	—PETER WILL VERBALIZE UNCOMFORTABLE FEELINGS AND LIST WAYS OF LIMITING MOTHERS INTRUSIVE BEHAVIOR IN 1 WEEK —PETER WILL BEGIN TO VERBALIZE VOID OF RELATIONSHIP WITH FATHER AND LIST ACTIVITIES TO PROMOTE RELATIONSHIP IN 2 WEEKS	2/8 BR

to tolerate physical or emotional stimulation. Peter's nurse asked Mrs. K. to call the nurses' station on the following day in order to titrate visits with Peter's emotional state. She also informed Mrs. K. that she, the social worker, and Mrs. K. would need to meet to discuss Peter's problems and ways to help. Mrs. K., although upset about the possibility of not visiting the next day, agreed to go along with these recommendations.

Peter's primary nurse and social worker met with his mother and father after asking Peter's permission. During that session and during subsequent family visits, Peter's parents showed a very distant relationship. Peter's father was also distant from his son and appeared to be very quiet and passive. Peter's mother focused a great deal of her energy and emotional life on Peter, her only child. Mrs. K. spoke of the loneliness she felt when Peter was at college and mentioned that at times she felt so sad that she wanted to die, although she affirmed that she would never do anything.

Peter continued to appear more agitated during family visits when his mother began to act intrusively. Consequently, Mrs. K. was encouraged to visit for briefer periods and to visit with Peter in a general area rather than his room. Mr. K. was encouraged to visit Peter alone at times, to foster a closer relationship with his son. Peter's mother was encouraged to take care of herself by developing some activities of her own. Peter's parents were encouraged to spend more time together and to attend a weekly support group at the local community mental health center for families of clients with a mental illness. Mrs. K. was instructed to encourage her husband and son to spend time alone together. The nursing care plan was revised at this time. (See *Revised Nursing Care Plan*, pages 128-129.)

After Peter had been in the hospital for 3 weeks, he was able to attend a regular group schedule that focused on the development of skills for daily living. He attended a communication skills group, a leisure interest group, and a medication education group, as well as various activity groups. He continued to express ambivalence about taking medication. With that in mind, he and his family decided to begin injections of fluphenazine (Prolixin) on a once-every-2-week schedule on an outpatient basis, rather than adhere to a daily pill schedule.

After 4 weeks, Peter's acute psychotic symptoms subsided greatly. He no longer believed that the FBI was out to harm him under command from God. He appeared to be eating and drinking without problem, and his weight was steadily increasing. His hygiene had improved to the point that he would shower each morning without a reminder. Family visits no longer caused an increase in agitation, although his mother and father needed reminders to become less and more involved, respectively. Peter continued to be very quiet in groups. Although his anxiety was greatly reduced, he did not seem to know how to behave in social situations on the unit. His affect was blunted, and he did not form any close ties. He was cooperative with the staff and in activities, but he did not express any strong interests. He was, however, able to participate successfully in structured activities that required gross motor coordination without strong social and verbal skills. For instance, he participated in an exercise group and appeared to enjoy walks with the staff and other clients. And in the communication group, which was organized around practicing basic social skills in a very structured manner, he was able to respond appropriately.

Although Peter expressed an interest in returning to a job after his discharge, he was encouraged to delay this for approximately 1 month. Staff assessment of Peter's functioning suggested that he would not succeed at a job at the present time, and that his compliance with outpatient treatment might allow him to function at a higher level eventually. Peter was disappointed that he would not be looking for a job immediately after discharge. But the staff encouraged him to recognize his success in the hospital program and the potential for continued success in a similar program after discharge.

Peter was urged to attend a community day program for individuals with chronic psychiatric disorders. This program would provide him with structured activities, monitoring of psychotic symptoms, opportunities to develop supportive relationships with individuals outside his family, and a continued assessment and maximization of his ability to function. In this setting, the staff could conduct a long-term assessment of Peter's employment potential and perhaps link him with a rehabilitation program that would help him develop skills commensurate with his ability. Peter agreed to receive his fluphenazine injection from the nurse at the community day treatment program. He took three passes before discharge to meet the staff at the day program and begin the activities.

Peter's parents were encouraged to meet with a counselor at the clinic associated with the day treatment center for support in coping with their son's illness and guidance in following through with the suggestions to spend more time together. Also, Mrs. K. was encouraged to use these meetings to explore and identify her needs, fears, and wishes for her son.

Peter's primary nurse talked with him regularly about his leaving the unit to help him prepare for discharge. Together, they summarized what he had accomplished on the unit in terms of learning to trust the staff and clients, complying with his medication schedule, meeting new people, and experiencing group situations to which he contributed positively. The nurse gave Peter positive feedback about his ability to work with the staff in helping himself and encouraged him to work with the community day treatment program staff as he had done with the hospital nursing staff. She encouraged him to let the staff know if he was having any difficulties—if the voices were bothering him, if he began to sleep or eat poorly, or if he felt nervous about people wanting to hurt him. She explained that he might require hospitalization in the future and, if so, to remember that the hospital was a safe place where he could feel more comfortable and get better. Finally, she told Peter that she was glad she got to know him and was sad to say good-bye, even though she was happy to see him feeling better and ready to go home.

SELECTED BIBLIOGRAPHY

Almond, R. *The Healing Community: Dynamics of the Therapeutic Milieu.* New York: Jason Aronson, 1974.

Arnold, H. "Working with Schizophrenic Patients—Four A's: A Guide to One-to-One Relationships," *American Journal of Nursing* 76(6):941-43, 1976.

Ayd, F. "The Major Tranquilizers," *American Journal of Nursing* 65(4):70-78, 1965.

Bateson, D., et al. "Towards a Theory of Schizophrenia," *Behavioral Sciences* 1:251-64, 1956.

Billett, G. "Nursing Care Study: Sam—A Long-Term Psychiatric Patient," *Nursing Times* 75(7):277-79, 1979.

Burgess, A., and Lazare, A. *Psychiatric Nursing in Hospital and Community.* Englewood Cliffs, N.J.: Prentice-Hall, 1976.

Coburn, D.C. "The Experience of Schizophrenia," *Journal of Psychiatric Nursing and Mental Health Services* 15(6):9-13, 1977.

Davis, D.R. "The Family Processes in Schizophrenia," *British Journal of Hospital Medicine* 20(5):524-31, 1978.

Diagnostic and Statistical Manual of Mental Disorders, 3rd ed. Washington, D.C.: American Psychiatric Association, 1980.

Engle, R.P., and Semrad, E.V. "Brief Hospitalization, the Recompensation Process," in *The New Hospital Psychiatry.* Edited by Abrams, G.M., and Greenfield, N.S. New York: Academic Press, 1971.

Grough, H. "Nursing Care Study, Schizophrenia: Silence Filled with Sound," *Nursing Mirror* 151(6):42-46, 1980.

Kreigh, H.A., and Perko, J.E. *Psychiatric and Mental Health Nursing: A Commitment to Care and Concern,* 2nd ed. Reston, Va.: Reston Publishing Co., 1983.

Lancaster, J. "Schizophrenic Patients: Activity Groups as Therapy," *American Journal of Nursing* 76(6):947-49, 1976.

Lawton, K. "Nursing Care Study, Schizophrenia: Laura Learns to Make Friends," *Nursing Mirror* 148(24):32-33, 1979.

Lidz, T.S., et al. *Schizophrenia and the Family*. New York: International University Press, 1965.

Mellow, J. "The Experiential Order of Nursing Therapy in Acute Schizophrenia," *Perspectives in Psychiatric Care* 6(6):249-55, 1968.

Melzer, M. "Group Treatment to Combat Loneliness and Mistrust in Chronic Schizophrenics," *Hospital and Community Psychiatry* 30(1):18-20, 1979.

Murray, R.B., and Heulskoetter, M.M.W. *Psychiatric/Mental Health Nursing: Giving Emotional Care*. Englewood Cliffs, N.J.: Prentice-Hall, 1983.

Paul, G.L., and Lentz, R.J. *Psychosocial Treatment of Chronic Mental Patients: Milieu vs. Social Learning Program*. Cambridge, Mass.: Harvard University Press, 1977.

Rawat, G.M. "Schizophrenia: Nursing Care Study," *Nursing Mirror* 145(22):18, 1977.

Robinson, A. "Communicating with Schizophrenic Patients," *American Journal of Nursing* 60(8):1120-23, 1960.

Rogers, C.R. *The Therapeutic Relationship and Its Impact*. Madison, Wis.: University of Wisconsin Press, 1967.

Schroder, P.J. "Nursing Intervention with Patients with Thought Disorders," *Perspectives of Psychiatric Care* 17(9):329, 1979.

Sederer, L.I. "Schizophrenic Disorders," in *Inpatient Psychiatry: Diagnosis and Treatment*. Edited by Sederer, L.I. Baltimore: Williams & Wilkins Co., 1983.

Sullivan, H.S. *The Interpersonal Theory of Psychiatry*. New York: W.W. Norton & Co., 1953.

Sullivan, H.S. "The Language of Schizophrenia," in *Language and Thought in Schizophrenia*. Berkeley, Calif.: University of California Press, 1964.

Topalis, M., and Aguilera, D.C. *Psychiatric Nursing*. St. Louis: C.V. Mosby Co., 1978.

Wilson, H.S., and Kneisl, C.R. *Psychiatric Nursing*, 2nd ed. Menlo Park, Calif.: Addison-Wesley Publishing Co., 1983.

Carolyn:
Safety and Independence with the Borderline Adult

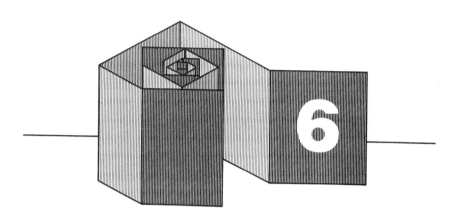

Barbara R. Garson, MSN, RN, CS

Individuals with a diagnosis of Borderline Personality Disorder have significant long-term impairment in their ability to cope with affect mediation. They generally have suffered deprivation as children and express feelings of profound emptiness, often with depression. These individuals tend to exhibit impulsive and unpredictable behavior, resorting to a variety of self-destructive behaviors as a way to cope with negative affect and to secure attention and care-taking. Their interpersonal relationships are often characterized as unstable and intense with frequent rapid shifts in attitudes toward others, ranging from intense anger and devaluation to idealization. Identity disturbance may be present and, in some individuals, psychotic symptoms may occur during periods of extreme stress. The primary reason for hospitalization is suicide potential.

The goals of inpatient hospitalization of an individual with Borderline Personality Disorder are to provide a safe, contained, and positive therapeutic environment without promoting regression, which will encourage greater dependency and hinder the transition to outpatient status. As the following case study demonstrates, nursing plays a vital role in achieving these goals.

CASE STUDY

This was the third psychiatric hospitalization for Carolyn White, a 32-year-old white, Protestant housewife who lived in an affluent suburb with her husband and two children. During her admission interview, Carolyn stated that she has come to the hospital "against my will" at her husband's insistence after threatening to take an overdose of her prescribed antidepressant medication.

Carolyn stated that she began to feel more depressed about 10 days before admission, when her outpatient therapist went on vacation. In therapy, she had been talking about her mother's death, which had occurred around this time 7 years ago, and her anxiety about her youngest child's impending kindergarten attendance. (She was afraid that she would have "nothing to do all day" while her child was in school.) Her recent symptoms included increased eating with a 5-pound weight gain, decreased sleep (2 hours per night over the past 6 days), and feelings of agitation.

Carolyn reported smoking one marijuana cigarette a day and expressed concerns about drug addiction. She denied using other drugs or alcohol. She described herself as "usually a very loving mother," but admitted she occasionally got very angry with her children, ages 5 and 7, at times hitting them when they irritated her.

Carolyn described feeling better when in the company of an adult who would help her plan her time and listen to her problems. Even at these times, however, she admitted feeling intense anxiety. She often would call her sister and ask her to come over when she "felt awful" and "didn't know what to do." In the weeks before admission, however, her sister seemed to be busier than usual and less able to visit. Carolyn also would call her husband at work many times each day, at times asking him to leave work and come home.

On the day of her admission, Carolyn had called her husband's office (for about the fifth time that day) and was told by his secretary that he was in a meeting and left strict instructions not to be disturbed, but that he would call her back. Carolyn then called her sister and told her that "life is not worth living anymore and I guess I'm going to have to do something to put an end to all the misery." At that point, Carolyn's sister called Carolyn's husband at work; he arrived home to find Carolyn watching television with a capped bottle of antidepressants in her hand. She hadn't taken any pills. He told Carolyn that he was taking her to the hospital. She argued with him, but finally complied.

During her admission interview, Carolyn insisted she was angry about her hospitalization; however, the interviewer noted that her affect was actually somewhat cheerful. When asked what she hoped to get out of the hospitalization, Carolyn stated that she wanted to end her feelings and thoughts about suicide, resolve her feelings about her mother's death, and reduce conflicts with her husband and her sister and her anxiety about her children.

Carolyn had been hospitalized twice before. Her first hospitalization occurred at age 19. While she was visiting home from college one weekend, her boyfriend told her he wanted to start seeing other people. In a rage, Carolyn ran to her mother's medicine cabinet and swallowed an entire bottle of Valium in front of her boyfriend. She was taken to the local hospital emergency room for medical treatment, then admitted to a private psychiatric hospital. She remained in the hospital for 5 weeks and was discharged 1 week before the planned discharge date because of her repeated infractions of unit rules. Records from that facility indicated that Carolyn was diagnosed as having an Adjustment Disorder with Mixed Emotional Features with a rule-out of Borderline Personality Disorder. She was treated with individual and group psychotherapy (no medication) and referred to individual therapy in the town where she was attending school. She did not follow through with outpatient therapy plans, however.

Carolyn reported no formal psychiatric contact after this first hospitalization. She described herself as feeling "always depressed" and admitted bouts of sexual promiscuity and heavy alcohol consumption during this period. She also cut her wrists several times, but received no required medical attention or subsequent psychiatric evaluation for these incidents.

Carolyn's second hospitalization occurred 7 years ago, shortly after her mother's death. While cleaning out her mother's home, Carolyn took an overdose of sleeping pills (unknown name and quantity) that she found in the house. She says that she had not contemplated killing herself in advance of this incident, but had been overwhelmed by feelings of anxiety and emptiness and impulsively took the pills to end those feelings. Her husband brought her to the emergency room of the local general hospital, where gastric lavage was performed. Later, she was admitted to the hospital's psychiatric unit.

During this hospitalization, Carolyn was treated with the antidepressant medication imipramine (Tofranil) and received individual, group, and, with her husband, couple's therapy. She again left the hospital earlier than planned, this time because "the doctors didn't really care about you there—all they wanted was your money." She was discharged with a diagnosis of Borderline Personality Disorder and was placed on imipramine 50 mg at hour of sleep and referred for individual therapy. She began to see her therapist shortly after discharge and had continued in individual therapy with the same therapist until the present time.

Carolyn reported receiving therapy with several different antidepressant medications over the last 7 years, most recently with a monoamine oxidase inhibitor. She expressed intense anger with her therapist for leaving on vacation at a time when she was feeling particularly depressed, and stated she would rather not ever see him again; he "had never helped," "only wanted her money," and "didn't really care."

During a telephone conference with the primary nurse, Carolyn's therapist reported having treated Carolyn for 7 years of once-a-week therapy, with two sessions a week during numerous times of crisis. According to the therapist, Carolyn often called between appointments with vague or concrete suicide threats. She frequently committed self-mutilation by cutting her arms with kitchen knives, and told him these acts helped her feel alive by feeling pain. Recently, the therapist had expressed concern to Carolyn about his ability to continue treating her, given her requests for more of his time than he was able to provide. He also expressed concern about her apparent inability to keep herself safe. At first, Carolyn had promised to stop cutting herself and to go to an emergency room if she felt she might take an overdose. But the evening before the therapist's scheduled departure for vacation, Carolyn called him and said that she was going to take an entire bottle of antidepressant medication because she couldn't make it through a week without him. The therapist spent 45 minutes with her on the telephone before she agreed not to harm herself.

Carolyn's medical history contained numerous gynecological complaints and workups, including two D & C's, intense menstrual cramping since menarche at age 13, and pain during intercourse. She claimed that her problems were hormonal in nature and that multiple medical opinions elicited from nationally known specialists suggested a slightly lower-than-normal estrogen level. However, estrogen replacement therapy, although it raised her estrogen level to within normal limits, had not improved her mood.

Her history also included poly-substance abuse. She experimented with "just about everything except heroin" and drank heavily between the ages of 19 and 24. Carolyn stated that she now avoided alcohol because she feared "losing control." She also denied using other drugs except marijuana, one cigarette per day for the past 2 weeks before admission.

Carolyn's family history revealed much relevant information. During her childhood, Carolyn considered her parents to be "perfect." Her father was a corporate executive; her mother always looked "beautiful" and was very active socially. But her mother also would occasionally "take to bed" for extended periods and would frequently direct "rage attacks" at Carolyn that consisted of severe verbal abuse. Carolyn re-

Continued on page 144

RECORDING THE DATA

After you have read the case, cluster significant data into functional health patterns.

Health management/health perception _____

_____

_____

_____

_____

Nutritional/metabolic _____

_____

_____

_____

Elimination _____

_____

_____

_____

Activity/exercise _____

_____

_____

_____

Cognitive/perceptual _____

_____

_____

_____

Sleep/rest _____

_____

_____

_____

Self-perception/self-concept _____

_____

_____

_____

Role relationship _____

_____

_____

_____

Sexuality/reproductive _____

_____

_____

_____

Coping/stress tolerance _____

_____

_____

_____

Value/belief _____

_____

_____

_____

ASSIGNING NURSING DIAGNOSES

Use your clustered data to select appropriate nursing diagnoses.

Health perception/health management

- ☐ Growth and Development, Altered (see Developmental Delay)
- ☐ Health Maintenance, Altered
- ☐ Infection, Potential for
- ☐ Injury (Trauma): Potential for
- ☐ Noncompliance (Specify)
- ☐ Poisoning: Potential for
- ☐ Suffocation: Potential for

Nutritional/metabolic

- ☐ Body Temperature, Potential Alteration in
- ☐ Developmental Delay: Physical Growth and Development
- ☐ Fluid Volume, Altered: Excess or Excess Fluid Volume
- ☐ Fluid Volume Deficit, Actual
- ☐ Fluid Volume Deficit, Potential
- ☐ Nutrition, Altered: Less Than Body Requirements or Nutritional Deficit (Specify)
- ☐ Nutrition, Altered: More Than Body Requirements or Exogenous Obesity
- ☐ Nutrition, Altered: Potential for More Than Body Requirements or Potential for Obesity
- ☐ Oral Mucous Membrane, Altered
- ☐ Skin Integrity, Impaired or Skin Breakdown
- ☐ Skin Integrity, Impaired or Potential Skin Breakdown
- ☐ Swallowing, Impaired or Uncompensated Swallowing Impairment
- ☐ Tissue Integrity, Impaired

Elimination

- ☐ Bowel Elimination, Altered: Constipation
- ☐ Bowel Elimination, Altered: Diarrhea
- ☐ Bowel Elimination, Altered: Incontinence
- ☐ Developmental Delay: Bowel/ Bladder Control
- ☐ Incontinence: Functional
- ☐ Incontinence: Reflex
- ☐ Incontinence: Stress
- ☐ Incontinence: Total
- ☐ Incontinence: Urge
- ☐ Urinary Elimination, Altered Patterns of
- ☐ Urinary Retention

Activity/exercise

- ☐ Activity Intolerance
- ☐ Activity Intolerance, Potential
- ☐ Airway Clearance, Ineffective
- ☐ Breathing Pattern, Ineffective
- ☐ Cardiac Output, Altered: Decreased
- ☐ Developmental Delay: Mobility
- ☐ Developmental Delay: Self-Care Skills
- ☐ Diversional Activity Deficit
- ☐ Gas Exchange, Impaired
- ☐ Home Maintenance Management, Impaired (Mild, Moderate, Severe, Potential, Chronic)
- ☐ Mobility, Impaired Physical
- ☐ Self-Care Deficit: Feeding
- ☐ Self-Care Deficit: Bathing/ Hygiene
- ☐ Self-Care Deficit: Dressing/ Grooming
- ☐ Self-Care Deficit: Toileting
- ☐ Self-Care Deficit: Total
- ☐ Tissue Perfusion, Altered: (Specify)

Sleep/rest

- ☐ Sleep Pattern Disturbance

Cognitive/perceptual

- ☐ Comfort, Altered: Pain
- ☐ Comfort, Altered: Chronic Pain

☐ Developmental Delay: (Specify Cognitive Area; attention, decision making, etc.)
☐ Hypothermia
☐ Hyperthermia
☐ Knowledge Deficit (Specify)
☐ Sensory-Perceptual Alteration: Input Excess or Sensory Overload
☐ Sensory-Perceptual Alteration: Input Deficit or Sensory Deprivation
☐ Thermoregulation, Ineffective
☐ Thought Processes, Altered
☐ Unilateral Neglect

Self-perception/self-concept

☐ Anxiety
☐ Body Image Disturbance
☐ Fear
☐ Hopelessness
☐ Personal Identity Confusion
☐ Powerlessness (Severe, Low, Moderate)
☐ Self-Esteem Disturbance

Role relationship

☐ Communication, Impaired Verbal
☐ Developmental Delay: Communication Skills
☐ Developmental Delay: Social Skills
☐ Family Processes, Altered
☐ Grieving, Anticipatory
☐ Grieving, Dysfunctional
☐ Parenting, Altered: 'Actual or Potential

☐ Role Performance, Disturbance in
☐ Social Interactions, Impaired
☐ Social Isolation (Rejection)

Sexuality/reproductive

☐ Rape-Trauma Syndrome: Compounded
☐ Rape-Trauma Syndrome: Silent Reaction
☐ Sexual Dysfunction
☐ Sexuality Patterns, Altered

Coping/stress tolerance

☐ Adjustment, Impaired
☐ Coping, Ineffective Individual
☐ Coping, Ineffective Family: Compromised
☐ Coping, Ineffective Family: Disabling
☐ Coping, Family: Potential for Growth
☐ Developmental Delay (Specify area)
☐ Post-Trauma Response
☐ Violence, Potential for (Self-Directed or Directed at Others)

Value/belief

☐ Spiritual Distress (Distress of Human Spirit)

You are now ready to develop a nursing care plan for this client. Use the following blank pages to do so. Then refer to the author's formulation, diagnostic summary, care plan, and summary.

NURSING CARE PLAN

Complete the chart below to develop a nursing care plan for this client.

Discharge outcomes/long-term goals	

Nursing diagnosis	Nursing intervention	

	Predicted outcomes/short-term goals (include time frame)	Date/signature

Return to Formulation, page 144

membered feeling very close to her father—much more so than to her mother—and recalled that he would occasionally sleep in her bed when "mom was too sick and needed to sleep alone." She did not recall any specific incidents of sexual abuse, however. She felt that most of her mother's attention was directed towards critiquing her appearance and criticizing her for not having enough friends and spending too much time at home. At the same time, she also remembers her mother becoming enraged if she stayed out with her friends for very long.

Carolyn frequently felt jealous of her sister Susan, 18 months younger, whom she perceived as their mother's favorite. Carolyn remembered caring for Susan frequently while they were growing up. She characterized their present relationship as stormy, with alternating periods of closeness and estrangement. Most recently, she had been turning to Susan for support. But she felt frustrated because Susan's husband discouraged Susan from spending time with her. According to Carolyn, Susan had a difficult marriage; her husband was an alcoholic who sometimes physically abused her.

On formal mental status examination, Carolyn presented as a 32-year-old white female who appeared slightly older than her stated age. She was neatly groomed and sat in a relaxed fashion during the interview. Her affect was generally calm and somewhat cheerful, although she became very angry when discussing her outpatient therapist and prior hospitalization experiences. Her content of speech reflected a preoccupation with suicide with no plan or intent, and feelings of anger toward her outpatient therapist and her husband. Although Carolyn stated that she was angry with her husband for bringing her to the hospital, her affect was not angry and her mood was calm when discussing this. No evidence of thought disorder or disturbance in perceptual state was apparent during her interview. Carolyn's coping strategies included impulsive self-destructive behavior, manipulative behavior, dependency, and anger. She was oriented to person, place, time, and situation; her memory and general fund of knowledge were good. Her abstraction capacity yielded a tendency to view all circumstances as revolving around herself. Carolyn's judgment was poor, as evidenced by her impulsive decisions to use suicide threats and attempts to cope with problems. Her perception and coordination appeared normal, and she was cooperative throughout the interview.

Reader may now complete Recording the Data, Assigning Nursing Diagnoses, and Nursing Care Plan.

FORMULATION

Masterson (1976) proposes that "abandonment depression" plays an important role in the behavioral manifestations of a borderline personality disorder as described in this case study. A matrix of interwoven emotions make up abandonment depression, including rage, fear, passivity, lability, and an overwhelming feeling of emptiness. Abandonment depression grows out of the incompletion of the separation/individuation stage of development at an early age. Since the separation does not occur, the child is unable to internalize or obtain "object constancy." Object constancy "is the capacity to evoke a stable, consistent mental image of the mother, whether she is there or not" (Kerr, 1987). It is the mother's inability to render the child free from her symbiotic relationship that prevents separation. The mother, instead of lending support when the child ventures toward separation and individuality, withdraws this support, warmth, and protection. She essentially "abandons" the child, withdrawing the care and concern that has been part of the relationship. An internal conflict, which involves the child's fear of seeking individuation in light of the fact that the mother abandons the child if he does so, is born at this point. This fear of abandonment follows the child into adulthood, and, as we see in this case, representative abandonments deeply affect the adult.

This client presented as at-risk for self-harm through impulsive self-destructive behavior. She was intensely angry with her outpatient therapist for his "abandonment" of her at a time when she was also coping with other major losses: her youngest child's anticipated school enrollment, the seventh anniversary of her mother's death, and the decreased availability of her sister. Initially, she responded to her feelings of loss and abandonment by becoming more dependent and demanding of attention from her sister and husband. During times when this attention was unavailable, she likely experienced intense feelings of emptiness, rejection, and depression and became more desperate in her maneuvers to obtain attention. Her threats to "put an end to all the misery" can be seen as both a strategy to get immediate attention and an expression of the serious, life-threatening nature of her emotional state.

During hospitalization, treatment would focus on reducing the imminent threat to Carolyn's life and on helping her develop more effective coping strategies. Extensive depth work to help her resolve issues surrounding losses and childhood deprivation would be inappropriate goals for a brief, crisis-oriented hospitalization. (This type of therapy would be considered only if resources were available for a lengthy hospitalization and if safety could be maintained during prolonged periods of regression when the client would be unable to control self-destructive impulses.) During this hospitalization, Carolyn needed help with focusing on realistic, short-term goals.

Continued on page 150

DIAGNOSTIC SUMMARY FOR CAROLYN

Data	Functional health pattern	Nursing diagnosis
—Recently took an overdose of antidepressants —On admission, stated that "Life was not worth living anymore... I guess I'm going to have to do something to put an end to all the misery" —Previously took an overdose of Valium after becoming enraged with her boyfriend —After her mother's death, took an overdose of pills (unknown name and quantity) —History includes numerous incidents of self-mutilation by cutting her arm with kitchen knives	Coping/Stress Tolerance	Potential violence directed at self related to depression and manipulative coping pattern
—Experiences symptoms of increased appetite with 5-pound weight gain, decreased sleep, and feelings of agitation —Would call husband several times each day, asking him to leave work to be with her at home	Role Relationship	Dysfunctional grieving related to death of mother, temporary loss of therapist, decreased availability of sister, and anticipated separation from youngest child
—Reports decreased sleep (2 hours per night over the past 6 days)	Sleep/Rest	Sleep pattern disturbance related to anxious state
—Experienced anxious feelings about her youngest child going to kindergarten; fears that she would have "nothing to do all day"	Activity/Exercise	Diversional activity deficit related to open nest syndrome and lack of community resource linkage

NURSING CARE PLAN

Complete the chart below to develop a nursing care plan for this client.

Discharge outcome/long-term goals		3. CAROLYN WILL BEGIN PROCESS OF	
1. CAROLYN WILL RE-ESTABLISH SELF-CONTROL. 2. CAROLYN WILL ESTABLISH AND UTILIZE MORE EFFECTIVE COPING STRATEGIES.		RESOLVING LOSSES.	
Nursing diagnosis	Nursing intervention	Predicted outcome/short-term goals (include time frame)	Date/signature
POTENTIAL VIO-LENCE DIRECTED AT SELF RELAT-ED TO DEPRES-SION AND MA-NIPULATIVE COPING PATTERN	—CONTRACT WITH CAROLYN TO MAINTAIN SAFETY AND TO LET STAFF KNOW IF SHE IS NOT FEELING IN CONTROL; ESTABLISH 15-MINUTE CHECK-INS AT NURSING STATION —ASSIST CAROLYN IN DEVELOPING ALTERNATIVE COPING STRATEGIES TO DEAL WITH DEPRESSION AND THE NEED FOR ATTENTION: ENCOURAGE HER TO TALK WITH OTHER PATIENTS AND TO UTILIZE GROUP AND INDIVIDUAL THERAPIES FOR SUPPORT AND TO ENGAGE IN ACTIVITIES TO ASSIST WITH TEM-PORARY RELIEF OF ANXIETY. ALSO ENCOUR-AGE HER TO ASK FOR ATTENTION AND TO EXPRESS ANGER VER-BALLY/DIRECTLY —ASSIST CAROLYN IN DIFFERENTIATING BETWEEN SUICIDAL THOUGHTS AND ACTIONS —CONDUCT A FAMILY MEETING TO SUPPORT DEVELOPING MORE EFFECTIVE COPING STRATEGIES WITHIN THE FAMILY SYSTEM AND TO EVALUATE THE WELFARE OF THE CHILDREN	—CAROLYN WILL HAVE DECREASED POTENTIAL FOR HARM TO HERSELF AS EVIDENCED BY: ABSENCE OF HARM TO SELF, DECREASED REPORTS OF FEELING OUT OF CONTROL —CAROLYN WILL EMPLOY ALTERNATIVE COPING STRATE-GIES (e.g., SEEK ASSISTANCE FROM STAFF BEFORE CUTTING HERSELF). PREDICTED TIME: 10 DAYS	9/5 BR
DYSFUNCTIONAL GRIEVING, RE-LATED TO DEATH OF MOTHER, TEM-PORARY LOSS OF THERAPIST, DECREASED	—ASSIST CAROLYN IN GROUPS AND IN INFOR-MAL MILIEU ACTIVITIES TO IDENTIFY OTHER INDIVIDUALS WITH WHOM SHE CAN SHARE THOUGHTS AND FEELINGS ABOUT LOSSES	—CAROLYN WILL VERBALIZE COGNITIVE UNDERSTANDING OF EXISTENCE OF LOSSES AND PATTERNS OF REACTIONS TO LOSSES —CAROLYN WILL IDENTIFY MORE CONSTRUCTIVE WAYS OF REACTING WITHIN HOSPITAL	9/5 BR

Continued

Nursing Care Plan *continued*

Nursing diagnosis	Nursing intervention	Predicted outcome/short-term goals (include time frame)	Date/signature
AVAILABILITY OF SISTER, AND ANTICIPATED SEPARATION FROM YOUNGEST CHILD	AND OTHER ISSUES IN ONE-TO-ONE SESSIONS WITH PRIMARY NURSE, PERMIT CAROLYN TO VENTILATE FEELINGS ABOUT LOSSES OR OTHER ISSUES WHILE HELPING HER CONTAIN ANXIETY WITHIN TOLERABLE LEVELS — DO NOT ENCOURAGE CLIENT TO EXPLORE DEPTH ISSUES; RATHER FOCUS CLIENT ON THE PRESENT AND HELP HER IDENTIFY WAYS TO GET SUPPORT IN DEALING WITH FEELINGS IN HER LIFE AT HOME — TEACH CAROLYN THE PHASES OF GRIEF AND THE TIME-LIMITED NATURE OF GRIEF IF AN INDIVIDUAL PASSES THROUGH ALL THE PHASES OF DENIAL, ANGER, BARGAINING, DEPRESSION, AND ACCEPTANCE	SETTING AND AT HOME (VIA FAMILY MEETINGS AND PASSES) —CAROLYN WILL LIST PHASES OF GRIEF AND IDENTIFY: ·TASKS OF EACH PHASE ·FEELINGS ASSOCIATED WITH PHASE ·WHAT PHASE SHE'S PRESENTLY IN PREDICTED TIME: 10 DAYS	
SLEEP PATTERN DISTURBANCE RELATED TO ANXIOUS STATE	— ENCOURAGE LOW-STIMULATION ACTIVITY BEFORE HOUR OF SLEEP — ENCOURAGE CAROLYN TO BRING IN FAMILIAR OBJECTS SUCH AS A CLOCK AND PILLOW/S, TO INCREASE HER COMFORT AT NIGHT — TEACH HER RELAXATION TECHNIQUES(DEEP BREATHING, MUSCLE RELAXATION) — OFFER HER WARM MILK AND HOT BATH OR SHOWER BEFORE ADMINISTERING SLEEP MEDICATION — ADMINISTER MEDICATION AND NOTE ITS EFFECTIVENESS	—CAROLYN WILL SLEEP 6 TO 8 HOURS PER NIGHT WITHIN 1 WEEK — CAROLYN WILL SPONTANEOUSLY EMPLOY DEEP BREATHING AND MUSCLE RELAXATION EXERCISES BEFORE SLEEP WITHIN 2 WEEKS	9/5 BR
DIVERSIONAL ACTIVITY DEFICIT RELATED	— AFTER REFERRING TO OCCUPATIONAL THERAPY FOR VOCATIONAL ASSESS-	— CAROLYN WILL BE ASSESSED FOR POSSIBLE EMPLOYMENT/ VOLUNTEER JOB WHILE HER	9/5 BR

Nursing diagnosis	Nursing intervention	Predicted outcome/short-term goals (include time frame)	Date/signature
TO "OPEN NEST" SYNDROME AND LACK OF COMMUNITY RESOURCE LINKAGE	MENT, ENCOURAGE CAROLYN'S PARTICIPATION IN RECREATION THERAPY AND OCCUPATIONAL THERAPY TO LEARN NEW SKILLS — DISCUSS WAYS IN WHICH CAROLYN CAN BUSY HERSELF WHILE YOUNGEST CHILD IS IN SCHOOL	CHILD IS IN SCHOOL IN 2 DAYS — SHE WILL IDENTIFY ACTIVITIES THAT ARE PLEASING AND FOLLOW-THROUGH WITH ONE OT PROJECT WITHIN 1 WEEK — SHE WILL MAKE A TENTATIVE WEEKLY SCHEDULE OF DIVERSIONAL ACTIVITIES FOR WHEN SHE RETURNS HOME (BY DISCHARGE)	

SUMMARY

Carolyn responded quite well to nursing interventions, which were based on ensuring safety and fostering independence. Carolyn tended to become dependent on certain people, especially staff members, and had the potential to regress easily while in the hospital. She was also extremely rejection-sensitive and sometimes perceived relatively small denials of her interpersonal needs as major blows to her self-esteem. Consequently, nursing care focused on assisting her in maintaining clear boundaries and maximizing her independence. She quickly became aware of the fact that this hospitalization would be brief and would focus on her safety. She readily took responsibility for 15-minute check-ins and was taken off this precaution after 5 days. She identified her symptoms of suicidal ideation as a direct result of an assortment of events with a "loss" theme: the anniversary of her mother's death, the temporary absence of her therapist, decreased contact with her sister, and the anticipated school attendance of her youngest child. Carolyn believed that her ability to identify these links would help her deal with the issue on an outpatient basis. She was maintained on her MAOI and demonstrated knowledge of its dietary restrictions. Carolyn left the hospital 10 days after admission, after two sessions with her therapist after his return from vacation.

It is important to note that the primary therapeutic relationship (Carolyn and her therapist) was respected throughout the hospitalization by the treatment team. It is within this relationship that Carolyn delved deeply into the core issues of separation/individuation and object constancy. The abandonment once felt by the child was once again recreated when the therapist went on vacation. This hospitalization proved beneficial because it provided the safety and support needed during the time Carolyn felt "abandoned."

REFERENCES

Kerr, N.J. "Patterns of Interaction with Borderline Clients," in *Comprehensive Psychiatric Nursing*, 3rd ed. Edited by Haber, J., et al. New York: McGraw-Hill Book Company, 1987.

Masterson, J. *Psychotherapy of the Borderline Adult*. New York: Brunner-Mazel, 1976.

SELECTED BIBLIOGRAPHY

Adler, G. "Helplessness in the Helpers," *British Journal of Medical Psychology* 45:315-26, 1972.

Adler, G. "Hospital Management of Borderline Patients and Its Relation to Psychotherapy," in *Borderline Personality Disorders: The Concept, the Syndrome, the Patient*. Edited by Harticollis, P. New York: International University Press, 1977.

Adler, G. "Hospital Treatment of Borderline Patients," *American Journal of Psychiatry* 130:32-36, 1973.

Almond, R. *The Healing Community: Dynamics of the Therapeutic Milieu*. New York: Jasson Aronson, 1974.

Bursten, B. *The Manipulator: A Psychoanalytic View*. New Haven, Conn.: Yale University Press, 1973.

Diagnostic and Statistical Manual of Mental Disorders, 3rd ed. Washington, D.C.: American Psychiatric Association, 1980.

Friedman, H.J. "Some Problems of Inpatient Management with Borderline Patients," *American Journal of Psychiatry* 126:299-304, 1969.

Gruber, K., and Schniewind, H. "Letting Anger Work for You," *American Journal of Nursing* 76(9):1450-52, 1976.

Jensen, H., and Tillotson, G. "Dependency in Nurse-Patient Relationships," in *Psychiatric Nursing*, vol. 1, 2nd ed. Edited by Mereness, D. Dubuque, Iowa: William C. Brown, 1971.

Kübler-Ross, E. *On Death and Dying*. New York: MacMillan Publishing Co., 1969.

Loomis, M. "Nursing Management of Acting-Out Behavior," *Perspectives in Psychiatric Care* 8(4):168-73, 1970.

Murray, R.B., and Huelskoetter, M.M.W. *Psychiatric/Mental Health Nursing: Giving Emotional Care*. Englewood Cliffs, N.J.: Prentice-Hall, 1983.

Rogers, C.R. *The Therapeutic Relationship and Its Impact*. Madison, Wis.: University of Wisconsin Press, 1967.

Sadavoy, J., et al. "Negative Responses of the Borderline to Inpatient Treatment," *American Journal of Psychotherapy* 33:404-17, 1979.

Sederer, L.I. *Inpatient Psychiatry: Diagnosis and Treatment*. Baltimore: Williams & Wilkins Co., 1983.

Sullivan, H.S. *The Interpersonal Theory of Psychiatry*. New York: W.W. Norton & Co., 1953.

Topalis, M., and Aguilera, D.D. *Psychiatric Nursing*. St. Louis: C.V. Mosby Co., 1978.

Wilson, H.S., and Kneisl, C.R. *Psychiatric Nursing*, 2nd ed. Menlo Park, Calif.: Addison-Wesley Publishing Co., 1983.

Wishnie, H.A. "Inpatient Therapy with Borderline Patients," in *Borderline States in Psychiatry*. Edited by Mack, J.E. New York: Grune and Stratton, 1975.

Mary:
Atypical Psychosis

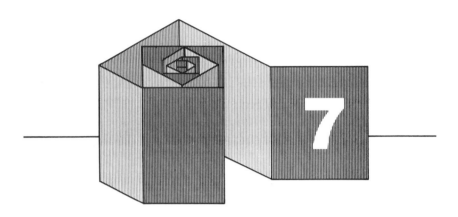

Sarah A. Roumanis, RN

An acutely psychotic client requires sensitive care in order to maintain psychophysiological functioning. Nurses treating such a client must come armed with skills in reality-orientation and maintenance of safety for client and caregiver. They must provide attention in many spheres, including activities of daily living as well as protection from overstimulation. But nursing interventions can be successful only if based on a thorough assessment of the client's abilities and needs, and only if implemented in a calm, nonjudgmental, and noncritical manner. Direct, clear communication is also vital, as the client interprets phenomena differently in the altered state. As demonstrated in this case study, this approach to intensive nursing care often can make the difference between success and failure when treating such a client.

CASE STUDY

Mary, an 18-year-old white, single, Irish Catholic female, had been admitted for her first psychiatric hospitalization. She was just completing her freshman year at college when she experienced her first psychiatric symptoms. At college, Mary lived in a dormitory with her roommate Patty. Her primary residence, however, was with her family—her parents and younger brother and sister—in their own home in a small town not far from the college.

Approximately a week-and-a-half prior to admission, Mary arrived home for a routine family visit to learn that her 16-year-old sister Kathy had just been admitted to the hospital with a diagnosis of an acute psychotic episode. According to her parents in a later interview, Mary became greatly distressed by this news. She informed her roommate and school officials that she needed a leave of absence until further notice, and stated she wanted to visit Kathy immediately.

Over the next week, Mary spent long periods of time with Kathy at the hospital, helping with her physical care and offering emotional support. All this began to take its toll on Mary; her parents and the staff noticed that she appeared very anxious and sometimes seemed confused. She would pace meaninglessly around Kathy's hospital room looking for objects she often already had in her hand.

Several days later, Mary began telling the staff that she thought the girl in Kathy's hospital bed might be an imposter; she asked them if Kathy was dead. She also expressed thoughts of harming Kathy and the belief that someone was inserting these and other thoughts into her head. During conversations, she would change topics abruptly, often asking whether it was Kathy or herself who was sick. Her speech became increasingly rambling and difficult to understand. She began believing that the nurses caring for Kathy were friends from school.

At times Mary would posture bizarrely, holding uncomfortable positions for long periods. The last few days prior to admission, she slept little, whereas she had typically slept uninterrupted for 8 hours per night. Mary's parents stated that even at home she appeared easily distracted and became disturbed by any changes in her environment. Her speech became pressured, intense, and more fragmented; sentences would be left uncompleted.

Mary's delusional thinking was now apparent. She believed that events happening to Kathy were really happening to herself. She repeatedly asked her parents "Why are they doing this to me?" but could not define clearly what she believed was being done to her.

At this point, Mary's parents made arrangements for Mary to be hospitalized. She was admitted to the same hospital as Kathy but to a different unit. At points throughout the admitting process, Mary appeared to understand that she was being hospitalized; at other moments she would ask plaintively, "What is happening, where am I?" Her parents were understandably distressed and overwhelmed at having both of their daughters hospitalized. They were clearly confused by the abrupt onset and severity of Mary's illness and seemed to find some relief in talking about her in an effort to understand what might have caused the psychotic break. But no clues were evident; Mary had no prior psychiatric history, and her medical history was normal.

Mary was the oldest of three children and the product of a normal labor and delivery. Her parents reported that she reached developmental milestones at normal times. They described her as an excellent student who maintained a high-B average throughout high school and her first year at college. She had a wide circle of friends, including several close ones and was active in several extracurricular activities in high school and college. According to her parents, she got along well with her roommate and had made several good friends at college. Mary dated throughout high school, and had one long-term relationship. At her mother's urging, she ended this relationship after revealing that he was pressuring her for sexual relations. Mary's mother, Mrs. Overland, believed that Mary dated occasionally at college but did not recall her mentioning anyone on a regular basis.

Mrs. Overland reported that Mary was always the most "nervous" of her three children. She and Mary always had a very close, dependent relationship. Mary would become anxious when faced with a major decision, seeking her mother's advice and guidance in most matters— from hairstyles to college courses—before making a final decision. Both parents admitted feeling quite concerned about how she would fare at college, where she would be forced to function more independently. They expressed relief that Mary's adjustment to college life had appeared to go so well, but questioned whether this was a superficial adjustment and whether being away from home was part of the stressor that precipitated the current episode.

Mary's relationship with her younger brother Michael was marked by a kind, nurturing quality. According to Mrs. Overland, they always got along well. In contrast, her relationship with her sister Kathy has been marked by constant arguments, bickering, and competition. They have never shared well and maintain different tastes in clothing and friends. Both Kathy and Michael still live in their parents' home and attend local schools. The parents report that Michael seems sad and somewhat confused by his sisters' hospitalizations.

Mr. and Mrs. Overland seemed to have difficulty discussing themselves and their relationship as a couple. The couple's style of interacting became more clear as the interview progressed. Mrs. Overland appeared to be the more emotionally reactive of the two. She cried easily throughout the interview, often turning to her husband for reassurance and support. Mr. Overland tended to give information in a more reserved fashion, but freely offered the reassurance and comfort Mrs. Overland sought. When asked if this was a consistent pattern, they concurred and stated that it was comfortable for both of them. They appeared committed to each other and reported being generally happy with their relationship.

When speaking of their children, the couple stated that they believed in "protecting the kids" from stress or hardship and did not argue openly in front of the children. They encouraged the children to come to them with their problems and actively helped them work out these problems. They did not view Kathy or Michael as being as dependent on them, as Mary is.

Mr. Overland, a self-employed auto mechanic, was an only child who emigrated from Ireland with his family at age 10. His father died of tuberculosis when Mr. Overland was 4 years old; his mother remarried 8 years after settling in the United States. There is no psychiatric history in Mr. Overland or his family of origin.

Mrs. Overland was born and raised in the town of current residence. Her father died in an auto accident, which the family labeled a suicide, when she was 5 years old. Mrs. Overland, her sister, and mother then moved into a two-family dwelling that they shared with Mrs. Overland's maternal grandparents.

At age 26, before her marriage to Mr. Overland, Mrs. Overland was hospitalized for an acute psychotic episode and treated with Insulin Shock Therapy. According to Mrs. Overland, the hospitalization was precipitated by the break-up of an important romantic relationship. Although she recovered from this episode within a month, she experienced several mini-psychotic episodes during the following year, which reportedly resolved spontaneously and did not require further hospitalization. Since that time, she had been symptom-free.

While Mary's parents were interviewed, Mary was admitted to the inpatient unit. She was described by the interviewer as a young, attractive woman appearing her stated age. She was very anxious and easily distracted. Her orientation to time and place fluctuated. She was aware of her situation intermittently, but admitted she was uncertain at times whether she was Mary or Kathy. Her affect was labile; at times she was smiling but then was quickly moved to tears. Her mood shifted from euphoria to irritability. Her speech and behavior exhibited an intense, pressured quality. She spoke rapidly, moving quickly from one topic to another in a disconnected fashion. During the interview, she would stand up abruptly and pace meaninglessly about the room. Her attention and concentration were clearly diminished; she refused to cooperate with any formal aspects of the psychological testing, quickly becoming irritable and standing up to pace. Although she denied experiencing hallucinations, delusional thinking was apparent in her assertions that others were placing thoughts in her head and her convictions that if only "they" would leave her alone, she could cure Kathy and herself. She also expressed thoughts

Continued on page 162

RECORDING THE DATA

After you have read the case, cluster significant data into functional health patterns.

Health management/health perception _____

_____

_____

_____

_____

Nutritional/metabolic _____

_____

_____

_____

Elimination _____

_____

_____

_____

Activity/exercise _____

_____

_____

_____

Cognitive/perceptual _____

_____

_____

_____

Sleep/rest _____

_____

_____

_____

Self-perception/self-concept _____

_____

_____

_____

Role relationship _____

_____

_____

_____

Sexuality/reproductive _____

_____

_____

_____

Coping/stress tolerance _____

_____

_____

_____

Value/belief _____

_____

_____

_____

ASSIGNING NURSING DIAGNOSES

Use your clustered data to select appropriate nursing diagnoses.

Health perception/health management

- ☐ Growth and Development, Altered (see Developmental Delay)
- ☐ Health Maintenance, Altered
- ☐ Infection, Potential for
- ☐ Injury (Trauma): Potential for
- ☐ Noncompliance (Specify)
- ☐ Poisoning: Potential for
- ☐ Suffocation: Potential for

Nutritional/metabolic

- ☐ Body Temperature, Potential Alteration in
- ☐ Developmental Delay: Physical Growth and Development
- ☐ Fluid Volume, Altered: Excess or Excess Fluid Volume
- ☐ Fluid Volume Deficit, Actual
- ☐ Fluid Volume Deficit, Potential
- ☐ Nutrition, Altered: Less Than Body Requirements or Nutritional Deficit (Specify)
- ☐ Nutrition, Altered: More Than Body Requirements or Exogenous Obesity
- ☐ Nutrition, Altered: Potential for More Than Body Requirements or Potential for Obesity
- ☐ Oral Mucous Membrane, Altered
- ☐ Skin Integrity, Impaired or Skin Breakdown
- ☐ Skin Integrity, Impaired or Potential Skin Breakdown
- ☐ Swallowing, Impaired or Uncompensated Swallowing Impairment
- ☐ Tissue Integrity, Impaired

Elimination

- ☐ Bowel Elimination, Altered: Constipation
- ☐ Bowel Elimination, Altered: Diarrhea
- ☐ Bowel Elimination, Altered: Incontinence
- ☐ Developmental Delay: Bowel/Bladder Control
- ☐ Incontinence: Functional
- ☐ Incontinence: Reflex
- ☐ Incontinence: Stress
- ☐ Incontinence: Total
- ☐ Incontinence: Urge
- ☐ Urinary Elimination, Altered Patterns of
- ☐ Urinary Retention

Activity/exercise

- ☐ Activity Intolerance
- ☐ Activity Intolerance, Potential
- ☐ Airway Clearance, Ineffective
- ☐ Breathing Pattern, Ineffective
- ☐ Cardiac Output, Altered: Decreased
- ☐ Developmental Delay: Mobility
- ☐ Developmental Delay: Self-Care Skills
- ☐ Diversional Activity Deficit
- ☐ Gas Exchange, Impaired
- ☐ Home Maintenance Management, Impaired (Mild, Moderate, Severe, Potential, Chronic)
- ☐ Mobility, Impaired Physical
- ☐ Self-Care Deficit: Feeding
- ☐ Self-Care Deficit: Bathing/Hygiene
- ☐ Self-Care Deficit: Dressing/Grooming
- ☐ Self-Care Deficit: Toileting
- ☐ Self-Care Deficit: Total
- ☐ Tissue Perfusion, Altered: (Specify)

Sleep/rest

- ☐ Sleep Pattern Disturbance

Cognitive/perceptual

- ☐ Comfort, Altered: Pain
- ☐ Comfort, Altered: Chronic Pain

☐ Developmental Delay: (Specify Cognitive Area; attention, decision making, etc.)
☐ Hypothermia
☐ Hyperthermia
☐ Knowledge Deficit (Specify)
☐ Sensory-Perceptual Alteration: Input Excess or Sensory Overload
☐ Sensory-Perceptual Alteration: Input Deficit or Sensory Deprivation
☐ Thermoregulation, Ineffective
☐ Thought Processes, Altered
☐ Unilateral Neglect

Self-perception/self-concept

☐ Anxiety
☐ Body Image Disturbance
☐ Fear
☐ Hopelessness
☐ Personal Identity Confusion
☐ Powerlessness (Severe, Low, Moderate)
☐ Self-Esteem Disturbance

Role relationship

☐ Communication, Impaired Verbal
☐ Developmental Delay: Communication Skills
☐ Developmental Delay: Social Skills
☐ Family Processes, Altered
☐ Grieving, Anticipatory
☐ Grieving, Dysfunctional
☐ Parenting, Altered: Actual or Potential

☐ Role Performance, Disturbance in
☐ Social Interactions, Impaired
☐ Social Isolation (Rejection)

Sexuality/reproductive

☐ Rape-Trauma Syndrome: Compounded
☐ Rape-Trauma Syndrome: Silent Reaction
☐ Sexual Dysfunction
☐ Sexuality Patterns, Altered

Coping/stress tolerance

☐ Adjustment, Impaired
☐ Coping, Ineffective Individual
☐ Coping, Ineffective Family: Compromised
☐ Coping, Ineffective Family: Disabling
☐ Coping, Family: Potential for Growth
☐ Developmental Delay (Specify area)
☐ Post-Trauma Response
☐ Violence, Potential for (Self-Directed or Directed at Others)

Value/belief

☐ Spiritual Distress (Distress of Human Spirit)

You are now ready to develop a nursing care plan for this client. Use the following blank pages to do so. Then refer to the author's formulation, diagnostic summary, care plan, and summary.

NURSING CARE PLAN

Complete the chart below to develop a nursing care plan for this client.

Discharge outcomes/long-term goals	

Nursing diagnosis	Nursing intervention	

	Predicted outcomes/short-term goals (include time frame)	Date/signature

Return to Formulation, page 162

of harming Kathy, but denied feeling suicidal. The interview was kept very brief, due to Mary's agitation and inability to cooperate fully. She was placed in a private room, and close staff observation was initiated.

Reader may now complete Recording the Data, Assigning Nursing Diagnoses, and Nursing Care Plans.

FORMULATION

As we began to go over the information and formulate an opinion about Mary's illness, we considered several diagnoses. Her presenting symptoms of agitation, confusion, delusions, and fragmented thought processes indicated an acute psychotic process, but additional features necessitated the diagnosis of acute manic episode with psychotic features. These included grandiosity; Mary felt she had been chosen to save the world, and that only she could adequately spread a message of love and peace to humankind. Another was hypersexuality; she was flirting in a sexually provocative fashion with the male staff, often undressing abruptly in their presence. She also had an increased energy level manifested by constant pacing and rapid, pressured speech.

Mary's parents had mentioned their concern about her ability to separate successfully from home and the stress this separation may have generated. Although we agreed that this stress may have contributed to Mary's psychosis, we felt it did not adequately explain such a severe episode. Rather, in light of her mother's psychiatric history and her sister Kathy's current psychotic episode, we considered that Mary might have a genetic vulnerability to psychotic decompensation under severe stress.

It would be months until the full severity and atypical features of Mary's illness became apparent. During this period she underwent multiple medication trials; severe side effects and idiosyncratic responses to medication necessitated many changes in medication dosage and type. She also required physical restraints for long periods to maintain her safety. Throughout Mary's hospitalization, nursing interventions would prove to be the single most important factor in managing Mary and helping her return to health.

SUMMARY

Mary remained in the hospital for a little more than 2 months. She spent more than half of that time in physical restraints. Her recovery was a slow, painful process marked by spurts of healthy progress followed by demoralizing relapses.

Continued on page 175

DIAGNOSTIC SUMMARY FOR MARY

Data	Functional health pattern	Nursing diagnosis
—Believes she hears voices calling to her and rushes down the hallway —Jumps from her bed to the windowsill —Has demonstrated that she can no longer safely be managed out of restraints —Medications are not effective in controlling her impulsive behavior	Health Perception/ Health Management	Potential for injury related to impulsivity and psychosis
—Experiences both visual and auditory hallucinations —Describes delusions of grandeur and paranoia and speaks of others placing thoughts in her head	Cognitive/Perceptual	Altered thought processes related to psychosis
—Exhibits pressured, intense, sometimes incoherent speech; disconnected and fragmented thoughts; and diminished attention span and concentration	Role Relationship	Impaired verbal communication related to psychotic, disorganized thinking
—Is unaware of her poor personal hygiene —Has sporadic eating patterns —Is incontinent of urine/stool while in restraints —Is unable to dress herself	Activity/Exercise	Self-care deficit: total, related to psychosis, delirium, and demoralization
—Experiences episodes of urinary/ fecal incontinence (but is not aware of this) —Exhibits an inability to provide self-care (hygiene, bathing, toileting)	Nutritional/ Metabolic	Potential impaired skin integrity related to extended period of time in restraints secondary to psychosis
—Periodically refuses or is unable to eat or drink	Nutritional/ Metabolic	Potential for altered nutrition, less than body requirements, related to psychosis, delirium, and demoralization
—Becomes anxious around times of decisionmaking —Has been restrained and out of milieu for approximately 1 month	Activity/Exercise	Diversional activity deficit related to prolonged confinement and poor tolerance to stimuli

Continued

Diagnostic Summary for Mary *continued*

Data	Functional health pattern	Nursing diagnosis
—Does not understand how poor her tolerance was for stimuli or change —Can still quickly disorganize when stressed or overwhelmed by even minimal activity —Admits much anxiety and apprehension with regard to her discharge date	Self-Perception/Self-Concept	Anxiety related to learning the hospital setting and possibility of relapse

NURSING CARE PLAN

Complete the chart below to develop a nursing care plan for this client.

Discharge outcome/long-term goals	
1. MARY WILL NOT HARM HERSELF DURING HOSPITALIZATION. 2. MARY WILL RECOGNIZE LIMITS AND WILL UNDERSTAND AND USE NEWLY LEARNED COPING TECHNIQUES.	

Nursing diagnosis	Nursing intervention	Predicted outcome/short-term goals (include time frame)	Date/signature
POTENTIAL FOR INJURY RELATED TO IMPULSIVITY AND PSYCHOSIS	—MONITOR MARY'S ROOM FOR ENVIRONMENTAL HAZARDS; e.g., GLASS, TACKS, SHARP OBJECTS —ARRANGE THE ROOM TO MINIMIZE RISKS; e.g., SIT IN A CHAIR IN FRONT OF THE DOOR SO MARY CANNOT EASILY RUSH FROM THE ROOM; PUSH THE BED AGAINST THE WALL AWAY FROM THE WINDOW —REDIRECT MARY FIRMLY AND CLEARLY, AWAY FROM POTENTIALLY HARMFUL BEHAVIORS; e.g., TELL HER SHE MAY NOT SIT ON THE WINDOW LEDGE —ENCOURAGE MARY TO VERBALIZE INTENDED ACTION PRIOR TO TAKING ACTION —ASSESS MARY FOR SUDDEN MOOD CHANGES THAT MAY PRESAGE DANGEROUS ACTIONS —ASSESS MARY FOR SUICIDAL OR HOMICIDAL IDEATION EVERY SHIFT —PROTECT MARY FROM HARM BY INITIATING PHYSICAL RESTRAINTS WHEN NECESSARY IF LESS RESTRICTIVE METHODS HAVE NOT BEEN EFFECTIVE —DO NOT REMOVE MARY FROM RESTRAINTS UNLESS SHE HAS DEMONSTRATED ADEQUATE CONTROL BY APPEARING CALM AND NOT ATTEMPTING TO REMOVE RESTRAINTS FOR MINIMUM OF 3 HOURS —REASSURE MARY THAT RESTRAINTS ARE FOR HER SAFETY AND NOT FOR PUNISHMENT	—MARY WILL VERBALLY CONTRACT WITH STAFF TO ALERT THEM WHEN SHE NEEDS HELP CONTROLLING BEHAVIOR WITHIN 3 WEEKS —MARY WILL DEMONSTRATE AN INCREASE IN HER ABILITY TO INDEPENDENTLY CONTROL BEHAVIOR AND ADHERE TO LIMITS WITHIN 4 WEEKS —MARY WILL DEMONSTRATE THE ABILITY TO BE OUT OF RESTRAINTS WITHOUT RISK OF INJURY WITHIN 24 HOURS	4/1 JM

Continued

Nursing Care Plan *continued*

Nursing diagnosis	Nursing intervention	Predicted outcome/short-term goals (include time frame)	Date/signature
	-REASSURE MARY THAT A STAFF MEMBER WILL BE PRESENT AT ALL TIMES WHILE SHE IS IN RESTRAINTS		
	-FREQUENTLY EXPLAIN TO MARY WHY HER BEHAVIOR HAS INDICATED THE NEED FOR RESTRAINTS; e.g., "YOU HAVE BEEN UNABLE TO ADHERE TO THE AGREED UPON LIMITS WITH JUST VERBAL REMINDERS"		
	-DOCUMENT ANY CONSISTENT PATTERNS OF BEHAVIOR		
	-AVOID ABRUPT, POSSIBLY FRIGHTENING ACTIONS		
	-REMOVE RESTRAINTS, ONE AT A TIME, WITH ADEQUATE CAREGIVERS PRESENT AND EVALUATE MARY'S CAPACITY TO CONTROL HERSELF		
	-RE-APPLY RESTRAINTS PROMPTLY IF MARY'S BEHAVIOR INDICATES A RISK FOR INJURY; e.g., TRYING TO STRIKE OUT AT NURSE OR HURT HERSELF WITH A DANGEROUS OBJECT		
	-ENCOURAGE THE DEVELOPMENT OF A RELATIONSHIP WITH THE PRIMARY NURSE BY MEETING FORMALLY WITH MARY, STARTING WITH 15-MINUTE MEETINGS AND INCREASING TO HOUR-LONG SESSIONS (IF TOLERATED)		
	-AVOID TAKING UNNECESSARY CONTROL OVER MARY'S BEHAVIOR		
	-INSTRUCT VISITORS ABOUT EXPECTATIONS AND LIMITATIONS REGARDING VISITS, AND ENSURE THEIR COMPLIANCE		

Discharge outcome/long-term goals	ORIENTED THOUGHTS.		
1. MARY WILL NO LONGER SHOW EVIDENCE OF HALLUCINATIONS OR DELUSIONS. 2. MARY WILL COMMUNICATE THOUGHTS CLEARLY, AS EVIDENCED BY REALITY—			
Nursing diagnosis	**Nursing intervention**	**Predicted outcome/short-term goals (include time frame)**	**Date/signature**
ALTERED THOUGHT PROCESSES RELATED TO PSYCHOSIS	—ASSIST MARY IN DISTINGUISHING HALLUCINATIONS AND DELUSIONS FROM REALITY —MAINTAIN A CALM, DIRECTIVE ATTITUDE IN HER PRESENCE --VERBALLY REASSURE MARY THAT THE VISIONS AND VOICES ARE NOT REAL —TEACH MARY THAT THE VISIONS AND VOICES ARE A PRODUCT OF HER ILLNESS	—MARY WILL ACKNOWLEDGE THROUGH WORDS AND ACTIONS THAT HALLUCINATIONS MIGHT NOT BE REAL WITHIN 1 TO 2 WEEKS —MARY WILL STATE THAT DELUSIONS AND HALLUCINATIONS ARE PART OF ILLNESS WITHIN 3 TO 4 WEEKS —MARY WILL DESCRIBE THE PURPOSE, ACTION, AND POTENTIAL SIDE EFFECTS OF HER MEDICATION WITHIN 2 WEEKS	4/1 SR
	—REASSURE MARY THAT SHE WILL BE SAFE —AVOID BEHAVIOR OR INTERACTIONS THAT MARY MIGHT INTERPRET AS VERIFYING HER PSYCHOTIC EXPERIENCES (i.e., WHISPERING) —AVOID ABRUPT, LOUD INTERACTIONS —KEEP EXTERNAL STIMULI LOW —ADMINISTER MEDICATION AS INDICATED AND EVALUATE RESPONSE —ORIENT MARY TO TIME, PLACE, PERSON, AND SITUATION AT REGULAR INTERVALS (q. SHIFT) —TEACH MARY PURPOSE, ACTION, AND POTENTIAL SIDE EFFECTS OF MEDICATION —REINFORCE HEALTHY BEHAVIORS AND THINKING PATTERNS —REDIRECT FOCUS FROM BIZARRE OR INAPPROPRIATE BEHAVIOR AND THOUGHTS TO MORE APPROPRIATE BEHAVIOR	—IN 3 TO 4 WEEKS, MARY WILL BE ABLE TO INTERACT WITH STAFF WITHOUT DISCUSSING DELUSIONS	

Continued

Nursing Care Plan *continued*

Discharge outcome/long-term goals			
1. MARY WILL COMMUNICATE CLEARLY AS EVIDENCED BY HER ABILITY TO STATE HER NEEDS AS WELL AS BY MAINTAINING A SOCIAL CONVERSATION WITH AT LEAST ONE OTHER PERSON.		2. MARY'S REGULAR BOWEL AND BLADDER HABITS WILL BE RESTORED BY DISCHARGE.	

Nursing diagnosis	Nursing intervention	Predicted outcome/short-term goals (include time frame)	Date/signature
IMPAIRED VERBAL COMMUNICATION RELATED TO PSYCHOTIC, DISORGANIZED THINKING	−ENCOURAGE CLEAR AND DIRECT COMMUNICATIONS −ASSIST MARY IN REPHRASING CONFUSING STATEMENTS OR QUESTIONS −REINFORCE ALL MARY'S EFFORTS AT CLEAR, DIRECT COMMUNICATION −ACKNOWLEDGE DIRECTLY WHEN MARY'S COMMUNICATION IS CLEAR AND REALITY-BASED −ROLE MODEL EFFECTIVE COMMUNICATION, GIVING SUGGESTIONS THAT PROMOTE EFFECTIVE COMMUNICATION −USE WORDS THAT ARE EASILY UNDERSTOOD AND BE CONCISE −ENCOURAGE CONSISTENCY BETWEEN WORDS AND ACTIONS −ENCOURAGE MARY TO EXPRESS ONLY ONE THOUGHT AT A TIME −CONTINUE TO TELL MARY WHAT IS BEING DONE AND WHY −GIVE ONLY BRIEF, CLEAR DIRECTIONS	−MARY WILL STATE CLEARLY WHEN SHE DOES NOT UNDERSTAND STAFF WITHIN 1 WEEK −MARY WILL ASK FOR ASSISTANCE IN COMMUNICATING THOUGHTS WITHIN 2 TO 3 WEEKS	4/1 JR
SELF-CARE DEFICIT: TOTAL RELATED TO PSYCHOSIS, DELIRIUM, AND DEMORALIZATION	−SEE INTERVENTIONS UNDER "POTENTIAL FOR ALTERED NUTRITION" −SEE INTERVENTIONS UNDER "POTENTIAL IMPAIRED SKIN INTEGRITY" −ENCOURAGE MARY TO ASSIST IN BATHING ROUTINES −ENCOURAGE MARY TO ASK FOR BEDPAN OR USE BATHROOM WHEN BEHAVIOR ALLOWS −ENCOURAGE MARY IN	−MARY WILL ASSIST IN BATHING SELF IN 1 WEEK −MARY WILL BATHE SELF IN 2 TO 3 WEEKS −MARY WILL ASSIST IN CLOTHING SELF IN 1 WEEK −MARY WILL SELECT OWN CLOTHES IN 3 WEEKS −MARY WILL BE CONTINENT OF URINE/FECES IN 1 WEEK	4/1 JR

Nursing diagnosis	Nursing intervention	Predicted outcome/short-term goals (include time frame)	Date/signature
	DRESSING SELF		
	—AVOID OFFERING CHOICES IN CLOTHING (THIS ADDS TO HER CONFUSION)		
	—ENCOURAGE TO PARTICI-PATE IN CLOTHING SELEC-TION WHEN CONFUSION IS IMPROVED (2 TO 3 WEEKS)		
	—DISCOURAGE INAPPRO-PRIATE REMOVAL OF CLOTHING		
	—TOILET ON A REGULAR BASIS		
	—ESTABLISH REGULAR TOILET PATTERNS; LIMIT FLUIDS AFTER 9 P.M.		
	—MONITOR FOR INCON-TINENCE, CONSTIPATION, OR URINARY RETENTION		
	—MAINTAIN BOWEL AND BLADDER RECORDS		
	—EVALUATE USE OF ADULT DISPOSABLE BRIEFS		
	—ENCOURAGE TO ASSUME RESPONSIBILITY FOR PERSONAL CARE AS TOLERATES		

Continued

Nursing Care Plan *continued*

Discharge outcome/long-term goals		
1. MARY WILL INITIATE AND SUSTAIN EFFORTS TO KEEP HER SKIN CLEAN, MOIST, AND INTACT.		

Nursing diagnosis	Nursing intervention	Predicted outcome/short-term goals (include time frame)	Date/signature
POTENTIAL IMPAIRED SKIN INTEGRITY RELATED TO EXTENDED PERIOD OF TIME IN RESTRAINTS SECONDARY TO PSYCHOSIS	—MONITOR MARY'S SKIN FOR POSSIBLE BREAKDOWN —BATHE MARY DAILY AND AFTER INCONTINENT EPISODES; ENCOURAGE HER TO ASSIST AS MUCH AS POSSIBLE —USE MILD SOAP TO MINIMIZE DRYING SKIN —MOISTURIZE MARY'S SKIN WITH LOTION —GENTLY MASSAGE MARY'S SKIN WHILE MOISTURIZING TO ENCOURAGE GOOD CIRCULATION. NOTE: SHE FINDS THIS MASSAGE RELAXING —TALK SOFTLY TO MARY ABOUT WHAT YOU ARE DOING AND ABOUT NORMAL DAILY EVENTS WHILE BATHING AND MOISTURIZING —TURN MARY EVERY 2 HOURS AS HER SKIN CONDITION INDICATES —POSITION MARY TO MAXIMIZE CIRCULATION AND MINIMIZE PRESSURE POINTS —UTILIZE ELBOW AND HEEL PADS OVER RED OR TENDER AREAS —UTILIZE SHEEPSKIN IF SKIN LOOKS RED OR TENDER —REMOVE LIMBS FROM RESTRAINTS AND DO R.O.M. EXERCISES (REMOVE ONLY ONE LIMB AT A TIME WITH STAFF ASSISTANCE) —ENCOURAGE MARY TO PARTICIPATE IN R.O.M. EXERCISES	—MARY WILL PARTICIPATE IN OWN CARE WITHIN 1 WEEK —MARY WILL DEMONSTRATE UNDERSTANDING OF WHY SKIN CARE MEASURES ARE IMPORTANT WITHIN 2 WEEKS —MARY'S SKIN WILL BE FREE OF SKIN BREAKDOWN THROUGHOUT HOSPITALIZATION	4/7 DA

Nursing diagnosis	Nursing intervention	Predicted outcome/short-term goals (include time frame)	Date/signature
	– REMOVE MARY FROM RESTRAINTS AND AMBULATE AS BEHAVIOR PERMITS – APPLY ADULT DIS- POSABLE DIAPERS IF INCONTINENCE WOR- SENS AND SKIN SHOWS EVIDENCE OF BREAK- DOWN		

Continued

Nursing Care Plan *continued*

Discharge outcome/long-term goals			
1. MARY WILL EAT A NUTRITIONALLY BALANCED DIET.			

Nursing diagnosis	Nursing intervention	Predicted outcome/short-term goals (include time frame)	Date/signature
POTENTIAL FOR ALTERED NUTRITION, LESS THAN BODY REQUIREMENTS RELATED TO PSYCHOSIS, DELIRIUM AND DEMORALIZATION	-ENCOURAGE ADEQUATE INTAKE OF HIGH-NUTRITION FOODS -UTILIZE DIETARY CONSULTATION; ASK PARENTS TO BRING IN MARY'S FAVORITE FOODS -ENCOURAGE PARENTS TO AVOID LEAVING SNACK FOODS OF LOWER NUTRITIONAL VALUE -DO NOT OFFER MARY A CHOICE OF FOODS OR DRINK; WILL ADD TO HER CONFUSION -OFFER ENSURE OR OTHER DIETARY SUPPLEMENT IF MARY WILL NOT TAKE SOLID FOODS -DO NOT OFFER FOODS AS REWARDS FOR GOOD BEHAVIOR -AVOID ASSOCIATING FOOD WITH BEHAVIOR OR MOOD STATE -MONITOR AND RECORD INTAKE EVERY SHIFT -MONITOR AND RECORD WEIGHT THREE TIMES PER WEEK -UTILIZE URINE SPECIFIC GRAVITY TO ASSESS HYDRATION -ALLOW MARY TO PARTICIPATE IN MENU SELECTION WHEN DISORGANIZATION CLEARS SIGNIFICANTLY	-MARY WILL ACKNOWLEDGE NEED FOR NUTRITIONALLY BALANCED DIET WITHIN 1 TO 2 WEEKS -MARY WILL PARTICIPATE IN MENU SELECTION WITHIN 2 TO 3 WEEKS -MARY'S WEIGHT WILL REMAIN AT BASELINE DURING HOSPITALIZATION	4/15

Discharge outcome/long-term goals			
1. MARY WILL UTILIZE A WELL-DEVELOPED DIVERSIONAL ACTIVITY PROGRAM WITHOUT ASSISTANCE AS PART OF HER DAILY ROUTINE POST-DISCHARGE.			
Nursing diagnosis	**Nursing intervention**	**Predicted outcome/short-term goals (include time frame)**	**Date/signature**
DIVERSIONAL ACTIVITY DEFICIT RELATED TO PROLONGED CONFINEMENT AND POOR TOLERANCE TO STIMULI	–EVALUATE MARY'S TOLERANCE FOR STIMULI DURING INTRODUCTION OF NEW ACTIVITIES	–MARY WILL VERBALIZE FEELINGS RELATED TO LIMITATIONS AND RESTRICTIONS IMMEDIATELY	5/5 DR
	–EXPLAIN TO MARY THE NEED TO PROCEED SLOWLY IN TAKING ON NEW ACTIVITIES	–MARY WILL ASSIST STAFF TO PLAN DIVERSIONAL PROGRAM WITHIN 2 TO 3 DAYS	
	–ALLOW MARY TO VERBALIZE HER FEELINGS ABOUT RESTRICTIONS	–MARY WILL ENGAGE IN EVALUATION PROCESS WITHIN 1 WEEK	
	–ENGAGE MARY AND FAMILY IN PLANNING SESSIONS	–MARY WILL HAVE A DAILY SCHEDULE OF ACTIVITIES DEVELOPED BEFORE DISCHARGE	
	–INTRODUCE ONE NEW ACTIVITY EVERY 2 TO 3 DAYS		
	–CONSIDER GAMES, VISITS, AND TIME OUTSIDE OF ROOM AS ONE ACTIVITY EACH		
	–COMPLIMENT MARY ON CREATIVE THINKING AND PLANNING		
	–SUPPORT MARY WHEN SYMPTOMS RETURN		
	–REASSESS MARY IF HER CONFUSION OR ANXIETY WORSENS AND DO NOT INTRODUCE NEW ACTIVITY UNTIL SYMPTOMS SUBSIDE		
	–DISCOURAGE USE OF EATING AS DIVERSION WHEN BORED		
	–OPENLY ACKNOWLEDGE AND PRAISE MARY'S STRENGTHS AND LIMITS		
	–INVOLVE MARY IN THERAPY GROUPS LAST		
	–INTRODUCE ONLY ONE NEW GROUP AT A TIME		
	–EDUCATE MARY REGARDING NEED FOR STRUCTURE AND ITS ROLE IN THE RECOVERY PROCESS		
	–EDUCATE HER REGARDING HOW TO PURSUE A SIMILAR PROGRAM ON AN OUTPATIENT BASIS		

Continued

Nursing Care Plan *continued*

Discharge outcome/long-term goals	SHE USES TO DECREASE ANXIETY.
1. MARY WILL RECOGNIZE SOURCE OF ANXIETY AND UTILIZE NEWLY LEARNED COPING SKILLS. 2. MARY WILL BE ABLE TO DESCRIBE A PROBLEM-SOLVING APPROACH	

Nursing diagnosis	Nursing intervention	Predicted outcome/short-term goals (include time frame)	Date/signature
ANXIETY RE-LATED TO LEAVING THE HOSPITAL SET-TING AND POS-SIBILITY OF RELAPSE	-ASSESS SOURCES OF MARY'S ANXIETY -DISPEL MYTHS ABOUT HER ILLNESS -TEACH HER THE FACTS ABOUT HER ILLNESS -TEACH HER THE VALUE OF APPROPRIATE MED-ICATION -TEACH HER HOW TO CONTINUE PREVENT-ATIVE TECHNIQUES AT HOME (i.e, RELAXATION TAPES, DEEP BREATHING, PROBLEM SOLVING) -DISCUSS THE BENEFITS OF INVOLVEMENT IN SUPPORT GROUPS -REVIEW HER LIMITA-TIONS AND STRENGTHS -REVIEW APPROPRIATE UTILIZATION OF OUT-PATIENT THERAPIST -INCLUDE MARY'S FAM-ILY IN YOUR TEACHING EFFORTS -CONVEY A SENSE OF UNDERSTANDING BY ACKNOWLEDGING DI-RECTLY THAT THERE ARE THINGS OVER WHICH SHE HAS LIM-ITED CONTROL -ENCOURAGE MARY TO FOCUS ON AREAS WHERE SHE HAS CONTROL (i.e, ADLs, CHOICES ABOUT DIVERSIONAL ACTIVITIES) -REVIEW HER CONDITION ON ADMISSION AND HER PRESENT PHYSICAL/ EMOTIONAL STATE	-MARY WILL IDENTIFY ANX-IETY AND SEEK ASSISTANCE FROM STAFF WITHIN 1 TO 2 DAYS -MARY WILL INVOLVE HER-SELF IN IDENTIFYING COP-ING MECHANISMS WITHIN 1 WEEK -MARY WILL VERBALIZE PURPOSE, ACTION, AND SIDE EFFECTS OF ALL DIS-CHARGE MEDICATIONS PRIOR TO DISCHARGE DATE	5/25 JA

Within the first week of hospitalization, Mary's impulsivity had increased. She would leap from a chair to the windowsill or somersault off her bed to the floor. She pushed nurses and other clients out of her way as she raced down the hallway looking for her parents, whom she believed were calling her. She also experienced visual hallucinations—insects crawling from the walls and blood on her clothing—and heard voices accusing her of "bad things."

Initially, our nursing care plans focused on maintaining Mary's safety, skin integrity, and nutritional status. We continued our attempts to engage her in dialogue, but she was still too disorganized to understand much of what was being said to her.

Mary was restricted to a private room with one-on-one staff contact. The plan was to decrease external stimuli and provide her with continual reminders of what behavior was appropriate. Our overriding goal was to maintain her safety, hopefully without the use of physical restraints. We consistently provided reality testing by assuring Mary that the voices she heard and visions she saw were not real, but merely a product of her illness.

Within a few days, however, we realized that Mary lacked sufficient internal controls and was too easily distracted and internally driven to be safely managed in this manner. Moreover, medications were proving ineffective, and some side effects were actually aggravating her condition. Therefore, we initiated physical restraints, with much better success.

Mary was not able to understand the need for her restraints, continually asking "Why are you doing this to me?" In accordance with our plan, we reminded her that the restraints were for her safety and not a punishment. We offered frequent reassurance that she would not be left alone in the restraints, and that a nurse would always be present.

Because the restraints proved demoralizing for both Mary and the staff, we would remove them periodically to evaluate her ability to control her behavior. In order to avoid inconsistency among the nursing staff, we established clear guidelines for determining when to remove the restraints. Before removal, Mary had to demonstrate control by remaining calm for at least 2 to 3 hours and not attempting to remove the restraints herself. If she demonstrated poor control at any time after removal, she was to be placed back in restraints for no less than 4 hours. We used the time in restraints to help Mary reorganize and try to understand what was being expected of her. We continually shared the reasoning behind our interventions with Mary to help provide her with a feeling of control and participation in her treatment, even though she clearly did not comprehend most of what was said.

At times, Mary became delirious due to idiosyncratic medication responses. Also, at times, due to medication side effects, she was incontinent of urine and stool but seemed unaware of this. Consequently, we initiated a care plan to protect her skin integrity. Her response to this made us aware that touch helped her, unlike some psychotic clients, to focus on reality. While bathing Mary, we would talk to her softly and encourage her to assist when able. While applying lotion, we would discuss normal events and gently massage her skin. Besides maintaining skin integrity, these techniques helped calm Mary and focus her on normal tasks.

At times, Mary either refused or was unable to eat or drink. Whether this was the result of delirium, psychosis, or a demoralization process was difficult to assess. Because we found that offering her a choice from a tray of foods only added to her disorganization, we asked her parents to identify her favorite foods and also encouraged them to bring these foods from home. (We discouraged them from bringing snack foods of low nutritional value, however.) We monitored Mary's weight and the specific gravity of her urine to ascertain her general physical condition.

Approximately 6 to 7 weeks into her hospitalization, Mary began to improve. She required restraints less frequently and began to experience fewer hallucinations and become more reality-oriented. The medication seemed to be taking effect, and the side effects became less severe.

Our nursing interventions changed as Mary's condition improved. Gradually, we allowed her to take more responsibility for her own activities of daily living. But with her improvement came a new problem. Mary decided that she no longer wanted to remain in her room alone or with a nurse; now that she was in more control, she wanted to join the other clients informally and in the treatment groups. Although we understood her desire, we also knew that she did not understand her poor tolerance for stimuli or change. Her thoughts still could quickly become disorganized when she was stressed or overwhelmed by even minimal activity.

With Mary's input, we outlined a structured activity program that introduced one new activity every several days. We began with puzzles and board games, and gradually allowed her to have visitors and spend some time out of her room. If she showed signs of disorganization or anxiety, we would stop the program for a day or two until she stabilized, then resume. We involved both Mary and her parents in this planning and evaluation process.

During the last 2 weeks of hospitalization, Mary made rapid progress. She began to demonstrate better interpersonal skills, no longer experienced hallucinations, and seemed well organized. She did, however, admit much anxiety and apprehension with regard to her discharge date.

As Mary's discharge date approached, the focus of nursing interventions changed once again. Most of the interactions with Mary were now geared towards teaching her about her illness and how to prevent a relapse. As she began to spend more time off the unit with her family, we discussed how to structure her time at home and explored support groups.

The termination process involved a review of her hospitalization and an assessment of her strengths and limitations. We discussed how Mary could best utilize an outpatient therapist.

Mary left the hospital with plans to return home, see an outpatient therapist, and join a support group. When we heard from her several months later, she was symptom-free.

In conclusion, appropriate nursing care clearly played a pivotal role in Mary's recovery. During the period when medication and verbal therapies were ineffective, nursing provided a safe, stable environment. And nursing set the expectations for appropriate behavior, provided a structure that enabled her to achieve those expectations, and supported her through the process of recovery.

SELECTED BIBLIOGRAPHY

Bernstein, L.R. "Patterns of Dysfunctional Reality Orientation," in *Comprehensive Psychiatric Nursing,* 3rd ed. Edited by Haber, J., et al. New York: McGraw-Hill Book Co., 1987.

Carpenito, L.J. "Altered Thoughts or Altered Perceptions," *American Journal of Nursing* 85(11):1283, 1985.

Feinsilver, D. "The Suicidal Patient: Clinical and Legal Issues," *Hospital Practice* 18(10):48E-48F, 48J, 48L, 1983.

Field, W.E., and Ruelke, W. "Hallucinations and How to Deal with Them," *American Journal of Nursing* 73:638, 1973.

Gluck, M. "Learning a Therapeutic Verbal Response to Anger," *Journal of Psychiatric Nursing and Mental Health Services* 19(3):9-11, 1981.

Knowles, R.D. "Disputing Irrational Thought," *American Journal of Nursing* 81:735, 1981.

Schroder, R.J. "Nursing Intervention with Patients with Thought Disorders," *Perspectives in Psychiatric Care* 17(1):32-39, 1979.

Schwartzman, S.T. "The Hallucinating Patient and Nursing Intervention," *Journal of Psychiatric Nursing and Mental Health Services* 13(6):23-28, 33-36, 1976.

Theresa:
An Adolescent with Anorexia Nervosa

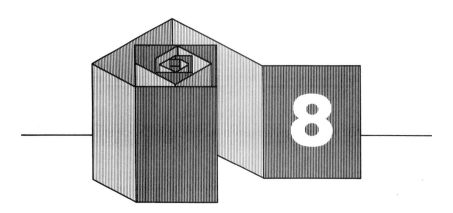

Ellen Bowen, MN, RN, CS

Clinicians in all mental health disciplines have struggled to identify effective therapeutic strategies for the client with anorexia nervosa, a disorder that typically affects functioning in interpersonal, social, familial, and academic spheres. Of the many approaches attempted, an appropriate mixture of behavioral, individual, and family therapy techniques has generally proven the most effective. Although one person enters the mental health delivery system, the "identified patient" becomes the family unit with its inherent dynamics. The following case study exemplifies this approach to therapy.

CASE STUDY

This was the first psychiatric admission for Theresa, a 13-year-old Caucasian female. An eighth-grade student at a private Catholic school, Theresa resided with her biological parents, three sisters, and two younger brothers in a suburb of Los Angeles. She was referred by her private psychiatrist because of a weight loss of 30 pounds over the previous 6 months. She was 5′1″ tall and weighed 70 pounds on admission.

On the day of admission, Theresa and her parents were interviewed together by the psychiatrist, social worker, and nurse. Most of the questions were directed to Theresa, but she frequently deferred to her parents.

Theresa stated that she felt "chubby" the previous autumn, when she weighed approximately 100 pounds, but that now at 70 pounds she felt she was looking her best. She was afraid that a gain of even a pound would make her "fat."

Theresa related that she hated food but was unable to elaborate on the reasons for this hatred. She refused to consume any foods that contained sweeteners, even artificial sweeteners, or any carbohydrates. She admitted to postprandial vomiting when she felt she had eaten too much.

Theresa also related that she had been very active recently. She swam and played tennis and golf competitively, and used the family pool and tennis court daily. Her parents reported that she spent several hours a day in vigorous activity and that if she didn't finish her exercise regimen during the day she would complete it at night before going to bed.

Her parents stated that last autumn their oldest daughter, Susan, had returned from a trip abroad 20 pounds heavier. They had encouraged Susan to lose weight and had even tried to "bribe" her to do so (with money for clothes and movies) without success. They wondered whether Susan's experience was a precipitant to Theresa's illness, and also mentioned that, in the past, Theresa's siblings had called her "chubby" even though she actually was thin.

Theresa had no goals for her hospitalization, although she was aware that she was admitted because her doctor felt that her low weight was a health hazard. She was satisifed that she looked just fine and was convinced that if she put on any weight she would be "fat."

Theresa first saw a psychiatrist, as an outpatient, 3 months before this hospitalization, after her parents had become alarmed at her accelerating weight loss. Theresa was puzzled about their concern. She attended her psychiatric sessions regularly, but would not identify any problems or concerns of her own. Because she continued to lose weight, hospitalization was recommended.

The medical history was essentially noncontributory; no allergies, no previous hospitalization, and no history of significant illnesses. Prior to her hospitalization, Theresa was seen by an endocrinologist and a gastroendocrinologist; neither found any specific abnormalities which could have caused her weight loss. Theresa had not begun her menstrual cycle.

Theresa was a product of a full-term normal pregnancy, labor, and delivery. She had no eating problems during her first years of life. She was bottle-fed and progressed to solid foods with no difficulty. Her developmental landmarks were normal; she walked and talked well within usual time frames, and was toilet-trained at age 2 without difficulty.

Theresa's parents described her as having been a "perfect child"—perfectionistic, orderly, and obedient—until her current difficulties began. She was active in school and athletic activities but had few friends, depending primarily on her family for emotional and social needs. Her parents characterized the family as nearly ideal and very close-knit, with the children all engaging in the same or similar activities much of the time. They described all of their children as being well-liked, yet with few friends; in the family, "the kids have each other." However, they reported that Theresa had become increasingly irritable and withdrawn in the 6 months prior to hospitalization, and had frequently excused herself from family activities in order to pursue her exercise regimen.

Theresa described her family as "perfect." She characterized her oldest sister, Susan, as both bright and popular and said that she would be attending college the following September; her sister Lisa as a very talented tennis player who was going to spend the summer in France; and her youngest sister, Nicole, as not only the most attractive of the girls but also the best student in this family of high achievers. When asked to talk about herself, Theresa consistently described the accomplishments of family members.

Mr. and Mrs. Montrose were equally difficult to interview, since both presented everything as being fine and "normal." Although superficially an "ideal" couple, they seemed excessively concerned with external appearances. They used nearly identical expressions in talking about themselves or each other ("They all had meant well and everybody did the best they could"). They showed little spontaneous display of emotion.

Mr. Montrose, a 48-year-old, immaculately dressed attorney, had established his own successful law firm. No history of mental illness was present in his family. He seemed reluctant to talk about himself, but not about his children. He did relate a desire to spend more time with his children but explained that his 10- to 12-hour workdays made this impossible.

Although college-educated, Mrs. Montrose had not worked since her marriage. Although pleasant and cooperative during the interview, she also seemed cautious and guarded. She seemed at a loss when pressed for details about personalities and feelings. She did state that "I find it difficult not to direct the lives of my children" even though they were now in their teens and no longer needed close direction.

The parents described each of their other children as extremely talented in at least one specialty, and stated that although Theresa did very well in school and was a good athlete, her accomplishments did not rival those of her sisters. They characterized Susan, age 17, as an "ideal" daughter—accomplished, well-behaved, and with a "super personality." She was gifted at languages and music. They described Lisa, age 15, as bright but tense and competitive, excelling at tennis, swimming, and schoolwork. She also had a gift for languages and was scheduled to visit France for the summer to study French. They characterized 11-year-old Nicole as a beautiful child and possibly the brightest of them all. A concert pianist, Nicole, like Theresa, was a perfectionist. As for 8-year-old Eric, "Four older sisters made him suffer but somehow he maintained himself very well." An avid golfer, he had just won a trophy the preceding week. They depicted their youngest child, 4-year-old Randy, as a bright, charming boy, who, although slow to adapt and not too sure of himself in new situations, eventually becomes secure.

During her admission interview, Theresa was cooperative and polite when questioned, but she offered little information spontaneously. She was dressed appropriately in a skirt and blouse, and her attractive shoulder-length blonde hair was neatly groomed. Her face was thin, drawn, and pale, and appeared older than her 13 years; her short, thin body looked younger.

Although she was invited to sit down, she stood quietly and almost motionless throughout the interview except for a slight rocking movement and occasional gestures and facial expressions. Her flow of speech and comprehension were normal. She laughed twice at appropriate times, but otherwise her mood was sad and depressed and her affect somewhat blunted, although appropriate.

On mental status examination, Theresa exhibited no manifestations of a thought disturbance. Her thought content was appropriate; she wanted to know when she would see her parents again, what her daily routine would be, how long she would be in the hospital, and other information related to her admission. She was able to respond adequately to the abstraction of proverbs and similarities. Her perception seemed normal, with the exception of her distorted body image. She was oriented in four spheres (time, place, person, situation). Her concentration, memory, retention, and recall were all normal. She performed quickly on all tasks. Her intellectual abilities were estimated as above-average, with a fund of general information consistent with her education, age, and intelligence. Her judgment was mostly normal, as measured by responses to typical situations; however, her judgment about eating was impaired. Theresa had little or no insight about her extremely low weight. She knew she was in the hospital because of her low weight, but insisted "I don't want to be fat."

Reader may now complete Recording the Data, Assigning Nursing Diagnoses, and Nursing Care Plan.

Continued on page 188

RECORDING THE DATA

After you have read the case, cluster significant data into functional health patterns.

Health management/health perception _____

_____

_____

_____

_____

Nutritional/metabolic _____

_____

_____

_____

Elimination _____

_____

_____

_____

Activity/exercise _____

_____

_____

_____

Cognitive/perceptual _____

_____

_____

_____

Sleep/rest _____

_____

_____

_____

Self-perception/self-concept _____

_____

_____

_____

Role relationship _____

_____

_____

_____

Sexuality/reproductive _____

_____

_____

_____

Coping/stress tolerance _____

_____

_____

_____

Value/belief _____

_____

_____

_____

ASSIGNING NURSING DIAGNOSES

Use your clustered data to select appropriate nursing diagnoses.

Health perception/health management

☐ Growth and Development, Altered (see Developmental Delay)
☐ Health Maintenance, Altered
☐ Infection, Potential for
☐ Injury (Trauma): Potential for
☐ Noncompliance (Specify)
☐ Poisoning: Potential for
☐ Suffocation: Potential for

Nutritional/metabolic

☐ Body Temperature, Potential Alteration in
☐ Developmental Delay: Physical Growth and Development
☐ Fluid Volume, Altered: Excess or Excess Fluid Volume
☐ Fluid Volume Deficit, Actual
☐ Fluid Volume Deficit, Potential
☐ Nutrition, Altered: Less Than Body Requirements or Nutritional Deficit (Specify)
☐ Nutrition, Altered: More Than Body Requirements or Exogenous Obesity
☐ Nutrition, Altered: Potential for More Than Body Requirements or Potential for Obesity
☐ Oral Mucous Membrane, Altered
☐ Skin Integrity, Impaired or Skin Breakdown
☐ Skin Integrity, Impaired or Potential Skin Breakdown
☐ Swallowing, Impaired or Uncompensated Swallowing Impairment
☐ Tissue Integrity, Impaired

Elimination

☐ Bowel Elimination, Altered: Constipation
☐ Bowel Elimination, Altered: Diarrhea
☐ Bowel Elimination, Altered: Incontinence
☐ Developmental Delay: Bowel/Bladder Control
☐ Incontinence: Functional
☐ Incontinence: Reflex
☐ Incontinence: Stress
☐ Incontinence: Total
☐ Incontinence: Urge
☐ Urinary Elimination, Altered Patterns of
☐ Urinary Retention

Activity/exercise

☐ Activity Intolerance
☐ Activity Intolerance, Potential
☐ Airway Clearance, Ineffective
☐ Breathing Pattern, Ineffective
☐ Cardiac Output, Altered: Decreased
☐ Developmental Delay: Mobility
☐ Developmental Delay: Self-Care Skills
☐ Diversional Activity Deficit
☐ Gas Exchange, Impaired
☐ Home Maintenance Management, Impaired (Mild, Moderate, Severe, Potential, Chronic)
☐ Mobility, Impaired Physical
☐ Self-Care Deficit: Feeding
☐ Self-Care Deficit: Bathing/Hygiene
☐ Self-Care Deficit: Dressing/Grooming
☐ Self-Care Deficit: Toileting
☐ Self-Care Deficit: Total
☐ Tissue Perfusion, Altered: (Specify)

Sleep/rest

☐ Sleep Pattern Disturbance

Cognitive/perceptual

☐ Comfort, Altered: Pain
☐ Comfort, Altered: Chronic Pain

☐ Developmental Delay: (Specify Cognitive Area; attention, decision making, etc.)
☐ Hypothermia
☐ Hyperthermia
☐ Knowledge Deficit (Specify)
☐ Sensory-Perceptual Alteration: Input Excess or Sensory Overload
☐ Sensory-Perceptual Alteration: Input Deficit or Sensory Deprivation
☐ Thermoregulation, Ineffective
☐ Thought Processes, Altered
☐ Unilateral Neglect

Self-perception/self-concept

☐ Anxiety
☐ Body Image Disturbance
☐ Fear
☐ Hopelessness
☐ Personal Identity Confusion
☐ Powerlessness (Severe, Low, Moderate)
☐ Self-Esteem Disturbance

Role relationship

☐ Communication, Impaired Verbal
☐ Developmental Delay: Communication Skills
☐ Developmental Delay: Social Skills
☐ Family Processes, Altered
☐ Grieving, Anticipatory
☐ Grieving, Dysfunctional
☐ Parenting, Altered: Actual or Potential

☐ Role Performance, Disturbance in
☐ Social Interactions, Impaired
☐ Social Isolation (Rejection)

Sexuality/reproductive

☐ Rape-Trauma Syndrome: Compounded
☐ Rape-Trauma Syndrome: Silent Reaction
☐ Sexual Dysfunction
☐ Sexuality Patterns, Altered

Coping/stress tolerance

☐ Adjustment, Impaired
☐ Coping, Ineffective Individual
☐ Coping, Ineffective Family: Compromised
☐ Coping, Ineffective Family: Disabling
☐ Coping, Family: Potential for Growth
☐ Developmental Delay (Specify area)
☐ Post-Trauma Response
☐ Violence, Potential for (Self-Directed or Directed at Others)

Value/belief

☐ Spiritual Distress (Distress of Human Spirit)

You are now ready to develop a nursing care plan for this client. Use the following blank pages to do so. Then refer to the author's formulation, diagnostic summary, care plan, and summary.

NURSING CARE PLAN

Complete the chart below to develop a nursing care plan for this client.

Discharge outcomes/long-term goals	

Nursing diagnosis	Nursing intervention	

	Predicted outcomes/short-term goals (include time frame)	Date/signature

Return to Formulation, page 188

FORMULATION

Theresa was hospitalized for treatment of anorexia nervosa. The clinical syndrome of anorexia nervosa involves a relentless pursuit of thinness with body image disturbances of delusional proportions; a deficit in accurate perception of body sensations, with inaccurate hunger awareness as the most pronounced deficiency; and a pervasive, paralyzing sense of ineffectiveness (Bruch, 1973).

Theresa had both cognitive and affective components to her disorder. She was excessively anxious about making mistakes and tended to believe herself a failure if she was not always successful. Such unrealistic expectations caused her to erect strict defenses against the possibility of failure. To preserve ego integrity, she maintained a self-critical and guarded attitude, which interfered with and constricted her range of perception, cognition, and judgment. She viewed expectations from her social environment and everyday interpersonal experiences as threats to her self-esteem, in response to which she erected a rigid, maladaptive defense system.

Theresa had difficulty expressing affect and was unable to deal with her impulses and painful inner conflicts. Thus, anxiety-arousing situations tended to threaten her equilibrium, causing her to retreat behind narrow and rigid internal boundaries. As a result, she appeared shallow and superficial in interpersonal situations. She did not achieve a sense of preadolescent confidence and competence and as a result was left without the ego strength necessary to experience the affectivity of adolescence without being overwhelmed by its emergence.

In summary, Theresa's superior level of cognitive functioning was impaired by excessive inhibition and perfectionistic traits, especially when she experienced anxiety in her interpersonal life. Rigid defense mechanisms, emotional overconstriction, and the maintenance of interpersonal distance interfered with adaptive reality testing. For example, Theresa would frequently misinterpret social interactions to be positive and deny all negative aspects of the interaction. She disregarded all situations that did not conform to her perceptual image.

The origin of Theresa's illness appeared to stem from a pattern of overcompliance and strenuous efforts toward achievement with little expression of personal feelings and desires—a pattern encouraged by her parents. Her efforts toward defining herself (individuation) were complicated by the pressure she felt to appear as others expect her to be, by an enmeshed family system, and by her own lack of confidence in her ability to think for herself. Dieting was one area in which she sought to gain control and counteract her feelings of ineffectiveness and low self-esteem.

Theresa described her family in ideal terms and was unwilling to acknowledge negative affect toward any member or any family problems or conflicts. Mr. and Mrs. Montrose also described their family as nearly ideal and very close-knit. While all family members interviewed emphasized their congeniality, each person tended to speak not for himself or herself but rather in the name of another family member, constantly modifying, correcting, or invalidating what the other had said. They functioned as if they could read each other's mind, explaining what the other truly meant.

Typically, the family of an anorexic client is intact, seems happy, and is financially and socially successful. Family members commonly present their family life as more harmonious than it actually is, or deny difficulties altogether. Such features commonly lead to a denial of illness or of the need for change (Bruch, 1978).

Enmeshment is one of the most glaring characteristics of these families. The family members are poorly individuated, with the primary group concern being the maintenance of overt harmony and closeness. Loyalty, self-sacrifice, and anticipation of others' needs are highly valued, but independence, disagreement, and conflict are viewed as threats to cohesion, if not as acts of hostility. Inevitably conflicts exist, but they are denied or remain suppressed (Minuchin, et al., 1978).

Evidence of enmeshment in the Montrose family was the family's polite indecisiveness, which led to dissatisfaction for each person. For example, the Montroses had great difficulty deciding what to do on their visits. The parents were frustrated that Theresa would not state how she wanted to spend the time during the visit; at the same time, they perceived her to be quietly disapproving of their decisions. Theresa had little experience stating a preference and so she continued, begrudgingly, to go along with parental decisions.

In most anorexic families, the facade of harmony conceals dissatisfied marital partners who strive for fulfillment in other areas—the mother in her children and the father in his occupation. The lines along which the family communicates are narrow, and attention is channeled toward the children so that the mother becomes excessively involved with them, perhaps overdirective, while at the same time unable to acknowledge their individuality and somewhat fearful of their adolescent psychosexual development and impending separation (Bruch, 1978). Parental overinvestment in and overdirectiveness of the children leads to high achievement orientation, in which the vulnerable child becomes more concerned with parental approval than with personal goals.

This situation was clearly evident in Theresa's case. Indeed, because of her parents' overdirectiveness and disregard of her individuality, Theresa developed a very fragile self-image and felt no real areas for self-control.

From a developmental perspective, Theresa had not learned to discriminate her own needs from her parents' needs and thus became a devoted, compliant, "perfect" child with little capacity to function autonomously. She was unprepared for the normal separation and individuation process of adolescence, and so took refuge in obsessively controlling her body through starvation and acted out her adolescent rebellion in a primitive, hostile-dependent fashion. However ruthless and brutalizing it may seem to others, self-starvation is positively valued by an anorexic client; it serves as an affirmation of discipline and self-determination, dampens threatening signals of physical change, and greatly simplifies matters of existence (Crisp, 1980).

This developmental focus suggests guidelines for the therapeutic process and foci of change relevant to the anorexic client. Specifically, an effective therapeutic program addresses such issues as acceptance of impulses and openness to affective experience; greater tolerance of the uncertainties of change and growth; encouragement of introspection, abstraction of thought, and realistic appraisal of limitations, competencies, and potentials; and increased understanding of experiential and dynamic factors inhibiting separation and individuation (Strober, 1985).

The inpatient milieu as a therapeutic program provides a supportive and realistic exposure to age- and gender-appropriate standards of behavior to encourage identity formation and individuation. The nursing staff utilizes group discussions and activities to develop appropriate social skills and to assist teenagers in overcoming their reluctance to deal with adolescent-related issues. These small group experiences provide a measured and safe environment for developmentally mature attempts at assertion, genuine self-expression, and discussion of interpersonal and psychosexual concerns.

The nursing staff endeavors to project patience, sensitivity, tact, genuine caring, and a desire to understand. They emphasize an overriding interest in the client's individual thoughts and feelings rather than in her ability to follow explicit rules and instructions. Therapeutic interventions focus on self-reflection and self-appraisal by the client to establish a sense of self and to decrease dependence on external objects for guidance and affirmation of self. Through this introspective exploration, any distorted sense of personal worth and inadequacy and an extreme dependence on external standards of performance and accomplishment are examined. Progress is heralded by increasing initiative in milieu activities, greater social engagement, and more assertive and genuine affective expression.

Because the nursing staff must force a changed eating pattern on a client who sees no need for change, the client typically reacts with hostility toward the nurse. In such circumstances, the nurse must be empathetic to the distress of the client, but also must maintain control of both that empathy and any reaction of anger or frustration to the client's hostility.

The nurse's feelings of anger and frustration are a genuine and intrinsic part of the treatment process and may be an element of countertransference. Generally, these feelings are based on the nurse's empathetic reaction to the client's plight. The client usually interprets the nurse's efforts at understanding as a sign of interest and concern.

The nurse must be able to keep in check any impulse to blame or scold—to see the client as stubborn, spoiled, or manipulative—or to act precipitously to alleviate the client's suffering with promises or quick remedies. The nurse must also be intuitive when monitoring and pacing interventions, knowing when to probe gently and when to hold back and wait patiently.

While the major focus of this treatment is on developmental issues, successful treatment of anorexia nervosa also includes weight restoration. The effects of starvation must be alleviated for the client to truly benefit from psychotherapy. Many of the symptoms regularly ascribed to the anorexic nervosa syndrome result directly from the physiological effects of starvation and will remit following weight restoration. In addition, maintenance of low weight through rigid dieting serves to reinforce the client's phobic posture toward weight as well as her tendency to avoid dealing realistically with significant life problems (Garfinkel and Garner, 1982).

The weight management program must be nonnegotiable. While the majority of anorexic clients strongly protest abdication of this control, most eventually admit that being relieved of this responsibility helps decrease food-related anxieties to more manageable proportions, and in the long run actually facilitates progress of the therapeutic program.

Family therapy represents another component of this multimodal treatment plan. Because family dynamics such as enmeshment, overprotectiveness, rigidity, and avoidance of conflict are pathogenic or help sustain anorexic symptoms, a determined effort to alter these operations promises therapeutic benefit (Strober, 1985). During therapy, the staff endeavors to provide "parenting" responses that support the family's role in encouraging the client to define herself from within. Like the parents of an individuating child, the staff ideally should offer a combination of protection, firm structure, reliability, support of initiative, and tolerance of regression (Stern, et al., 1981). Family therapy strives to help each family member become more autonomous and less enmeshed—a change

Continued on page 197

DIAGNOSTIC SUMMARY FOR THERESA

Data	Functional health pattern	Nursing diagnosis
—Presents with extremely poor weight-to-height ratio (weight—70 lbs., height—5′1″) —Demonstrates manipulation around food intake; e.g., concealing food in napkins —Vomits after meals	Nutritional/Metabolic	Altered nutrition: less than body requirements, related to 30-pound weight loss secondary to psychological factors
—Expresses a belief that a gain of 1 pound would make her "fat"	Self-Perception/Self-Concept	Body image disturbance related to inaccurate perception of self as obese, secondary to cognitive perceptual distortions as part of anorexia nervosa
—Constantly talks about food issues —States she has obsessive thoughts about her weight	Cognitive/Perceptual	Altered thought processes related to starvation secondary to anorexia nervosa
—Exhibited a slight rocking movement during the interview —Engages in excessive, inappropriate exercise (e.g., doing jumping jacks in the dayroom)	Self-Perception/Self-Concept	Moderate anxiety related to irrational thoughts of being overweight secondary to anorexia nervosa
—Expresses feelings of inadequacy and ineffectiveness (e.g., inability to make decisions or to express her own opinion)	Coping/Stress Tolerance	Ineffective individual coping related to low self-esteem secondary to personal vulnerability during a maturational crisis
—Lacks a sense of identity: expresses poor self-knowledge; seems unsure of how to act or react; compares herself to others; demonstrates overcompliance; and relies on external rather than internal cues, e.g., constantly seeks feedback about her behavior —Exhibits family problems: states she needs to excel to be accepted by parents; lacks self-identity (e.g., when asked to state a preference says "we," referring to her family, rather than "I"); and experiences anxiety and guilt over breaking with "family tradition" to do "something different"	Self-Perception/Self-Concept	Personal identity confusion related to an enmeshed family system secondary to rigid structures and unspoken rules dictating conformity and compliance by family members

NURSING CARE PLAN

Complete the chart below to develop a nursing care plan for this client.

Discharge outcome/long-term goals	
1. THERESA WILL ATTAIN A WEIGHT COMPATIBLE WITH THE PHYSIOLOGICAL NEEDS OF A 13-YEAR-OLD AND WILL VERBALIZE NEUTRALIZED ATTITUDE TOWARDS HER WEIGHT.	

Nursing diagnosis	Nursing intervention	Predicted outcome/short-term goals (include time frame)	Date/signature
ALTERED NUTRITION: LESS THAN BODY REQUIREMENTS, RELATED TO 30-POUND WEIGHT LOSS SECONDARY TO PSYCHOLOGICAL FACTORS	–DIET MANAGEMENT PROGRAM: • WEIGH THERESA TWO TIMES A WEEK IN THE MORNING BEFORE BREAKFAST, WHILE SHE'S DRESSED IN A HOSPITAL GOWN • ENCOURAGE HER TO CONSUME 600 CALORIES PER MEAL. ENSURE THAT NUTRITIONALLY BALANCED TRAYS ARE PREPARED BY THE DIETARY DEPARTMENT. ALLOW THERESA INPUT ON THE MENU, BUT ALLOW NO SUBSTITUTIONS ONCE THE MEALS ARE PLANNED • GIVE HER ½-HOUR TO EAT; OBSERVE HER CLOSELY DURING THE MEAL. RECORD CALORIC INTAKE • MAKE UP ANY CALORIC DEFICITS IMMEDIATELY AFTER A MEAL WITH A HIGH-CALORIC SUPPLEMENT. GIVE THERESA 15 MINUTES TO DRINK THE SUPPLEMENT • ENSURE THAT THERESA REMAINS WITHIN SIGHT OF STAFF FOR 3 HOURS AFTER EACH MEAL. SHOULD SHE VOMIT, OR BE OUT OF STAFF'S SIGHT, REPLACE THE ENTIRE MEAL WITH A SUPPLEMENT • IF SHE REFUSES TO MEET THE CALORIC INTAKE REQUIREMENT, AUTOMATICALLY INSTITUTE TUBE FEEDING	–THERESA WILL GAIN 1½ TO 2 POUNDS PER WEEK, BEGINNING IMMEDIATELY –THERESA WILL CONSUME 600 CALORIES PER MEAL BEGINNING IMMEDIATELY –THERESA WILL EAT HER MEAL WITHIN A ½-HOUR TIME ALLOTMENT, BEGINNING IMMEDIATELY –WITHIN 1 MONTH, THERESA WILL NOT VOMIT AFTER MEALS	12/4 EB
BODY IMAGE DISTURBANCE RELATED TO INACCURATE PERCEPTION OF SELF AS OBESE SECOND-	–PROVIDE THERESA WITH REALITY ORIENTATION WITH REGARD TO HER NEED TO MAINTAIN AN ADEQUATE WEIGHT FOR SURVIVAL DO NOT DISCUSS	–THERESA WILL ADMIT SEVERE WEIGHT LOSS AS BEING UNDESIRABLE WITHIN 3 TO 4 MONTHS	12/4 EB

Continued

Nursing Care Plan *continued*

Nursing diagnosis	Nursing intervention	Predicted outcome/short-term goals (include time frame)	Date/signature
ARY TO COGNITIVE PERCEPTUAL DISTORTIONS AS PART OF ANOREXIA NERVOSA	PARTICULAR WEIGHT STANDARDS OR OTHER SPECIFIC ISSUES INVOLVING WEIGHT OR FOOD		
ALTERED THOUGHT PROCESSES RELATED TO STARVATION SECONDARY TO ANOREXIA NERVOSA	–DO NOT DISCUSS FOOD, WEIGHT, EXERCISE, OR THE DIET MANAGEMENT PROGRAM WITH THERESA. ENSURE THAT THE FOOD IS A PRESCRIPTION WRITTEN FOR HER SO THE PROCEDURE SHOULD BE CARRIED OUT WITH A "MATTER-OF-FACT" ATTITUDE	–WITHIN 3 MONTHS, THERESA WILL TALK LESS ABOUT FOOD (2 TO 3 TIMES PER WEEK) –THERESA'S PERCEPTION AND JUDGMENT REGARDING SITUATION WILL RESOLVE BY DISCHARGE	12/4 EB
MODERATE ANXIETY RELATED TO IRRATIONAL THOUGHTS OF BEING OVERWEIGHT SECONDARY TO ANOREXIA NERVOSA	–SET LIMITS ON EXERCISING. ALLOW HER SOLITARY EXERCISE UNLESS SHE IS NOT GAINING WEIGHT –ENCOURAGE HER INVOLVEMENT IN LEISURE PLANNING ACTIVITIES IN OCCUPATIONAL THERAPY –PROMOTE EXPRESSION OF HER FEELINGS THROUGH ART PROJECTS	–WITHIN 2 MONTHS, THERESA WILL BEGIN TO USE OTHER MEANS THAN EXERCISE TO COPE WITH ANXIETY (e.g., TALKING TO STAFF) –THERESA WILL COMPLETE ONE ART PROJECT WITHIN 3 WEEKS	12/4 EB

Discharge outcome/long-term goals	MAKING.	
1. TO DECREASE ASSOCIATIONS BETWEEN FOOD AND STRESS AND DEVELOP NON-FOOD RELATED COPING MECHANISMS, e.g. VERBALIZATION OF INDEPENDENT PROBLEM-SOLVING SKILLS AND DECISION		

Nursing diagnosis	Nursing intervention	Predicted outcome/short-term goals (include time frame)	Date/signature
INEFFECTIVE INDIVIDUAL COPING, RELATED TO LOW SELF-ESTEEM SECONDARY TO PERSONAL VULNERABILITY DURING A MATURATION CRISIS	−FOSTER SUCCESSFUL EXPERIENCES; IDENTIFY AND UTILIZE HER STRENGTHS −TEACH HER ASSERTION SKILLS THROUGH ROLE MODELING −DO NOT ALLOW HER TO ELICIT OTHERS TO MAKE DECISIONS FOR HER; RATHER, ENCOURAGE HER TO REACH HER OWN CONCLUSIONS	−WITHIN 2 WEEKS, THERESA WILL BE ABLE TO VERBALIZE HER OWN OPINIONS 40% OF THE TIME IN INDIVIDUAL SESSIONS AND 20% OF THE TIME IN GROUPS	12/4 EB
PERSONAL IDENTITY CONFUSION RELATED TO ENMESHED FAMILY SYSTEM SECONDARY TO RIGID STRUCTURES AND UNSPOKEN RULES DICTATING CONFORMITY AND COMPLIANCE BY FAMILY MEMBERS	−ENCOURAGE THERESA TO IDENTIFY AND EXPRESS HER FEELINGS. INCREASE HER AWARENESS OF FEELINGS THAT ORIGINATE WITHIN HERSELF −ENCOURAGE INTROSPECTION AND SELF-APPRAISAL BY ASKING QUESTIONS THAT FOSTER EXPLORATION −AVOID MAKING EVALUATIVE STATEMENTS ABOUT HER PROGRESS −DO NOT REDUCE COGNITIVE CONFLICT BY GIVING ANSWERS, MAKING INTERPRETATIONS, OR STATING HOW SHE FEELS. DO NOT REINFORCE COMPLIANCE; ALLOW HER TO TRY OUT "NEW" BEHAVIORS −DO NOT MAKE INTERPRETATIONS OR JUDGMENTS ABOUT FAMILY RELATIONSHIPS; RATHER ENCOURAGE HER TO EXPLORE HER ROLE IN THE FAMILY BY REFLECTING COMMENTS BACK TO HER −HELP HER DISCRIMINATE HER FAMILY'S STYLE AND FEELINGS AS DISTINCT FROM HER OWN BY REDIRECTING THE	−OVER THE NEXT 2 WEEKS, THERESA WILL DEMONSTRATE INCREASED SELF-ASSURANCE BY MAKING "I FEEL" STATEMENTS 50% OF THE TIME DURING ONE-TO-ONE SESSIONS, AND BY ONCE A DAY DEMONSTRATING LESS NEED TO CONFORM TO RULES AND REGULATIONS AND EXPECTATIONS OF OTHERS; e.g., MAKING AGE-APPROPRIATE PROTEST TO RULES −BY THE TIME OF DISCHARGE, THERESA WILL VERBALIZE INSIGHT INTO FAMILY DYNAMICS AND HER ROLE IN THE FAMILY	12/4 EB

Continued

Nursing Care Plan *continued*

Nursing diagnosis	Nursing intervention	Predicted outcome/short-term goals (include time frame)	Date/signature
	CONVERSATION TO HER OWN INDIVIDUAL EXPERIENCE AS SEPARATE FROM HER FAMILY —WHEN SHE EXPRESSES FEELINGS OF GUILT AND RESPONSIBILITY TOWARDS HER PARENTS, HELP HER EXPLORE THE SOURCE OF THOSE FEELINGS AND RELATED FEARS		

that allows the adolescent to develop autonomy, to individuate, and to function independently.

SUMMARY

Theresa was assigned a primary nurse on the day shift and an associate staff for the evening shift. These staff members were responsible for developing a care plan specific to Theresa's needs as well as coordinating her nursing care needs with the rest of the nursing team.

Within a week of hospitalization, the primary nurse presented the anorexic regimen outlined in the nursing care plan to Theresa in a non-threatening, concise manner. In doing so, the nurse avoided ambiguity, pointed out the seriousness of her illness, communicated concern, and explained clearly the expectations and plan of action should these expectations not be met.

During the first phase of hospitalization, Theresa alternated periods of crying, screaming, and threatening with periods of quiet pleading for a reduced caloric intake. She was in constant movement—hopping, jumping, pacing—and sat only when required to. She was also getting insufficient sleep; she would stay up late at night and get up early in the morning to exercise. Because of this, she was moved into a room near the nurses' station to enable closer observation.

Due to Theresa's constant activity, her caloric intake was increased periodically to ensure an adequate weight gain. She eventually required 3,000 calories per day to ensure a weight gain of 1½ to 2 pounds per week. She ate a variety of foods but her eating pattern was characterized by frequent trips to the food line to "look," watching what peers ate and following suit, frequent spitting up of vitamin supplements, and hiding food in napkins. On two occasions, she stuffed her mouth with bread until she choked; staff had to apply the Heimlich maneuver to dislodge the bread. She did not vomit or require tube feeding. Only after 8 months was weight restoration achieved and her caloric intake reduced to maintenance level.

Working with Theresa required much patience during the first 3 months of hospitalization. The only affect she displayed towards staff was anger, and all of her conversation centered around food and weight. During this period, the nursing staff tried to listen in a nonjudgmental manner until Theresa demonstrated increased insight into the issues underlying her eating disorder.

On the unit, Theresa was remote and only a passive participant in activities. She rarely initiated conversation or interactions with other people, although she would respond when others approached her. As she established close relations with staff that did not lead to overdependence or a lost sense of self, she became more available to positive peer interactions.

Theresa had great difficulty conceptualizing her conflicts and putting feelings into words. Initially, she put great effort into trying to act in accordance with her perception of staff expectations. She relied on external rather than internal cues to give direction and to determine her feelings about herself and her experiences. When she was stressed by situations that had no clear guidelines for her behavior, she panicked and became desperate for guidance. She would pace, wring her hands, and go from staff to staff asking what she should do. She would then perseverate on all of her options. In order to help increase her awareness of her own subjective experience, staff avoided interpretations or evaluative statements about her behavior. As she decreased her dependence on others for self-definition, she found that her sense of self was vague. When left to define herself from within, she was bewildered.

Small group experiences helped Theresa negotiate social interactions in a measured and safe environment, as well as explore the impact of her behavior on others. Milieu activities such as community meetings, client-staff meetings, and girls' group provided reinforcement for successful peer interactions. She became a group leader (President of the Community) and began working through her overwhelming feelings of self-doubt with the feedback she received on her performance in this position. Near the end of her hospitalization, she became more decidedly "adolescent": she was more humorous, more provocative, and took risks to challenge staff and overstep rules—the signs of an incipient sense of identity and mastery and of a more internalized self-esteem.

As Theresa neared discharge, her methods of dealing with life situations remained somewhat rigid, but she was beginning to show signs of tolerating the anxiety that comes with change and the long, slow process of identity-building. She had begun to challenge some of the implicit family values and resist the effect of these values on her. While she remained sensitive to her parents' wishes and fearful of displeasing them, she had progressed in her ability to define her own wishes and to feel less concern with their expectations.

She also gained insight into the way she displaced her psychological struggles onto her body. Because interpersonal conflicts were threatening to her, she turned negative feelings towards others back onto herself; to battle with herself was less anxiety-producing than to battle with others. With her new insight, she expressed more of a desire to be her own person, different from her family when she desired, and more willingness to confront others as part of the normal process of growing up.

At the time of discharge, Theresa demonstrated the capability to mediate her eating and maintain her weight at an appropriate level. She was able to link emotions and interpersonal problems with disturbances in her eating and maintain a more normal eating pattern. She manifested no significant distortions of her body image and was able to maintain a reasonable level of physical exercise.

During her hospitalization, Theresa made sustained and steady progress towards individuation and psychological separation from her parents. Over the course of treatment, she became more realistic in her perception of both of her parents. Because she was able to identify their strengths and weaknesses, at the time of discharge, she had developed a more positive and realistic relationship with them. Whereas in the past she had experienced great difficulty displaying any critical attitudes about her parents, during therapy she became adamant in her criticisms, especially towards her mother. On the one hand, she observed that her mother was very tight emotionally and unavailable to her for real closeness, and also perceived her mother as treating her in a less relaxed and more cautious manner than the other children. On the other hand, Theresa expressed concern that she herself was overly critical and reactive towards her mother. In discussing these issues, Theresa achieved insight into her own fluctuating needs for independence and dependence in her relationship with her mother.

For their part, Theresa's parents made considerable progress in loosening parental expectations and allowing her more room for individual growth and expression. Theresa became more able to identify and respond to her own internal experience and began to develop a sense of her own individual identity. She continued to be slightly rigid and obsessive and to have somewhat excessive needs for external validation; her increased self-confidence and more autonomous sense of identity remained fragile personality constellations requiring continued psychotherapeutic intervention upon discharge. Towards this end, Theresa was assigned an outpatient therapist for weekly sessions. In addition, she and her family were referred to a family therapist for once-a-week sessions.

REFERENCES

Bruch, H. *Eating Disorders: Obesity, Anorexia Nervosa, and the Person Within*. New York: Basic Books, 1973.

Bruch, H. *The Golden Cage*. Cambridge, Mass.: Harvard University Press, 1978.

Crisp, A.H. *Anorexia Nervosa: Let Me Be*. New York: Grune & Stratton, 1980.

Garfinkel, P., and Garner, D. *Anorexia Nervosa, a Multidimensional Perspective*. New York: Brunner-Mazel, 1982.

Minuchin, S., et al. *Psychosomatic Families: Anorexia Nervosa in Context*. Cambridge, Mass.: Harvard University Press, 1978.

Stern, S., et al. "Anorexia Nervosa: The Hospital's Role in Family Treatment," *Family Practice* 20:395-408, 1981.

Strober, M. "The Treatment of Anorexia Nervosa in Adolescents: Theoretical and Clinical Strategies," in *Handbook of Psychotherapy for Anorexia Nervosa and Bulimia*. Edited by Garner, D., and Garfinkel, P. New York: Guilford, 1985.

SELECTED BIBLIOGRAPHY

Dresser, R. "Legal and Policy Considerations in Treatment of Anorexia Nervosa Patients," *International Journal of Eating Disorders* 3:40-52, 1984.

Garner, D., and Garfinkel, P. *Handbook of Psychotherapy for Anorexia Nervosa and Bulimia*. New York: Guilford, 1985.

Kagan, D., and Squires, R. "Dieting, Compulsive Eating, and Feelings of Failure Among Adolescents," *International Journal of Eating Disorders* 3:15-26, 1983.

Kim, M.J. *Classification of Nursing Diagnosis: Proceedings of the Fifth National Conference*. St. Louis: C.V. Mosby Co., 1984.

Levenkron, S. *Treating and Overcoming Anorexia Nervosa*. New York: C. Scribner's Sons, 1982.

Palazzoli, M.S. *Self Starvation*. New York: Jason Aronson, 1978.

Swift, W., et al. "Ego Development in Anorexic Inpatients," *International Journal of Eating Disorders* 3:73-80, 1984.

Philip:
Attention Deficit Disorder

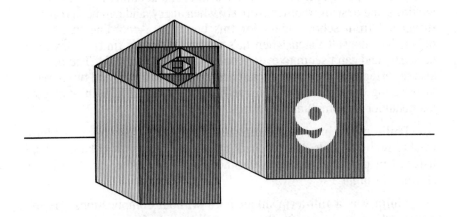

Diane Moreau, MN, RN, CNA

Attention deficit disorder (ADD) is a clinical syndrome characterized in children by symptoms of inattention, restlessness, and impulsivity. ADD is the term once used to refer to clients who were "hyperactive" or suspected of suffering from "minimal brain syndrome." More frequently found in males than females, ADD is differentiated from conduct disorders, where behavior is clearly antisocial.

Treatment for a client with ADD with hyperactivity involves both medication and a highly structured environment (such as inpatient hospitalization) with individual supervision and psychotherapy. Nursing care for such a client involves a behavioral approach and teaching more adaptive, affective coping strategies. Nurses are also influential in evaluating drug efficacy.

CASE STUDY

Philip, a 12½-year-old Caucasian boy, was brought to the hospital by his parents for evaluation and treatment of his hyperactive, oppositional, and disruptive behavior. He lived at home, in a heavily populated suburban area, with his biological parents and two siblings, a 16-year-old sister and a 7-year-old brother. Philip's father, a mechanic, and his mother, a homemaker, both completed high school and frequently attended the local Protestant church.

At admission, Philip was described by his parents as having excess energy, with difficulty in attending to and completing tasks and severe behavioral problems at school. Over the last few years, he had been involved in repeated physical fights at school and at home. He had broken windows and destroyed other property when angry, and had been recently suspended from school again for this behavior. According to Philip's father, he "doesn't listen when he's spoken to, never finishes anything he starts, and can't seem to ever keep his hands to himself." The parents also reported that Philip seems sad and irritable at times, and often made disparaging comments about himself. They asked for help in managing his behavior at home and at school.

Philip, when interviewed directly, stated, "I'm here because I have trouble with the kids and teachers at school. I guess I'm bad. I don't listen to my parents, and I hit my brother a lot." He also reported difficulty sleeping at night.

Philip was a full-term infant born without complications. He experienced no problems in the neonatal period. His parents reported developmental milestones within the normal limits, but remembered him as being more active and restless than his siblings. His attention span was always poor, and he seemed to have difficulty sitting still. He often ran out into the street and was constantly climbing and falling, sustaining minor injuries. His mother stated that he was always hard to comfort, was a light eater, and that he cried excessively.

Philip's past medical history included the usual childhood diseases. His immunizations were up-to-date, and he had no known allergies to foods or medication. At age 4 he experienced a loss of consciousness secondary to head trauma, with no known sequelae. He was tried on Ritalin at age 8 by the family pediatrician, but the parents reported no observable change in his behavior while he was on the medication. They stated that dosage increases or adjustments were not made at that time. Philip was not on any medications at time of admission, and denied any alcohol or drug use. He reported no specific health problems and no somatic complaints.

This was the first inpatient evaluation for Philip, although he had come to the attention of various school psychologists and counselors at a young age. According to school reports, as early as first grade Philip was labeled a "management problem" and was placed in classes for the educationally handicapped. He never was a good student, demonstrating variable performance and low frustration tolerance in the classroom. Although tests revealed normal intelligence, he consistently demonstrated underachievement—especially in reading, spelling, and arithmetic. In educationally handicapped classes, he earned primarily Ds for his coursework. His parents received frequent calls from the school concerning his behavior.

Socially, Philip never had many friends. His interactions with peers at school and in the neighborhood were frequently provocative and resulted in verbal and physical fights. He did not belong to any clubs or play any organized sports; his favorite activities were swimming and bicycle riding. Philip said that he had one friend at school with whom he liked to spend time. He also stated that he liked girls but did not have a girlfriend.

Philip's parents stated that they had tried "everything" to control his behavior, including lecturing, spanking with an open hand and a belt, and sending him to his room. They reported that even when he did "settle down," he invariably engaged in some sort of disruptive behavior within 30 minutes. They stated that no one had ever suggested psychiatric intervention before, and that they were seeking help now at the recommendation of Philip's school counselor.

Philip's family had resided in the same middle-class neighborhood for the past 10 years. Philip and his brother shared a bedroom in their three-bedroom home; their sister had a room of her own. The parents reported that financial demands had created a strain for them, and that they had experienced some marital discord. They contemplated separation in the past, but stayed together to try to "work it out." They reported that the tension between them had recently eased somewhat, except for arguments about how best to manage Philip. Although they enjoyed family outings and trips, these often resulted in fighting, Philip's misbehavior, and "everyone having a horrible time." Philip was seen as the catalyst for the family arguments and fighting. According to the parents, Philip had a positive relationship with his sister, whom he "feels close to." He had a poor relationship with his brother, marked by constant fighting.

Philip's father reported that as a child, Philip was somewhat "hyper" and mischievous in school, and frequently got caught at pranks and cheating. He related no family history of psychiatric disturbances or medical problems. None of the other children had experienced behavioral, learning, or psychiatric problems.

On direct interview, Philip presented as an attractive, well-oriented 12½-year-old who appeared younger than his stated age. He responded willingly and spontaneously to questions asked. His speech was normal in rate, rhythm, and tone. His mood was slightly anxious, with some sadness noted when discussing his problems. Philip admitted feeling sad at times, but stated that he usually felt "bored." His intellect and memory were adequate, and his fund of knowledge seemed average. He was able to stay seated throughout the interview and appeared attentive to the

Continued on page 210

RECORDING THE DATA

After you have read the case, cluster significant data into functional health patterns.

Health management/health perception _____

_____

_____

_____

_____

Nutritional/metabolic _____

_____

_____

_____

Elimination _____

_____

_____

_____

Activity/exercise _____

_____

_____

_____

Cognitive/perceptual _____

_____

_____

_____

PHILIP: ATTENTION DEFICIT DISORDER

Sleep/rest _____

_____

_____

_____

Self-perception/self-concept _____

_____

_____

_____

Role relationship _____

_____

_____

_____

Sexuality/reproductive _____

_____

_____

_____

Coping/stress tolerance _____

_____

_____

_____

Value/belief _____

_____

_____

_____

ASSIGNING NURSING DIAGNOSES

Use your clustered data to select appropriate nursing diagnoses.

Health perception/health management

- ☐ Growth and Development, Altered (see Developmental Delay)
- ☐ Health Maintenance, Altered
- ☐ Infection, Potential for
- ☐ Injury (Trauma): Potential for
- ☐ Noncompliance (Specify)
- ☐ Poisoning: Potential for
- ☐ Suffocation: Potential for

Nutritional/metabolic

- ☐ Body Temperature, Potential Alteration in
- ☐ Developmental Delay: Physical Growth and Development
- ☐ Fluid Volume, Altered: Excess or Excess Fluid Volume
- ☐ Fluid Volume Deficit, Actual
- ☐ Fluid Volume Deficit, Potential
- ☐ Nutrition, Altered: Less Than Body Requirements or Nutritional Deficit (Specify)
- ☐ Nutrition, Altered: More Than Body Requirements or Exogenous Obesity
- ☐ Nutrition, Altered: Potential for More Than Body Requirements or Potential for Obesity
- ☐ Oral Mucous Membrane, Altered
- ☐ Skin Integrity, Impaired or Skin Breakdown
- ☐ Skin Integrity, Impaired or Potential Skin Breakdown
- ☐ Swallowing, Impaired or Uncompensated Swallowing Impairment
- ☐ Tissue Integrity, Impaired

Elimination

- ☐ Bowel Elimination, Altered: Constipation
- ☐ Bowel Elimination, Altered: Diarrhea
- ☐ Bowel Elimination, Altered: Incontinence

- ☐ Developmental Delay: Bowel/Bladder Control
- ☐ Incontinence: Functional
- ☐ Incontinence: Reflex
- ☐ Incontinence: Stress
- ☐ Incontinence: Total
- ☐ Incontinence: Urge
- ☐ Urinary Elimination, Altered Patterns of
- ☐ Urinary Retention

Activity/exercise

- ☐ Activity Intolerance
- ☐ Activity Intolerance, Potential
- ☐ Airway Clearance, Ineffective
- ☐ Breathing Pattern, Ineffective
- ☐ Cardiac Output, Altered: Decreased
- ☐ Developmental Delay: Mobility
- ☐ Developmental Delay: Self-Care Skills
- ☐ Diversional Activity Deficit
- ☐ Gas Exchange, Impaired
- ☐ Home Maintenance Management, Impaired (Mild, Moderate, Severe, Potential, Chronic)
- ☐ Mobility, Impaired Physical
- ☐ Self-Care Deficit: Feeding
- ☐ Self-Care Deficit: Bathing/Hygiene
- ☐ Self-Care Deficit: Dressing/Grooming
- ☐ Self-Care Deficit: Toileting
- ☐ Self-Care Deficit: Total
- ☐ Tissue Perfusion, Altered: (Specify)

Sleep/rest

- ☐ Sleep Pattern Disturbance

Cognitive/perceptual

- ☐ Comfort, Altered: Pain
- ☐ Comfort, Altered: Chronic Pain

☐ Developmental Delay: (Specify Cognitive Area; attention, decision making, etc.)

☐ Hypothermia

☐ Hyperthermia

☐ Knowledge Deficit (Specify)

☐ Sensory-Perceptual Alteration: Input Excess or Sensory Overload

☐ Sensory-Perceptual Alteration: Input Deficit or Sensory Deprivation

☐ Thermoregulation, Ineffective

☐ Thought Processes, Altered

☐ Unilateral Neglect

Self-perception/self-concept

☐ Anxiety

☐ Body Image Disturbance

☐ Fear

☐ Hopelessness

☐ Personal Identity Confusion

☐ Powerlessness (Severe, Low, Moderate)

☐ Self-Esteem Disturbance

Role relationship

☐ Communication, Impaired Verbal

☐ Developmental Delay: Communication Skills

☐ Developmental Delay: Social Skills

☐ Family Processes, Altered

☐ Grieving, Anticipatory

☐ Grieving, Dysfunctional

☐ Parenting, Altered: Actual or Potential

☐ Role Performance, Disturbance in

☐ Social Interactions, Impaired

☐ Social Isolation (Rejection)

Sexuality/reproductive

☐ Rape-Trauma Syndrome: Compounded

☐ Rape-Trauma Syndrome: Silent Reaction

☐ Sexual Dysfunction

☐ Sexuality Patterns, Altered

Coping/stress tolerance

☐ Adjustment, Impaired

☐ Coping, Ineffective Individual

☐ Coping, Ineffective Family: Compromised

☐ Coping, Ineffective Family: Disabling

☐ Coping, Family: Potential for Growth

☐ Developmental Delay (Specify area)

☐ Post-Trauma Response

☐ Violence, Potential for (Self-Directed or Directed at Others)

Value/belief

☐ Spiritual Distress (Distress of Human Spirit)

You are now ready to develop a nursing care plan for this client. Use the following blank pages to do so. Then refer to the author's formulation, diagnostic summary, care plan, and summary.

NURSING CARE PLAN

Complete the chart below to develop a nursing care plan for this client.

Discharge outcomes/long-term goals	

Nursing diagnosis	Nursing intervention	

	Predicted outcomes/short-term goals (include time frame)	**Date/signature**

Return to Formulation, page 210

discussion; he fidgeted at times, apparently due to anxiety. Finally, he denied suicidal or homicidal thoughts, delusions, or hallucinations.

Reader may now complete Recording the Data, Assigning Nursing Diagnoses, and Nursing Care Plan.

FORMULATION

Philip presented with a cluster of symptoms typical of attention deficit disorder (ADD) with hyperactivity (APA, 1980). More common in males, this syndrome begins early in life and is characterized by hyperactivity, impulsivity, attentional difficulties, and excitability. Other symptoms that are often considered part of the syndrome include deficits in academic performance despite normal intelligence, low self-esteem, sleep-related problems, difficulties in social interaction, aggression, and variability of mood and performance (Ross and Ross, 1982).

Philip's pervasive dysfunction had seriously affected all areas of his life. Because of his difficulties in attending and poor concentration, he had trouble persevering with tasks and suffered learning impairment. His impulsivity and excitability affected his relationships with parents, siblings, teachers, and peers. Peers disliked his behavior and tended to avoid or reject him. Parents and teachers respond with critical statements, punishments, and negative judgments—all typical responses (Cunningham and Barkley, 1979). Noting that he repeatedly failed at tasks his peers accomplished easily, and that he consistently was unable to exert self-control, Philip internalized a sense of powerlessness and worthlessness. Cantwell (1975) reports that this internalization results in chronic low self-esteem and depression, resulting in the development of defense mechanisms designed to preserve psychological equilibrium (Gardner, 1975). Use of negative attention-seeking behavior at home and at school typically served as a means to increase feelings of power and self-worth, as well as to discharge anger and frustration (Ross and Ross, 1982). In this case, the result was continued negative response from Philip's environment. In addition, the resulting stress on his family system caused a decreased ability to cope with Philip's behavior, leading to a pattern of response that intensified his problems (Ross and Ross, 1982).

Philip's hospitalization focused on treatment of several major areas: a medication trial of stimulants, to attempt to decrease the symptoms of hyperactivity and inattention; the use of pre- and post-medication rating forms by nursing staff, teachers, and parents, to provide an objective measure of change or improvement in selected target symptoms; and individual and family therapy to address emotional and behavioral problems. After an initial and careful assessment of Philip's behavioral rep-

Continued on page 220

DIAGNOSTIC SUMMARY FOR PHILIP

Data	Functional health pattern	Nursing diagnosis
—Devalues self through criticism and self-deprecating statements —Is unable to verbalize strengths —Verbalizes sadness about not being able to compete effectively with peers —Lacks ability to initiate and complete simple tasks —Frequently loses self-control and verbalizes resulting guilt	Self-Perception/Self-Concept	Self-esteem disturbance related to feelings of worthlessness and failure secondary to Attention Deficit Disorder
—Has difficulty making and keeping friends at home and school —Frequently exhibits inappropriate attention-seeking behaviors with peers (e.g., interrupts, talks loudly, touches peers, teases and mimics others)	Role Relationship	Impaired social interactions related to inattention and impulsivity secondary to Attention Deficit Disorder
—Is unfamiliar with his drug trial —Is on a routine, prescribed stimulant medication	Cognitive/Perceptual	Knowledge deficit: stimulant medication related to newly prescribed drug trial
—Experiences loss of appetite as a side effect of stimulants	Nutritional/Metabolic	Potential altered nutrition: less than body requirements related to anorexia secondary to stimulant therapy
—Has difficulty sleeping; is a restless sleeper. —Sleeps 2 to 3 hours a night	Sleep/Rest	Sleep pattern disturbance related to hyperactivity secondary to Attention Deficit Disorder
—Has a history of intense acting-out behaviors (e.g., temper tantrums, physical and verbal aggression, property destruction —Has a history of repeated expulsion from school due to his behavior —Has a history of impulsive behavior with no thought to potential consequences	Coping/Stress Tolerance	Ineffective individual coping related to low self-esteem and low frustration tolerance secondary to Attention Deficit Disorder
—Family has a history of tension and discord over management of Philip's behavior —Family has a history of inconsistent and ineffectual use of punishment techniques in response to behavioral problems.	Coping/Stress Tolerance	Ineffective family coping: compromised, related to client's severe behavior and attentional problems secondary to Attention Deficit Disorder

NURSING CARE PLAN

Complete the chart below to develop a nursing care plan for this client.

Discharge outcome/long-term goals	
1. BY DISCHARGE, PHILIP WILL DEMON-STRATE DECREASED FREQUENCY OF SELF-DEPRECATING STATEMENTS.	

Nursing diagnosis	Nursing intervention	Predicted outcome/short-term goals (include time frame)	Date/signature
SELF-ESTEEM DISTURBANCE RELATED TO FEELINGS OF WORTHLESSNESS AND FAILURE SECONDARY TO ATTENTION DEF-ICIT DISORDER	–ASSIST IN THE IDENTIFI-CATION OF STRENGTHS: ·AVOID JUDGMENTAL COMMENTS ·DISCOURAGE EMPHASIS ON FAILURE ·GIVE VERBAL PRAISE FOR NEAT APPEARANCE, ACTIVITIES WELL DONE, AND OTHER SUCCESSES	–IN 2 WEEKS, PHILIP WILL BE ABLE TO STATE ONE POSITIVE ACCOMPLISHMENT HE ACHIEVED EACH DAY	10/1 DM
	–FOSTER SUCCESSFUL EX-PERIENCES BY: ·BREAKING TASKS INTO SMALL, ACHIEVABLE COMPONENTS ·PRESENTING TASKS IN SEQUENCE FROM EASIEST TO MORE DIFFICULT ·USING SIMPLE INSTRUC-TIONS TO FACILITATE UNDERSTANDING ·PROVIDING VERBAL PRAISE FOR THE SUCCESS-FUL COMPLETION OF COMPONENT PARTS OF TASKS ·DEVISING AND IMPLE-MENTING A BEHAVIORAL PROGRAM THAT REWARDS TASK COMPLETION (e.g., PHILIP WILL EARN 10 POINTS FOR COMPLETING 10 MINUTES OF COOPER-ATIVE PLAY WITH A PEER. HE CAN TRADE THESE POINTS FOR 30 MINUTES OF FREE PLAY TIME IN THE SWIMMING POOL ·STRUCTURING COOPERA-TIVE RATHER THAN COM-PETITIVE PLAY WITH PEERS ·PROVIDE EMOTIONAL SUP-PORT WHEN FAILURES OCCUR	–IN 1 MONTH, PHILIP WILL BE EARNING 75% OF AVAILABLE POINTS FOR TASK COMPLETION PERFORMANCE	

Discharge outcome/long-term goals			
1. BY DISCHARGE, PHILIP WILL DEMON-STRATE THE ABILITY TO APPROACH A PEER, INITIATE A CONVERSATION OR ACTIVITY, AND COMPLETE THE CONVER-SATION OR ACTIVITY.			

Nursing diagnosis	Nursing intervention	Predicted outcome/short-term goals (include time frame)	Date/signature
IMPAIRED SOCIAL INTERACTIONS RELATED TO IN-ATTENTION AND IMPULSIVITY SECONDARY TO ATTENTION DEF-ICIT DISORDER	-PROVIDE SPECIFIC DAILY TIME FOR ESTABLISHING A ONE-TO-ONE RELATION-SHIP. INITIALLY, PROVIDE FREQUENT CONTACTS OF SHORT DURATION IN AN ATMOSPHERE OF WARM, SUPPORTIVE ACCEPTANCE	-IN 1 MONTH, FREQUENCY OF PHILIP'S TEASING AND OTHER PROVOCATIVE BEHAVIOR WITH PEERS WILL DECREASE BY 50%	10/1 RM
	-SET LIMITS ON INAPPRO-PRIATE BEHAVIORS THAT INTERFERE WITH OTHERS:	-IN 1 MONTH, PHILIP WILL BE CONSISTENTLY EARNING POINTS FOR PARTICIPATION IN SOCIAL SKILLS TRAINING SESSIONS	
	·POINT OUT BEHAVIORS THAT PEERS DISLIKE		
	·SUGGEST AND MODEL APPROPRIATE WAYS TO IN-TERACT WITH PEERS		
	·PROVIDE OPPORTUNITIES FOR STRUCTURED COOPER-ATIVE PLAY		
	·REDUCE STIMULI IN THE ENVIRONMENT (INCLUDING NUMBER OF PEOPLE, AMOUNT OF NOISE, NUM-BERS OF CHOICES) WHEN HYPERACTIVITY IS ES-CALATING		
	·GIVE VERBAL PROMPT TO STOP TEASING AND NAME-CALLING BEHAVIORS. IF BEHAVIOR CONTINUES, PROVIDE PHILIP WITH A 5-MINUTE TIME OUT FOR POSITIVE REINFORCEMENT IN A QUIET CORNER OF THE WARD. SET TIMER FOR 5 MINUTES, ALLOW TO RETURN TO THE AC-TIVITY WHEN THE TIME HAS ELAPSED		
	-PROVIDE A STRUCTURED ENVIRONMENT WITH CONSISTENT ROUTINE, RULES, AND BEHAVIORAL CONSEQUENCES		
	-IMPLEMENT SOCIAL SKILLS TRAINING. PROVIDE POSITIVE REINFORCEMENT (e.g., PRAISE AND TOKENS, POINTS, TREATS) FOR AC-	-PHILIP WILL DEMONSTRATE A NEWLY LEARNED SOCIAL SKILL WEEKLY (WITHIN 2 WEEKS)	

Continued

Nursing Care Plan *continued*

Nursing diagnosis	Nursing intervention	Predicted outcome/short-term goals (include time frame)	Date/signature
	TIVE PARTICIPATION IN SESSIONS. INITIALLY, STRUCTURE THE SESSIONS TO INCLUDE ONLY STAFF AND PHILIP; AS PHILIP'S SKILL INCREASES, INTRO- DUCE ONE OTHER AND THEN MULTIPLE PEERS — TEACH PHILIP ONLY ONE SKILL WEEKLY; KEEP SKILL PROGRESSION FROM SIMPLE TO MORE COMPLEX (e.g., EYE CONTACT, GREET- ING ANOTHER, STARTING A CONVERSATION, EXPRESS- ING AN OPINION, EXPRESS- ING A FEELING)		

Discharge outcome/long-term goals	TIMES.		
1. BY DISCHARGE, PHILIP WILL BE ABLE TO STATE THE NAME, DOSAGE, AND FREQUENCY OF HIS PRESCRIBED MEDICATION. 2. BY DISCHARGE, PHILIP WILL APPROACH STAFF TO TAKE MEDICATIONS AT DESIGNATED			

Nursing diagnosis	Nursing intervention	Predicted outcome/short-term goals (include time frame)	Date/signature
KNOWLEDGE DEFICIT: STIMU- LANT MEDICA- TION RELATED TO NEWLY PRE- SCRIBED DRUG TRIAL	— TEACH PHILIP ABOUT PRE- SCRIBED MEDICATION: · NAME, DOSAGE, AND FREQUENCY · SIDE EFFECTS TO BE A- WARE OF AND WHAT TO DO IF THEY OCCUR · REASON FOR TAKING MED- ICATION AND BENEFITS — REINFORCE LEARNING BY ASKING PHILIP TO STATE THE FACTS ABOUT HIS MED- ICATION WHILE ADMINISTER- ING MEDICATIONS — PROVIDE POSITIVE REIN- FORCEMENT FOR HIS DEM- ONSTRATED ABILITY TO ANSWER CORRECTLY ANY QUESTIONS ASKED ABOUT THE INFORMATION TAUGHT (FACTS ABOUT MEDICATION) — AS DATE OF DISCHARGE NEARS, INITIATE A POSITIVE REINFORCEMENT PROGRAM FOR PHILIP APPROACHING AND ASKING FOR MEDICA- TIONS AT THE DESIGNATED TIME — INSTRUCT PHILIP'S PAR- ENTS IN ADMINISTRATION OF MEDICATIONS — CLARIFY ANY MISCONCEP- TIONS HELD BY EITHER PARENTS OR PHILIP ABOUT WHAT THE MEDICATIONS WILL AND WILL NOT DO	— IN 1 MONTH, PHILIP WILL TAKE MEDICATION AS ORDERED — IN 1 MONTH, PHILIP WILL STATE NAME, DOSAGE, AND FREQUENCY AND SIDE EFFECTS OF MEDICA- TION WITHOUT VERBAL PROMPTS — IN 1 MONTH, PARENTS WILL BE ABLE TO STATE NAME, DOSAGE, FREQUENCY, AND SIDE EFFECTS OF MEDICATIONS	10/1 DM

Continued

Nursing Care Plan *continued*

Discharge outcome/long-term goals	
1. AT DISCHARGE, PHILIP WILL MAINTAIN ADE-QUATE WEIGHT-FOR-HEIGHT NORMS. 2. AT DISCHARGE, PHILIP WILL BE SLEEPING ADEQUATELY TO PROVIDE FOR REST AND BODILY RESTORATION.	

Nursing diagnosis	Nursing intervention	Predicted outcome/short-term goals (include time frame)	Date/signature
POTENTIAL ALTERED NUTRI-TION: LESS THAN BODY RE-QUIREMENTS RELATED TO ANOREXIA SEC-ONDARY TO STIM-ULANT THERAPY	– MONITOR ADEQUATE FOOD AND FLUID INTAKE BY RECORDING WEEKLY WEIGHTS AT INITIATION OF STIMULANT THERAPY – PROVIDE PHILIP WITH THE OPPORTUNITY TO SELECT PREFERRED FOODS	– IN 3 WEEKS, PRESENCE OR ABSENCE OF WEIGHT LOSS WILL BE DOCUMENTED	10/1 DM
SLEEP PATTERN DISTURBANCE RELATED TO HY-PERACTIVITY SECONDARY TO ATTENTION DEFI-CIT DISORDER	– ASSESS AMOUNT OF AND CHARACTER OF SLEEP – EVALUATE AND DOCUMENT ANY CHANGES IN SLEEP PATTERN BEFORE AND AF-TER STIMULANT MEDICA-TIONS ADMINISTERED – PROVIDE A QUIET, NON-STIMULATING ENVIRON-MENT FOR SLEEP – OFFER A WARM BATH, WARM MILK, AND OTHER RELAXANTS AT BEDTIME – ATTEMPT TO RECREATE THE NORMAL NIGHT ROU-TINE EMPLOYED AT HOME – ENCOURAGE QUIET STORY-TELLING	– IN 1 WEEK, AMOUNT AND CHAR-ACTER OF SLEEP WILL BE ASSESSED AND DOCUMENTED – IN 4 WEEKS, ANY CHANGES IN SLEEP PATTERN WITH STIMU-LANT MEDICATIONS WILL BE DOCUMENTED	10/1 DM

Discharge outcome/long-term goals	
1. BY DISCHARGE, PHILIP WILL DEMONSTRATE THE ABILITY TO VERBALIZE ANGRY FEELINGS WITH THE ASSISTANCE OF AN ADULT 2. BY DISCHARGE, PHILIP WILL DEMONSTRATE THE ABILITY TO REMOVE HIMSELF FROM	SITUATIONS CAUSING INCREASING STRESS OR ANGER 50% OF THE TIME.

Nursing diagnosis	Nursing intervention	Predicted outcome/short-term goals (include time frame)	Date/signature
INEFFECTIVE INDIVIDUAL COPING RELATED TO LOW SELF-ESTEEM AND LOW FRUSTRATION TOLERANCE SECONDARY TO ATTENTION DEFICIT DISORDER	—ASSIST PHILIP TO RECOGNIZE AND IDENTIFY FEELINGS BY: · PROVIDING FEEDBACK ON NONVERBAL BEHAVIOR AND POSSIBLE FEELING STATE · SUGGESTING HOW OTHER CHILDREN OR ADULTS MIGHT FEEL IN SIMILAR SITUATIONS · UTILIZING SMALL GROUP DISCUSSIONS WITH PEERS TO EXPLORE HOW PEERS FEEL IN SIMILAR SITUATIONS · ASSISTING IN IDENTIFYING SOURCES OR POTENTIAL SOURCES OF FEELINGS · PROVIDING POSITIVE REINFORCEMENT FOR ANY ATTEMPTS OR SUCCESSES IN IDENTIFICATION AND LABELING OF FEELINGS —HELP PHILIP TO DEAL WITH HIS FEELINGS BY: · HAVING HIM MODEL AND PRACTICE VERBALIZATION OF FEELINGS IN A MINIMALLY THREATENING SITUATION · HAVING HIM USE ROLEPLAY WITH PEERS TO IDENTIFY FEELINGS AND PRACTICE POSSIBLE COPING STRATEGIES · PROVIDING VERBAL PROMPTS TO HELP HIM RECOGNIZE ESCALATION OF FEELINGS · HELPING HIM RECOGNIZE HOW CURRENT EXPRESSION OF FEELINGS AFFECTS HIS LIFE AND CAUSES PROBLEMS AT HOME AND AT SCHOOL · UTILIZING POSITIVE-REINFORCEMENT FOR ALL ATTEMPTS TO DEAL WITH FEELINGS APPROPRIATELY	—IN 3 WEEKS, PHILIP WILL ACTIVELY PARTICIPATE IN ROLEPLAY WITH STAFF AND BE ABLE TO STATE ONE POSSIBLE REACTION OR FEELING IN THE SITUATION —IN 6 WEEKS, PHILIP WILL DEMONSTRATE THE ABILITY TO LEAVE A STRESSFUL SITUATION WHEN PROMPTED TO DO SO BY STAFF —IN 8 WEEKS, PHILIP WILL BE ABLE TO DESCRIBE A PROBLEMSOLVING APPROACH TO A HYPOTHETICAL SITUATION POSED BY HIS PRIMARY NURSE —IN 8 WEEKS, PHILIP WILL BE ABLE TO VERBALIZE HIS INCREASING TENSION AND DEMONSTRATE THE USE OF AN ADAPTIVE COPING STRATEGY IN AT LEAST ONE SITUATION —IN 6 WEEKS, THERE WILL BE A 50% DECREASE IN IMPULSIVE BEHAVIOR	10/1 RM

Continued

Nursing Care Plan *continued*

Nursing diagnosis	Nursing intervention	Predicted outcome/short-term goals (include time frame)	Date/signature
	eg, REMOVING HIMSELF FROM SITUATION, DIRECTLY STATING FEELINGS OR NEEDS, ASKING FOR STAFF ASSISTANCE IN THESE AREAS		
	· ANTICIPATING POTENTIALLY STRESSFUL SITUATIONS AND USING PROBLEM-SOLVING STRATEGIES WITH HIM PRIOR TO OCCURENCE		
	· REMAINING AVAILABLE TO HIM DURING PERIODS OF INCREASING TENSION		
	· TEACHING HIM TO REMOVE HIMSELF FROM SITUATIONS (eg, GO TO HIS ROOM OR TO CALL FOR TIME OUT) BEFORE LOSS OF CONTROL OCCURS		
	– SET CONSISTENT LIMITS ON BEHAVIOR		
	– INTERRUPT IMPULSIVE ACTS TO MAINTAIN CLIENT AND MILIEU SAFETY		

PHILIP: ATTENTION DEFICIT DISORDER

Discharge outcome/long-term goals			
1. BY DISCHARGE, FAMILY MEMBERS WILL BE ABLE TO ARTICULATE A STRUCTURED PLAN TO REINFORCE PHILIP'S APPROPRIATE BEHAVIOR AND CONSEQUENCES FOR HIS ACTING OUT BEHAVIORS			

Nursing diagnosis	Nursing intervention	Predicted outcome/short-term goals (include time frame)	Date/signature
INEFFECTIVE FAMILY COPING RELATED TO CLIENT'S SEVERE BEHAVIOR AND ATTENTIONAL PROBLEMS SECONDARY TO ATTENTION DEFICIT DISORDER	—COUNSEL FAMILY IN MANAGING PHILIP'S BEHAVIOR: · PROVIDE REASSURANCE, SUPPORT, AND POSITIVE FEEDBACK · TEACH PARENTS HOW TO GIVE POSITIVE REINFORCEMENT FOR ADAPTIVE, APPROPRIATE BEHAVIOR · MODIFY EFFECTIVE UNIT BEHAVIORAL MANAGEMENT PLAN TO FIT HOME ENVIRONMENT · ASSIST PARENTS IN PLANNING ACTIVITIES FOR PHILIP · TEACH PARENTS USE OF TIME OUT FOR TARGETED INAPPROPRIATE BEHAVIORS AND REASONABLE EXPECTATIONS FOR BEHAVIOR	—IN 8 WEEKS, PHILIP'S PARENTS WILL REPORT DECREASED TENSION AND CONFLICT IN THE HOME WHEN PHILIP VISITS	10/1 DM

Continued

ertoire, including antecedents and consequences of his behavior with peers and family members, the staff undertook behavioral interventions designed to decrease maladaptive behaviors, increase his sense of mastery and self-esteem, and teach him more effective coping strategies for use after hospitalization.

SUMMARY

Philip made significant progress during his 3-month course of hospitalization. The medication helped decrease his symptoms of hyperactivity and inattention, and a structured program helped decrease the teasing and mimicking of peers, interrupting, oppositional behavior, and aggression. Individual and family therapy, along with the therapeutic milieu of the unit itself, helped Philip make some gains in developing both a better understanding of his behavior and an increasing ability to cope with his environment. He began to show increased ability to delay gratification and to verbalize feelings rather than acting-out aggressively, and became able to take a "time out" on his own when he felt himself becoming upset. He was able to recognize and verbalize pride in his success with earning points on the unit and in accomplishing tasks. Both the frequency and duration of his participation in group activities and games with peers increased steadily.

Philip's family was actively involved throughout his hospitalization and recognized his improvement. Their participation in family therapy helped them better understand Philip's needs and recognize family interactional patterns that foster continued progress.

After discharge, Philip returned home to his parents and siblings. He continued outpatient therapy for medication management and family counseling, and attended a special education program with a highly structured and behaviorally oriented program. While continued progress was expected, Philip's problems are long-standing. At discharge, he still suffered from poor self-esteem and some degree of emotional and behavioral disturbance. But with continued outpatient therapy and a positive and well-structured school setting, the prognosis for continued improvement was good.

SELECTED BIBLIOGRAPHY

American Psychiatric Association. *Diagnostic and Statistical Manual of Mental Disorders,* 3rd ed. Washington, D.C.: American Psychiatric Association, 1980.

Bloomingdale, L.M., ed. *Attention Deficit Disorder.* New York: Spectrum, 1984.

Cantwell, D.P. *The Hyperactive Child: Diagnosis, Management, Current Research*. New York: Spectrum, 1975.

Carpenito, L.J. *Handbook of Nursing Diagnosis*. Philadelphia: J.B. Lippincott Co., 1985.

Cunningham, C.E., and Barkley, R.A. "The Interactions of Normal and Hyperactive Children with Their Mothers in Free Play and Structured Tasks," *Child Development* 50:217-24, 1979.

Gardner, R.A. "Psychotherapy in Minimal Brain Dysfunction," in *Current Psychiatric Therapies*, vol. 15. Edited by Masserman, J.H. New York: Grune & Stratton, 1975.

The Lippincott Manual of Nursing Practice. Philadelphia: J.B. Lippincott Co., 1982.

Loney, J. "Hyperkinesis Comes of Age: What Do We Know and Where Should We Go?" *American Journal of Orthopsychiatry* 50(1):28-42, 1980.

Ross, D.M., and Ross, S.A. *Hyperactivity: Current Issues, Research, and Theory*, 2nd ed. New York: John Wiley & Sons, 1982.

Satterfield, J.H., et al. "Multimodality Treatment: A One Year Follow Up of 84 Hyperactive Boys," *Archives of General Psychiatry* 36:965-74, 1979.

Satterfield, J.H., et al. "Multimodality Treatment: A Two Year Evaluation of 61 Hyperactive Boys," *Archives of General Psychiatry* 37:915-19, 1980.

Satterfield, J.H., et al. "Three Year Multimodality Treatment Study of 100 Hyperactive Boys," *The Journal of Pediatrics* 98(4):650-55, 1981.

Whalen, C.K., and Hanker, B., eds. *Hyperactive Children: The Social Ecology of Identification and Treatment*. New York: Academic Press, 1980.

Wolman, B.B., et al., eds. *Handbook of Treatment of Mental Disorders of Childhood and Adolescence*. Englewood Cliffs, N.J.: Prentice-Hall, 1978.

Joey:
Infantile Autism

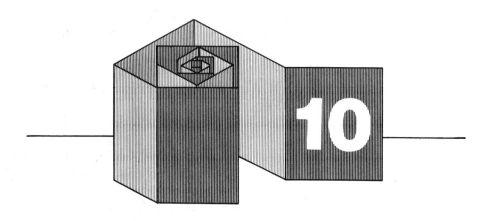

Joanne Thompson, MSN, RN

A child with infantile autism experiences serious developmental delays in several spheres, notably interpersonal and social functioning. Disruptions in parental functioning, family process, potential for social isolation, and potential for grieving generally occur at some point in the diagnosis and treatment of a child with a developmental disability. Certainly this is the case with infantile autism, a pervasive and profound disability affecting the child at an early age and involving disturbances in relating, motility, perception, language, and cognition. A primary behavioral approach, coupled with intensive family education, often represents the best hope for achieving some level of equilibrium in the child's life. While interventions are developed primarily for the child, the nurse also involves family members in a discussion and "working-through" of feelings associated with caring for a child with a poor prognosis. The nurse's anticipatory guidance in the grieving process assists the parents in putting a seemingly devastating illness into a more functional perspective. Thus, the nurse treats target behaviors in the hospital within a behavioral framework that can be implemented in the home after discharge. Continued family support is necessary to help the child achieve further developmental milestones. Ultimately, of course, the family must reach a decision about the need for the child's long-term placement outside the home.

CASE STUDY

Joey was 4 years, 8 months old when admitted to the child psychiatric unit for his first psychiatric hospitalization. He was referred by his treating psychologist for a diagnostic evaluation of behavioral problems, language delay, and "autistic" symptoms. At the time of admission, Joey lived with his biological parents and two younger sisters in a modest three-bedroom home that the family had purchased recently. This hospitalization represented the first psychiatric hospitalization for any member of Joey's immediate or extended family; naturally, his parents were quite anxious about the experience. The nurse, whose first contact with Joey and his parents occurred on the day of admission, devoted several hours to obtaining an accurate history, assessing Joey's behavior and adjustment to the unit, evaluating parent response, and developing goals for hospitalization.

The nurse identified these concerns and problems in Joey's behavior: running away, temper tantrums, hyperactivity, biting others, and noncompliance. Language delay, ritualistic and stereotypic behaviors, short attention span, and inconsistent performance of age-appropriate self-help skills were also identified as presenting problems. Joey's parents dated the onset of their concerns about Joey to approximately age 21 months, coincident with the mother's return home from the hospital following the birth of the youngest daughter. At this time, the parents noticed that Joey began to withdraw, stopped speaking (he had been speaking in single words since age 1), developed tantrums, and seemed to lose interest in relating to others around him, including decreased interaction with his environment. He also began to exhibit intense preoccupations with and attachments to strange objects, such as human hair, bright lights, and running water. He expressed an intense dislike at having certain articles of his clothing removed.

By age 2½, Joey had begun to run off from his yard and to flee from his parents when out in public. This constant "elopement" from his surroundings was coincidental with his general activity level, which his parents described as having a "driven" quality with no seeming purpose or direction. Joey seemed to have no sense of danger; he would climb out unlocked windows, unlock simple window locks and climb out, climb bookcases and high fences, and unlock doors and run outside. The most disturbing aspect of these behaviors to his parents was the potential for danger to Joey; to ensure his safety, the family had resorted to installing special locks on all windows and doors and providing close supervision at all times. Joey's nocturnal wandering and running off while the family slept represented another problem. In an attempt to solve this problem, the parents had Joey sleep with them in their bed. Despite these efforts at preventing opportunities for Joey to flee, Joey still managed to do so, necessitating calls to the local police for help on an average of one to three times a week. Joey's mother described Joey as "sneaky," relating to the nurse that he would "watch to see if you are looking at him" and run off as soon as he had diverted attention.

The nurse's assessment of Joey's behavioral history revealed that Joey's temper tantrums, running off, handbiting, and noncompliance with demands were the most stressful behaviors for his family and the most recalcitrant to any behavior modification technique they used. The tantrums occurred as often as 20 times a day and as little as once a day, most often in the context of demands but also sometimes without known antecedents. Joey's parents found this inconsistency in frequency and duration perplexing; it resulted in inconsistent parental responses to the tantrum behavior. Tantrum duration was described as from a few minutes to more than 2 hours; tantrums consisted of intense, loud screaming and running frantically around an area, often with handbiting. The running away–darting off behavior appeared related to Joey's "driven" need to be on the move, since he seemed interested only in the act of running off and never went to any particular location. In his parents' words, Joey seemed "obsessed" with "getting out" of "wherever" he was. Joey's parents considered him to be problematical because he rarely complied with their demands or directions; in fact, demands often seemed to trigger tantrums. A closer look at the noncompliance revealed that most of the demands presented to Joey involved the cessation of his ritualistic behaviors or the interruption of his preoccupying activities and behavior. Additionally, the nurse noted that Joey's parents described noncompliance in terms such as "He pretends not to hear; he doesn't seem to listen to directions or demands."

The nurse's assessment also included a review of Joey's health and his developmental, social, and self-adaptive living skills. Joey's medical history revealed that complete neurologic, audiologic, and physical examinations beginning at age 2½ had revealed no abnormalities. (Audiology and neurology evaluations were done because of his delayed language and because of diagnostic questions centering around the possibility of hearing loss or neurological disturbance.) Aside from recurring ear infections as an infant, Joey had enjoyed good physical health. His early developmental history showed that he was an irritable baby who did not like much cuddling. His motor milestones were all within normal limits; in fact, gross motor skills were excellent for his age. His parents reported no feeding problems; however, even though he could use utensils well, he preferred to eat with his fingers and was careless in his self-feeding. Joey had begun toilet-training at age 2½ and, apart from nocturnal enuresis, he managed his toileting needs independently. He needed supervised assistance in the areas of hygiene, however. Socially, Joey had never expressed much interest in toys or playing—aside from tickle or chase games, which he enjoyed immensely. He had never been interested in playing with other children and did not interact with his siblings, except in aggressive ways. He was quite attached to his mother and would protest violently at any separation from her; yet, he rarely noticed his mother when she was with him. Joey's language milestones were deviant; babbling was present at 8 months followed by single words at 1 year, with all words and use of speech absent by 21 months. At age 4 years, 8 months, he had no speech and did not gesture to communicate his needs.

The nurse's assessment of Joey's family revealed a young Hispanic couple who had married in their teens. Both were high school graduates and held full-time jobs. Until their recent purchase of a new home, the couple had resided with Joey's maternal grandmother, whom Joey's mother described as strict and somewhat critical of her mothering. The couple's marriage, although intact, was strained; they had discussed separation at one time. Their sources of strain and conflict centered around financial pressures, disagreements among extended family members about Joey, Joey's chronic and markedly dysfunctional behavior (which had a very disruptive effect on the family functioning), and the demands of caring for a growing family. Most of the couple's interaction within the marriage related to the problems with Joey; they rarely spent time alone with each other.

Although the parents had heard the word "autism" applied to their son, they were not fully informed, and in fact hoped the problems were related to Joey's language and "getting a handle" on Joey's behavior. Both parents appeared "afraid" of the diagnosis, and clearly were overwhelmed, burdened, and stressed by the demands of caring for their handicapped son. Joey's father tended to respond to the continual stressors by increasing his work hours, avoiding home life, and using alcohol to excess. Joey's mother stated she was attempting to cope with the situation. She was very involved with trying to manage her son, but felt alone and isolated from her husband and from her family. She expressed feelings of helplessness, guilt, anger, and depression.

The nurse's assessment of Joey revealed a healthy-looking, attractive boy who exhibited extreme withdrawal and marked hypoactivity. During the assessment, he did not seem to notice either the nurse's presence or her face. He quickly abandoned any toys given to him, and could not be engaged in any play activity. Although he accepted physical approach, his response to human touch was passive and characterized by clinging to the nurse's body, smelling the nurse's hair, or sitting passively on the nurse's lap. Joey did not speak and made no sounds except for occasional grunting and tongue-clicking; he responded inconsistently to simple one-step commands, whether presented with or without visual clues. He made no attempts to imitate sounds or behavior, and remained nearly oblivious to the nurse or her demands. Although he demonstrated good eye-hand coordination and visual motor skills in tasks such as manipulating puzzles and blocks, he did so with little attention to the activity and with only

Continued on page 232

RECORDING THE DATA

After you have read the case, cluster significant data into functional health patterns.

Health management/health perception _____

_____

_____

_____

_____

Nutritional/metabolic _____

_____

_____

_____

Elimination _____

_____

_____

_____

Activity/exercise _____

_____

_____

_____

Cognitive/perceptual _____

_____

_____

_____

Sleep/rest _____

_____

_____

_____

Self-perception/self-concept _____

_____

_____

_____

Role relationship _____

_____

_____

_____

Sexuality/reproductive _____

_____

_____

_____

Coping/stress tolerance _____

_____

_____

_____

Value/belief _____

_____

_____

_____

ASSIGNING NURSING DIAGNOSES

Use your clustered data to select appropriate nursing diagnoses.

Health perception/health management

- ☐ Growth and Development, Altered (see Developmental Delay)
- ☐ Health Maintenance, Altered
- ☐ Infection, Potential for
- ☐ Injury (Trauma): Potential for
- ☐ Noncompliance (Specify)
- ☐ Poisoning: Potential for
- ☐ Suffocation: Potential for

Nutritional/metabolic

- ☐ Body Temperature, Potential Alteration in
- ☐ Developmental Delay: Physical Growth and Development
- ☐ Fluid Volume, Altered: Excess or Excess Fluid Volume
- ☐ Fluid Volume Deficit, Actual
- ☐ Fluid Volume Deficit, Potential
- ☐ Nutrition, Altered: Less Than Body Requirements or Nutritional Deficit (Specify)
- ☐ Nutrition, Altered: More Than Body Requirements or Exogenous Obesity
- ☐ Nutrition, Altered: Potential for More Than Body Requirements or Potential for Obesity
- ☐ Oral Mucous Membrane, Altered
- ☐ Skin Integrity, Impaired or Skin Breakdown
- ☐ Skin Integrity, Impaired or Potential Skin Breakdown
- ☐ Swallowing, Impaired or Uncompensated Swallowing Impairment
- ☐ Tissue Integrity, Impaired

Elimination

- ☐ Bowel Elimination, Altered: Constipation
- ☐ Bowel Elimination, Altered: Diarrhea
- ☐ Bowel Elimination, Altered: Incontinence
- ☐ Developmental Delay: Bowel/Bladder Control
- ☐ Incontinence: Functional
- ☐ Incontinence: Reflex
- ☐ Incontinence: Stress
- ☐ Incontinence: Total
- ☐ Incontinence: Urge
- ☐ Urinary Elimination, Altered Patterns of
- ☐ Urinary Retention

Activity/exercise

- ☐ Activity Intolerance
- ☐ Activity Intolerance, Potential
- ☐ Airway Clearance, Ineffective
- ☐ Breathing Pattern, Ineffective
- ☐ Cardiac Output, Altered: Decreased
- ☐ Developmental Delay: Mobility
- ☐ Developmental Delay: Self-Care Skills
- ☐ Diversional Activity Deficit
- ☐ Gas Exchange, Impaired
- ☐ Home Maintenance Management, Impaired (Mild, Moderate, Severe, Potential, Chronic)
- ☐ Mobility, Impaired Physical
- ☐ Self-Care Deficit: Feeding
- ☐ Self-Care Deficit: Bathing/Hygiene
- ☐ Self-Care Deficit: Dressing/Grooming
- ☐ Self-Care Deficit: Toileting
- ☐ Self-Care Deficit: Total
- ☐ Tissue Perfusion, Altered: (Specify)

Sleep/rest

- ☐ Sleep Pattern Disturbance

Cognitive/perceptual

- ☐ Comfort, Altered: Pain
- ☐ Comfort, Altered: Chronic Pain

☐ Developmental Delay: (Specify Cognitive Area; attention, decision making, etc.)
☐ Hypothermia
☐ Hyperthermia
☐ Knowledge Deficit (Specify)
☐ Sensory-Perceptual Alteration: Input Excess or Sensory Overload
☐ Sensory-Perceptual Alteration: Input Deficit or Sensory Deprivation
☐ Thermoregulation, Ineffective
☐ Thought Processes, Altered
☐ Unilateral Neglect

Self-perception/self-concept

☐ Anxiety
☐ Body Image Disturbance
☐ Fear
☐ Hopelessness
☐ Personal Identity Confusion
☐ Powerlessness (Severe, Low, Moderate)
☐ Self-Esteem Disturbance

Role relationship

☐ Communication, Impaired Verbal
☐ Developmental Delay: Communication Skills
☐ Developmental Delay: Social Skills
☐ Family Processes, Altered
☐ Grieving, Anticipatory
☐ Grieving, Dysfunctional
☐ Parenting, Altered: Actual or Potential

☐ Role Performance, Disturbance in
☐ Social Interactions, Impaired
☐ Social Isolation (Rejection)

Sexuality/reproductive

☐ Rape-Trauma Syndrome: Compounded
☐ Rape-Trauma Syndrome: Silent Reaction
☐ Sexual Dysfunction
☐ Sexuality Patterns, Altered

Coping/stress tolerance

☐ Adjustment, Impaired
☐ Coping, Ineffective Individual
☐ Coping, Ineffective Family: Compromised
☐ Coping, Ineffective Family: Disabling
☐ Coping, Family: Potential for Growth
☐ Developmental Delay (Specify area)
☐ Post-Trauma Response
☐ Violence, Potential for (Self-Directed or Directed at Others)

Value/belief

☐ Spiritual Distress (Distress of Human Spirit)

You are now ready to develop a nursing care plan for this client. Use the following blank pages to do so. Then refer to the author's formulation, diagnostic summary, care plan, and summary.

NURSING CARE PLAN

Complete the chart below to develop a nursing care plan for this client.

Discharge outcomes/long-term goals	

Nursing diagnosis	Nursing intervention	

	Predicted outcomes/short-term goals (include time frame)	Date/signature

Return to Formulation, page 232

fleeting interest.

One brief tantrum and handbiting episode occurred when the nurse persisted with getting him to remain with completing a puzzle. The nurse noticed that immediately upon commencing the tantrum, Joey looked to her for a response, seemingly indicating a wish that the demand be withdrawn. When she did not immediately withdraw the demand, he began to shriek and bite his hand, while at the same time maintaining eye contact with her. Such eye contact was the only actual indication of relatedness she noted.

Joey's affect was almost entirely blunted and without much facial expression aside from the angry affect of verbal commands as different from other forms of noise or sound. He could build a tower of nine cubes, scribble spontaneously, follow one-step commands, and imitate some tasks when food was presented as a reward. His general behavior in receptive language and comprehension skills was consistent with those of a 15- to 18-month-old child. Finally, throughout the nurse's assessment, Joey displayed a profound disinterest in or ability to attend meaningfully to sensory information presented to him, regardless of the type of sensory input—visual, tactile, or auditory.

Reader may now complete Recording the Data, Assigning Nursing Diagnoses, and Nursing Care Plan.

FORMULATION

After a thorough evaluation, Joey was diagnosed as having infantile autism and moderate mental retardation, with significant deficits in many parameters of adaptive functioning. His behaviors, although characteristically observed in children with a diagnosis of autism, nevertheless represented unmanageable, unsocialized sources of potential danger and presented serious impediments to the acquisition of more adaptive, socialized, and appropriate behavior and functioning. His profound delays in language development, lack of meaningful language (receptively or expressively), and mental retardation also complicated the task of formulating a nursing and teaching care plan. The complicating variables arose from Joey's high volume of presenting problems, low level of functioning, decreased behavioral responsiveness, and poor prognostic indicators.

In Joey's case, clearly his maladaptive and potentially dangerous and isolating behaviors needed to be decreased and brought under manageable control. Only then could the nurse devote the necessary time and energy to addressing behaviors and functioning that would enhance his acquisition of more appropriate adaptive skills and learning.

Treatment of the family and parental dyad also formed a vital part of nursing intervention. For Joey, the nurse believed that hospitalization represented the first major diagnostic evaluation effort and a source of stress, but also of hope, for the parents. The nurse anticipated that the parental goals—whether realistic or unrealistic—needed to be dealt with sensitively, and realistic feedback gently introduced and integrated. At this point, Joey's parents appeared extremely vulnerable and scared, yet also somewhat hopeful. The nurse recognized the need for care in preserving family functioning while dealing effectively with Joey's behavioral and diagnostic realities.

SUMMARY

During Joey's 2-month hospital stay, he received interdisciplinary evaluations (psychiatric and psychological tests, speech and language therapies, occupational therapy, recreational therapy) and individualized nursing treatment interventions. Interdisciplinary team evaluations, together with ongoing nursing assessments, confirmed the diagnosis of infantile autism and severe mental retardation. (*Note:* Mental retardation accompanies the diagnosis of autism in two-thirds of all cases because of the effect of autism symptoms on learning and cognitive style.) In Joey's case, a separate diagnosis of severe mental retardation accompanied the primary diagnosis of autism because of the implications for behavioral and school management needs. Joey's profound disturbance in relating and his absence of meaningful language at nearly 5 years of age suggested a profound degree of autistic disturbance with a poor likelihood of improvement, particularly in social adjustment and independent living. The result? A guarded prognosis for Joey's future capacities.

By the time of discharge, Joey demonstrated significant behavioral improvement, with cessation of running away, decreased frequency of tantrums, and improved self-help skills. Although he continued to experience occasional tantrums, the episodes were brief and responsive to the prescribed interventions; handbiting was completely eliminated. At discharge, he consistently used utensils when he ate and dressed and undressed himself independently with minimal adult assistance. He no longer exhibited intense tantrum reactions to removal of his clothes, and would wear pajamas at night without incident. Overall, he appeared to have responded exceptionally well to the prescribed nursing interventions in a structured environment that featured consistent use of firm, structured limits and behavioral reinforcers. Only slight changes were made to the plan in an attempt to stimulate Joey's relatedness and attending skills. Joey's lack of improvement in relating and attending behaviors reflected both the severe degree of his autistic disturbance and the limited

Continued on page 245

DIAGNOSTIC SUMMARY FOR JOEY

Data	Functional health pattern	Nursing diagnosis
—Often runs away from supervising persons or supervised areas —Displays impulsive, excessive, and unpredictable behavior with no awareness of personal rules of safety (climbs dangerously high fences, cabinets, bookcases, etc., in a reckless manner) —Demonstrates self-injurious behavior (handbiting) while engaged in tantrum behavior	Health Perception/ Health Management	Potential for injury related to impulsivity and lack of knowledge of safety precautions
—Exhibits immediate tantrum behavior response to frustrating situations or events —Engages in tantrum behavior of excessive frequency and duration in relation to precipitating stressor or age-appropriate responses —Demonstrates self-injurious behavior, such as handbiting	Coping/Stress Tolerance	Ineffective individual coping related to diminished capacity for frustration tolerance secondary to Infantile Autism
—Demonstrates age-appropriate fine motor manipulation of eating utensils, but insists on eating with fingers —Demonstrates fine motor ability to dress and undress self, but may not comprehend directions and prefers adults to dress-undress him —Has fixations with certain items of clothing—refuses to wear pajamas, for example	Activity/Exercise	Self-care deficits: feeding and dressing/grooming related to sensorimotor/cognitive deficits secondary to Infantile Autism
—Engages in numerous ritualistic, stereotypic behaviors, consistent with diagnosis of autism —Displays delay in language development, with current language level of about age 1 year —Suffers moderate mental retardation —Demonstrates decreased relating, withdrawal, and nonuse of language, social interaction, or play objects	Role Relationship Cognitive/Perceptual	Developmental delay: communication skills, social skills, inattention, poor decision-making related to developmental disability secondary to Infantile Autism

Data	Functional health pattern	Nursing diagnosis
—Marital conflict exists between Joey's parents —Parents exhibit inconsistent behavioral intervention with Joey —Family relationship pressures exist (e.g., with grandmother and grandfather) —Parents acknowledge feeling overwhelmed, burdened, and depressed	Role Relationship	Altered parenting related to child's condition and economic and relationship problems
—Parents are not sure of the meaning of Joey's handicap —Parents are unaware of the steps of the grieving process (i.e. anger, denial, etc.) —Parents are not aware of the possible ramifications of an ill child vis-à-vis cultural background/beliefs	Role Relationship	Anticipatory parental grieving related to anticipated losses secondary to child's diagnosis/condition
—Conflictual relationships exist within the extended family —Only limited time/energy resources are available in the primary family unit —Economic instability exists	Activity/Exercise	Impaired home maintenance management related to inadequate resources and child's disability

NURSING CARE PLAN

Complete the chart below to develop a nursing care plan for this client.

Discharge outcome/long-term goals	
1 BY DISCHARGE, THERE WILL BE A 50% DECREASE IN THE MALADAP- TIVE BEHAVIORS CONTRIBUTING TO RISK FOR POTENTIAL INJURY. 2. BY DISCHARGE, JOEY'S PARENTS	WILL BE ABLE TO DESCRIBE THE USE OF 4 SAFETY PRECAUTIONS TO BE IMPLEMENTED AT HOME.

Nursing diagnosis	Nursing intervention	Predicted outcome/short-term goals (include time frame)	Date/signature
POTENTIAL FOR INJURY RELATED TO IMPULSIVITY AND LACK OF KNOWLEDGE OF SAFETY PRE- CAUTIONS	-DECREASE POTENTIAL FOR INJURY BY: ·MAINTAINING CLOSE SU- PERVISION AND PHYSICAL PROXIMITY AT ALL TIMES ·REGARDING ANY SUDDEN DARTING OFF FROM PRE- SCRIBED AREA OR PER- SON AS UNSAFE BEHAVIOR REQUIRING IMMEDIATE INTERVENTION (INCLUDES PUNISHMENT CONSE- QUENCE) ·PROVIDING STRONG VER- BAL DISAPPROVAL (e.g, "THERE IS NO RUNNING AWAY."), FOLLOWED WITH IMMEDIATE CORNER "TIME OUT" OF 2 MINUTES DURATION, AND FINISHED BY RESTATING BEHAVIOR EXPECTATION (i.e, JOEY REMAINS WITH NURSE) ·PROVIDING FIRM VERBAL/ PHYSICAL DEMAND (PROMPT) AT TIMES OF TRANSITION TO OR FROM ANY AREA ON/OFF UNIT, HOLDING JOEY'S HAND FIRMLY DURING ALL TRANSPORT SITUATIONS ·REDIRECTING IMMEDI- ATELY ANY FAILURE TO COMPLY WITH PREVIOUS INTERVENTION, BY FOL- LOWING INTERVENTION PRECEDING IT, AND RE- PEATING UNTIL COMPLI- ANCE WITH EXPECTATION IS DEMONSTRATED -TEACH JOEY SAFE BE- HAVIORS BY: ·ESTABLISHING BASELINE OF RUNNING AWAY/UN- SAFE BEHAVIOR, INCLUD- ING RESPONSE TO DECEL- ERATION INTERVENTIONS ·WHEN FREQUENCY OF UNSAFE BEHAVIOR IS DE-	-WITHIN 3 WEEKS OF HOSPITAL- IZATION, ACCURATE FREQUENCY AND RESPONSE TO INTERVEN- TION BASELINE WILL BE ESTAB- LISHED -WITHIN 3 WEEKS OF HOSPITAL- IZATION, JOEY WILL DEMON- STRATE COMPLIANCE WITH IN- TERVENTIONS, WITH FREQUEN- CY OF NONCOMPLIANCE DE- CREASED TO THREE TO FOUR TIMES PER WEEK -WITHIN 6 WEEKS OF HOSPITAL- IZATION, JOEY WILL DEMON- STRATE DECREASED UNSAFE BEHAVIOR IN ALL SITUATIONS -BY DISCHARGE, PARENTS WILL DEMONSTRATE COMFORT WITH AND SUCCESS IN IMPLE- MENTATION OF PRESCRIBED INTERVENTIONS 75% OF THE TIME	12/2 97

Nursing diagnosis	Nursing intervention	Predicted outcome/short-term goals (include time frame)	Date/signature
	CREASED TO A RATE OF TWO TO FOUR TIMES PER DAY, BEGINNING TO WITHDRAW NURSE HAND-HOLDING DURING TRANSPORT ON THE UNIT ONLY		
	· WHEN FREQUENCY OF UNSAFE BEHAVIOR IS DECREASED TO ZERO TO TWO TIMES PER DAY IN ALL SITUATIONS, BEGINNING TO GRADUALLY FADE HAND-HOLDING OFF-UNIT TRANSPORT TRANSITIONS, OBSERVING RESPONSE		
	· CONTINUING WITH ALL INTERVENTIONS UNTIL JOEY CEASES TO NEED HAND-HOLDING AND CAN REMAIN SAFELY WITH GROUP OR INDIVIDUAL		
	— ANTICIPATE DISCHARGE NEEDS BY:		
	· INCLUDING PARENTS IN DEMONSTRATION AND PRACTICE SESSIONS, WITH PARENTAL DISCUSSION/USE OF INTERVENTIONS WHILE WITH JOEY ON HOME VISITS		
	· ASSISTING PARENTS IN IDENTIFYING POTENTIAL SOURCES OF DANGER/ INJURY IN HOME OR NEIGHBORHOOD ENVIRONMENT AND CONSEQUENT BEHAVIORAL INTERVENTIONS		

Continued

Nursing Care Plan *continued*

Discharge outcome/long-term goals	
1. BY DISCHARGE, TANTRUM BEHAVIOR WILL BE REDUCED BY 75%. 2. JOEY'S SELF-INJURIOUS BEHAVIOR WILL BE ELIMINATED.	

Nursing diagnosis	Nursing intervention	Predicted outcome/short-term goals (include time frame)	Date/signature
INEFFECTIVE INDIVIDUAL COPING RELATED TO DIMINISHED CAPACITY FOR FRUSTRATION TOLERANCE SECONDARY TO INFANTILE AUTISM	—OBTAIN BEHAVIOR BASELINE, INCLUDING ANTECEDENT EVENTS/STIMULI, BEHAVIOR DESCRIPTIONS, FREQUENCY, AND DURATION —ISOLATE INCIDENCES OF DEMAND-RELATED TANTRUMS AND NONDEMAND-RELATED TANTRUMS —DEAL WITH DEMAND-RELATED TANTRUMS (COMPLIANCE SITUATION) BY: ·PASSIVELY IGNORING TANTRUM BEHAVIOR, INCLUDING SELF-INJURIOUS BEHAVIOR. NOTE: PASSIVE IGNORE REFERS TO WITHDRAWAL OF ATTENTION TO THE INTERVENING/DISRUPTIVE BEHAVIOR, WHILE ATTENTION REMAINS FOCUSED ON COMPLETION OF DEMAND ·PROVIDING VERBAL/PHYSICAL PROMPTS CONTINUOUSLY THROUGH COMPLETION OF DEMAND ·PROVIDING POSITIVE ATTENTION OR REWARD WHEN COMPLIANCE WITH DEMAND IS MET, CONTINUING TO PASSIVELY IGNORE TANTRUM IF PRESENT —NONDEMAND-RELATED TANTRUMS (NO EXTERNAL DEMAND PRESENT) BY: ·ACTIVELY IGNORING TANTRUM BEHAVIOR NOTE: ACTIVE IGNORE REFERS TO COMPLETE CESSATION AND WITHDRAWAL OF BOTH EYE CONTACT AND PHYSICAL CONTACT ·ACTIVELY IGNORING SELF-INJURIOUS BEHAVIOR ·RESUMING INTERACTION/ATTENTION FOLLOWING COMPLETE CESSATION OF TANTRUM BEHAVIOR	—WITHIN 4 WEEKS, JOEY WILL DEMONSTRATE COMPLIANCE WITH AT LEAST TWO OUT OF EVERY THREE DEMANDS —WITHIN 4 WEEKS, HE WILL DEMONSTRATE A CAPACITY TO COPE WITH NONDEMAND STRESSORS, BY DECREASING TANTRUMS TO A RATE OF ZERO TO THREE TANTRUMS PER WEEK, EACH WITH A DURATION OF LESS THAN 5 MINUTES PER TANTRUM	12/2 JT

Discharge outcome/long-term goals			
1. JOEY WILL FEED HIMSELF WITH MINIMAL ASSISTANCE AND WILL DRESS AND UNDRESS HIMSELF IN ACCORDANCE WITH AGE-APPROPRIATE NORMS BY DISCHARGE.			

Nursing diagnosis	Nursing intervention	Predicted outcome/short-term goals (include time frame)	Date/signature
SELF CARE DEFICITS: FEEDING AND DRESSING/GROOMING RELATED TO SENSORY-MOTOR/COGNITIVE DEFICITS, SECONDARY TO INFANTILE AUTISM	—FOR SELF-CARE DEFICITS, FEEDING: ·PROVIDE JOEY WITH A FORK AND/OR SPOON AS INDICATED AT ALL MEALS ·PROVIDE HIM WITH A FIRM VERBAL/PHYSICAL PROMPT AT BEGINNING OF EACH MEAL (e.g., "EAT WITH YOUR SPOON"). ACCOMPANY PROMPT BY PHYSICALLY PLACING UTENSIL IN JOEY'S HAND ·DO NOT ALLOW JOEY TO EAT WITH HIS FINGERS; IF HE ATTEMPTS TO DO SO REMOVE HIS PLATE OF FOOD IMMEDIATELY AND REPEAT PRECEDING INTERVENTION ·REPEAT AND CONTINUE ABOVE INTERVENTIONS UNTIL EXPECTED OUTCOME BEHAVIOR OCCURS ·RESPOND TO TANTRUMS, PROTESTS, OR OTHER MANIFESTATIONS OF INEFFECTIVE COPING AND FRUSTRATION TOLERANCE DIFFICULTIES ACCORDING TO INTERVENTIONS OUTLINED IN THE NURSING DIAGNOSIS "INEFFECTIVE INDIVIDUAL COPING" (PAGE 238) —FOR SELF-CARE DEFICITS, DRESSING/GROOMING: ·SELECT CLOTHES AND PLACE THEM BEFORE JOEY ON THE FLOOR HAVE JOEY SIT ON THE FLOOR ·PROVIDE VERBAL/PHYSICAL PROMPTS (e.g, PUT YOUR SHIRT ON) ·PROVIDE ASSISTANCE WHERE NECESSARY AND FOLLOW INTERVENTION FOR DEMAND-RELATED	—WITHIN 4 WEEKS OF HOSPITALIZATION, JOEY WILL FEED HIMSELF WITH UTENSILS 70% OF THE TIME AND WILL DRESS AND UNDRESS WITH VERBAL/PHYSICAL PROMPTS 80% OF THE TIME	12/2 J T

Continued

Nursing Care Plan *continued*

Nursing diagnosis	Nursing intervention	Predicted outcome/short-term goals (include time frame)	Date/signature
	TANTRUM (PAGE 238) · CONTINUE WITH PREVIOUS INTERVENTIONS THROUGH COMPLETION OF DRESSING ─FOR SELF-CARE DEFICITS, UNDRESSING: FOLLOW PREVIOUS INTERVENTIONS BUT REVERSE ORDER OF DEMANDS/PROMPTS (e.g., "TAKE YOUR SHIRT OFF")		

Discharge outcome/long-term goals			
1. AS A PRECURSOR TO LEARNING SPECIFIC SKILLS, JOEY WILL EXHIBIT INCREASED ATTENTION TO ENVIRON- MENTAL STIMULI PRESENTED TO HIM.			

Nursing diagnosis	Nursing intervention	Predicted outcome/short-term goals (include time frame)	Date/signature
DEVELOPMENTAL DELAY: SOCIAL SKILLS; COM- MUNICATION SKILLS; INATTEN- TION; POOR DE- CISION MAKING RELATED TO DE- VELOPMENTAL DISABILITY SEC- ONDARY TO IN- FANTILE AUTISM	—STRUCTURE JOEY'S EN- VIRONMENT WITH A MINIMUM OF "FREE TIME" TO DECREASE FREQUENCY OF RITUAL- ISTIC BEHAVIORS AND INCREASE ADAPTIVE BE- HAVIOR —ACCOMPANY ALL RE- QUESTS OF JOEY WITH VERBAL/PHYSICAL/ VISUAL CUES —STRUCTURE DAILY ROU- TINE TO INCLUDE HOURLY 10-MINUTE ONE-TO-ONE SESSION WITH NURSE REQUIRING ATTENDING BEHAVIOR AND FUNC- TIONAL USE OF OBJECTS	—JOEY WILL RESPOND APPRO- PRIATELY TO ENVIRONMENTAL STIMULATION IN 1 MONTH —JOEY WILL BE ABLE TO ATTEND TO/PARTICIPATE IN AT LEAST ONE AGE-APPRO- PRIATE STRUCTURED ACTIVITY WITH ONE-TO-ONE ASSISTANCE FROM NURSE IN 1 MONTH	12/2

Continued

Nursing Care Plan *continued*

Discharge outcome/long-term goals	
1. THE NUMBER AND INTENSITY OF FACTORS CONTRIBUTING TO ALTERATION IN PARENTING WILL BE REDUCED AS EVIDENCED BY: A) A PLAN TO DEAL WITH GRANDPARENTS AND B) INCREASED VERBALIZATION OF	PRESSURES BY BOTH PARENTS. 2. AT LEAST 2 SPECIFIC STRATEGIES AND COPING SKILLS WILL BE UTILIZED TO ENHANCE POTENTIAL FOR EFFECTIVE PARENTING AND RESTABILIZATION OF FAMILY FUNCTIONING.

Nursing diagnosis	Nursing intervention	Predicted outcome/short-term goals (include time frame)	Date/signature
ALTERED PARENTING RELATED TO CHILDS CONDITION AND ECONOMIC AND RELATIONSHIP PROBLEMS	—ESTABLISH REGULAR WEEKLY HOUR-LONG PARENTING SESSIONS TO FOCUS ON SPECIFIC PARENTAL CONCERNS AND PARENTING NEEDS/ISSUES —SUPPORT THE PARENTS' INVOLVEMENT WITH JOEY —PROVIDE REALISTIC INSTRUCTION ON SPECIFIC BEHAVIOR INTERVENTIONS APPROPRIATE TO THE FAMILY'S ABILITY TO FOLLOW-THROUGH AND ACHIEVE SUCCESS ON A GRADUAL BASIS —GRADUALLY INCREASE COMPLEXITY OF INSTRUCTIONS, PARTICULARLY THOSE INVOLVING BEHAVIORAL MANAGEMENT —COUNSEL RELATED TO MARITAL NEEDS FOR TIME ALONE AND AWAY FROM CHILD(REN) TO DEVELOP RELATIONSHIP	—WITHIN 1.5 MONTHS, JOEY'S PARENTS WILL BE ABLE TO IDENTIFY, LIST, AND DISCUSS 2 MAJOR SPECIFIC STRESSORS WHICH CONTRIBUTE TO PARENTING PROBLEMS —THEY WILL DEMONSTRATE KNOWLEDGE, COMFORT, AND SUCCESS IN IMPLEMENTING BEHAVIOR INTERVENTIONS WITHIN 1.5 MONTHS —THEY WILL BEGIN TO IDENTIFY MUTUAL NEEDS AND AREAS OF INTEREST APART FROM CHILD(REN) WITHIN 1.5 MONTHS	12/2 √

Discharge outcome/long-term goals			
1. JOEY'S PARENTS WILL VERBALIZE THE MEANING AND IMPLICATIONS OF JOEY'S DIAGNOSIS OF AUTISM AND SEVERE MENTAL RETARDATION. 2. THE PARENTS WILL BEGIN TO EXPRESS		BOTH POSITIVE AND NEGATIVE AFFECT WITH EACH OTHER AND WITH PRIMARY NURSE RELATIVE TO ISSUES OF GRIEVING, LOSS, ETC.	
Nursing diagnosis	Nursing intervention	Predicted outcome/short-term goals (include time frame)	Date/signature
ANTICIPATORY PARENTAL GRIEVING RE-LATED TO AN-TICIPATED LOSS-ES SECONDARY TO CHILD'S DIAG-NOSIS/CONDITION	-ENCOURAGE AND SUP-PORT THE PARENT'S EXPRESSION OF FEEL-INGS AND PROVIDE AN EMOTIONAL CLI-MATE OF ACCEPTANCE, UNDERSTANDING, AND SYMPATHY -ALLOW PARENTS TO EXPRESS GRIEF AND ANGER; PROVIDE THEM WITH OPPORTUN-ITIES FOR WORKING-THROUGH -ACKNOWLEDGE THE REAL FEELINGS OF "LOSS" PERCEIVED BY PARENTS FOLLOWING AC-CEPTANCE OF A DIAGNO-SIS OF SEVERE HANDICAP -SUPPORT/REINFORCE INTERVENTIONS BY OTHER DISCIPLINES/ AGENCIES	- BY WEEK 4, PARENTS WILL BEGIN TO VERBALIZE SPECIFIC FEELINGS ABOUT THE CHILD'S DIAGNOSIS - BY WEEK 8, THEY WILL BE ABLE TO ASK QUESTIONS RELATED TO LONG-TERM IMPLI-CATIONS OF DIAGNOSIS/HANDICAP	12/2

Continued

Nursing Care Plan *continued*

Discharge outcome/long-term goals	—STATE THE COMMUNITY RESOURCES / AGENCIES THEY PLAN TO UTILIZE.		
1. BY DISCHARGE, THE PARENTS WILL BE ABLE TO: —USE BEHAVIORAL MANAGEMENT SKILLS —STATE HOW AND WHEN THEY WILL BRING JOEY TO FOLLOW-UP VISITS			

Nursing diagnosis	Nursing intervention	Predicted outcome/short-term goals (include time frame)	Date/signature
IMPAIRED HOME MAINTENANCE MANAGEMENT RELATED TO INADEQUATE RESOURCES AND CHILD'S DISABILITY	—IDENTIFY ANTICIPAT-ED DISCHARGE NEEDS WITH FAMILY AND INITIATE COM-MUNITY REFERRALS (e.g., SCHOOL PLACE-MENT, SUPPORT AGENCIES) —PROVIDE PARENTS WITH IN DEPTH IN-STRUCTION IN BE-HAVIOR INTERVENTION FOR HOME MANAGE-MENT IN PREPAR-ATION FOR DIS-CHARGE NEEDS —ENCOURAGE PARENTS TO IDENTIFY ANTICIPATED TREATMENT CONCERNS AND NEEDS	—BY WEEK 4, PARENTS WILL IDENTIFY AND LIST SPECIFIC NEEDS OF FAMILY/CHILD IN RELATION TO RETURNING JOEY TO THE FAMILY —BY WEEK 8, PARENTS WILL DEMONSTRATE ABILITY TO MANAGE THREE OF JOEY'S MOST PROBLEMATIC BEHAVIORS —BY WEEK 8, PARENTS WILL HAVE MET WITH REPRESEN-TATIVES OF COMMUNITY REFERRAL AGENCY	12/2

level of his cognitive function. Although Joey appeared capable of learning some cognitive/adaptive skills, as well as capable of establishing some relatedness to the environment, such achievements would most likely be minimal and acquirable only to the extent that structure, consistency, and firm behavioral measures could be continually enforced.

During Joey's hospitalization, his parents made remarkable gains in their ability to pull together and reestablish effective relational and coping strategies. Nursing interventions—which focused on increasing parental knowledge and understanding of Joey's handicaps and problems, openly acknowledging and discussing the issues and concerns unique to a family with a handicapped child, and facilitating appropriate community referrals—succeeded in achieving the restabilization of family functioning, a major goal of hospitalization.

Both 2- and 4-month posthospitalization follow-ups with the family revealed that the family was actively utilizing available community resources (initiated during hospitalization) and that Joey's behavior at home was remaining stable. He was enrolled in special classes for autistic children, which he attended regularly. At the 1-year follow-up, however, his tantrums and dangerous behavior had returned; consequently, he was then placed in a long-term residential school facility specializing in the long-term needs of autistic children. Final contact with this family at 2 years posthospitalization revealed a stable, healthy adjustment to this residential placement by both Joey and his family.

SELECTED BIBLIOGRAPHY

Cantwell, D., et al. "Families of Autistic and Dysphasic Children: Family Life and Interaction Patterns," *Archives of General Psychiatry* 36:682-87, 1979.

Cantwell, D., et al. "Family Factors in the Syndrome of Infantile Autism," in *Autism: A Reappraisal of Concepts and Treatment.* Edited by Rutter, M., and Schopler, E. New York: Plenam Press, 1978.

Levin, D.S. *Developmental Experiences: Treatment of Developmental Disorders in Children.* New York: Aronson, 1985.

Morgan, S.B. *The Unreachable Child: An Introduction to Early Childhood Autism.* Memphis: Memphis State University Press, 1981.

Nelson, D.L. *Children with Autism and Other Pervasive Disorders of Development and Behavior: Therapy Through Activities.* Thorofare, N.J.: Slack, 1984.

Ward, A.J. *Childhood Autism and Structured Therapy: Selected Papers on Early Childhood Autism.* Chicago: Nelson-Hall, 1976.

Jana:
An Adult Client with an Eating Disorder

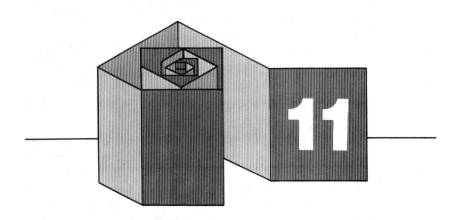

Johanna Ehlhardt, BSN, RN

The client with bulimia presents the nurse with a particular challenge in assessing the degree to which a mental disorder can interrupt an individual's functioning in interpersonal, academic, and family spheres. The evaluation process involves not only an observation of the severity of the client's maladaptive behaviors, but also an investigation and speculation into the underlying purpose of the specific behaviors. In this particular case, the nurse spent much time determining the meaning of the client's binging/vomiting and self-destructive behavior. This step, which actively involved the client, provided the nurse with insight into the client's maladapative coping behaviors and helped direct the development of the nursing assessment and the formulation of the nursing diagnoses and care plan.

CASE STUDY

Jana, a 25-year-old Caucasian, single, Catholic female, was brought into the emergency room (ER) after a suicide attempt, having taken an overdose of a prescribed antidepressant drug (desipramine [Norpramin]) with a large quantity of alcohol (a liter of wine). At the time of evaluation, she was clear and coherent in thought, but her speech was slurred and her memory and recall of recent events was impaired. Intervention at this time consisted of maintaining close observation of her vital signs and level of consciousness should an abrupt change occur due to ingestion of the substances.

During initial evaluation, Jana admitted to the psychiatrist that she had been in outpatient psychiatric care for 1 year for treatment of an eating disorder. She had sought the treatment after feeling out of control with her eating. More recently, she had been experiencing prevailing depression and overwhelming anxiety, which led to her suicide attempt.

After evaluation in the ER, Jana was admitted, voluntarily, to the adjacent acute care psychiatric facility for further observation and evaluation of her lethality and depression and for evaluation of any possible medical problems and functional impairments resulting from her eating disorder. On the unit, she was given extensive mental status and physical examinations.

Jana reported onset of self-destructive behaviors about 6 months prior to hospitalization. At first, these behaviors consisted of cutting her wrist with a razor blade about once every 10 to 12 weeks and drinking from one to three glasses of wine every night. At that time, her psychiatrist had been out of town on vacation for approximately 1 week. The psychiatrist had left Jana with the phone number of a colleague with whom she could connect should she begin to experience any difficulties. However, Jana chose not to call the other psychiatrist. Jana also admitted desiring death about once a day for about the past 3 months. She denied any concrete thought of death prior to that time. These impulsive behaviors seemed to be precipitated by stressful events and accompanied by alcohol ingestion.

Assessment of Jana's eating disorder revealed a long-standing history of eating difficulties and periods of significant obesity from age 17 to age 19. With severe dietary restriction, she was able to maintain a more acceptable weight of 100 pounds for a period of 3 years (from age 19 to 21). But then, coincident with pressures of college and social life, Jana began to feel increasingly anxious and out of control and began to binge—at first, one to two times a week, then increasing to one to two times each day. Often, she would combine these binges with increased alcohol use. Jana began to panic at sudden increases in her weight but seemed unable to control her binging. Looking back, she remembered feeling some relief from impulsive eating at first, but then experiencing overwhelming guilt and panic soon after the binge. Jana then began to use a laxative (Correctol) to control her weight—at first, five to ten tablets per day, escalating to up to 30 per day. She continued this pattern of use periodically over 1 year.

During this period, she began to experience bowel disturbances; she then began to use vomiting as a method of weight control. In addition to providing relief from the sensation of overeating, the vomiting also brought relief from the overwhelming guilt and shame brought on by binging. Jana's vomiting pattern emerged initially as after binges only, but gradually escalated to after every meal (whether or not a binge). Sometimes she would experience early morning anxiety and vomit on an empty stomach. She binged primarily at night but sometimes also in the late afternoon when she arrived home from work. Typically, she would stop at a store on her way home from work to shop for her binge. Her binge foods consisted primarily of sweets, pastas, and other carbohydrate-laden foods. Once home, Jana would quickly unplug the phone, pull the drapes shut, and then begin eating and drinking. Shortly afterwards she would vomit. At first, she needed a spoon or her finger to induce vomiting, but by the time of admission, she was able to elicit her own esophageal reflex and vomit without any aids. As a direct result of excessive vomiting, her potassium level had become significantly depleted (to a level of 1.6 mEq/ml—normal is 4 to 5 mEq/ml) on admission.

About 5 to 6 months prior to admission, she began to experience muscle cramping in her legs; she sought treatment for these cramps in a local ER. At that time, cardiopathy was noted on an electrocardiogram. She also began to develop some dental problems, particularly erosion of the enamel due to irritation from gastric secretions.

Over the 2 weeks prior to admission, Jana lost 10 pounds and experienced extreme fatigue. Her binging and purging had increased to three times a day. She complained of a tight, constricted feeling in her throat that made swallowing difficult and of an "enormous" twisting knot in her stomach. She began to experience vertigo upon standing; during her examination she displayed a severe drop in orthostatic blood pressure. In addition to her suicidal ideation and eating disorder, Jana reported chronic sleep difficulties, claiming to average only 3 to 4 hours of sleep per night over the past year. Otherwise, her medical history revealed no remarkable findings; she experienced the usual childhood diseases without significant incident. Although her menses had been normal in onset and initially in duration and cycle, at the time of admission she had not menstruated for 3 years. Upon admission, her weight was 117 pounds and height was 5'7".

Jana reported feelings of worthlessness, sadness, helplessness, hopelessness, lack of control, nervousness, anxiety, and decreased concentration. When questioned regarding her self-perceptions, Jana revealed much self-negation and derogatory ideation, overwhelming guilt, poor self-worth, and hyperresponsibility. She viewed herself as overweight, even though her body weight was certainly appropriate for her frame. Upon further questioning, she expressed rigid ideas about her weight and body image.

Regarding her social history, Jana had been living alone in a one-bedroom apartment for 3 years and employed as a paralegal secretary in a local law clinic for the same time period. Jana describes her work as boring; she "despises" her job, but has been reluctant to find another. It appears from her reports that she is quite perfectionistic, completing assignments compulsively and thoroughly. However, Jana had begun to take from 1 to 3 sick days a month (usually after nights of heavy binging, vomiting, and drinking). Although she was just 14 units shy of earning a B.A. degree in law (progress that had taken her 5 years of part-time school to accomplish), she stated that she had lost interest in completing her degree.

As for her family history, Jana was the eldest of three girls; her sisters were 3 and 5 years younger. Her mother and father lived together. The only significant emotional difficulty was her father's alcoholism. Jana denied any other known mental illness in her immediate or extended family. She described her relationship with her mother as being rather consonant and pleasant, but not supportive of any endeavors that Jana may have wanted to pursue. She had many altercations with her father during adolescence. She admitted to some episodes of sexual abuse during childhood; occasionally, her father attempted to fondle her and her sisters. These attempts ceased as the girls became older and resisted them. Jana was close only to one sister, who was somewhat debilitated with a physical handicap and lived in a board and care home.

Jana's social history included minimal dating in high school and a long-term relationship of 1½ years' duration while in college, but no other relationships since that time. When questioned about the nature of her long-term relationship and why it ended, she was rather vague and defensive, simply stating that she and her boyfriend had some arguments about her dietary habits. She claimed no sexual activity since the relationship's end. Jana spoke of two friends with whom she initiated social activities consisting mostly of dining out and going to movies. She described her relationships with her coworkers as pleasant, superficial, and distant. Regarding leisure interests, she had been quite active in tennis and had become sufficiently skilled to enter amateur competitions in her home town, and also enjoyed weaving and working with yarn.

On mental status examination, Jana presented as a woman appearing her stated age, appropriately and casually dressed, with good hygiene. She was cooperative with the interviewer, made good eye contact, and displayed clear, coherent speech and a depressed mood with restricted affect. Regarding thought processes, Jana appeared to have good knowledge, minimal abstraction ability, fair calculation ability, good judgment, no associational disturbances, and orientation in four spheres. Her insight was judged as fair. She presented without impairment in reality testing,

Continued on page 256

RECORDING THE DATA

After you have read the case, cluster significant data into functional health patterns.

Health management/health perception _____

_____

_____

_____

_____

Nutritional/metabolic _____

_____

_____

_____

Elimination _____

_____

_____

_____

Activity/exercise _____

_____

_____

_____

Cognitive/perceptual _____

_____

_____

_____

Sleep/rest _____

_____

_____

_____

Self-perception/self-concept _____

_____

_____

_____

Role relationship _____

_____

_____

_____

Sexuality/reproductive _____

_____

_____

_____

Coping/stress tolerance _____

_____

_____

_____

Value/belief _____

_____

_____

_____

ASSIGNING NURSING DIAGNOSES

Use your clustered data to select appropriate nursing diagnoses.

Health perception/health management

- ☐ Growth and Development, Altered (see Developmental Delay)
- ☐ Health Maintenance, Altered
- ☐ Infection, Potential for
- ☐ Injury (Trauma): Potential for
- ☐ Noncompliance (Specify)
- ☐ Poisoning: Potential for
- ☐ Suffocation: Potential for

Nutritional/metabolic

- ☐ Body Temperature, Potential Alteration in
- ☐ Developmental Delay: Physical Growth and Development
- ☐ Fluid Volume, Altered: Excess or Excess Fluid Volume
- ☐ Fluid Volume Deficit, Actual
- ☐ Fluid Volume Deficit, Potential
- ☐ Nutrition, Altered: Less Than Body Requirements or Nutritional Deficit (Specify)
- ☐ Nutrition, Altered: More Than Body Requirements or Exogenous Obesity
- ☐ Nutrition, Altered: Potential for More Than Body Requirements or Potential for Obesity
- ☐ Oral Mucous Membrane, Altered
- ☐ Skin Integrity, Impaired or Skin Breakdown
- ☐ Skin Integrity, Impaired or Potential Skin Breakdown
- ☐ Swallowing, Impaired or Uncompensated Swallowing Impairment
- ☐ Tissue Integrity, Impaired

Elimination

- ☐ Bowel Elimination, Altered: Constipation
- ☐ Bowel Elimination, Altered: Diarrhea
- ☐ Bowel Elimination, Altered: Incontinence
- ☐ Developmental Delay: Bowel/Bladder Control
- ☐ Incontinence: Functional
- ☐ Incontinence: Reflex
- ☐ Incontinence: Stress
- ☐ Incontinence: Total
- ☐ Incontinence: Urge
- ☐ Urinary Elimination, Altered Patterns of
- ☐ Urinary Retention

Activity/exercise

- ☐ Activity Intolerance
- ☐ Activity Intolerance, Potential
- ☐ Airway Clearance, Ineffective
- ☐ Breathing Pattern, Ineffective
- ☐ Cardiac Output, Altered: Decreased
- ☐ Developmental Delay: Mobility
- ☐ Developmental Delay: Self-Care Skills
- ☐ Diversional Activity Deficit
- ☐ Gas Exchange, Impaired
- ☐ Home Maintenance Management, Impaired (Mild, Moderate, Severe, Potential, Chronic)
- ☐ Mobility, Impaired Physical
- ☐ Self-Care Deficit: Feeding
- ☐ Self-Care Deficit: Bathing/Hygiene
- ☐ Self-Care Deficit: Dressing/Grooming
- ☐ Self-Care Deficit: Toileting
- ☐ Self-Care Deficit: Total
- ☐ Tissue Perfusion, Altered: (Specify)

Sleep/rest

- ☐ Sleep Pattern Disturbance

Cognitive/perceptual

- ☐ Comfort, Altered: Pain
- ☐ Comfort, Altered: Chronic Pain

☐ Developmental Delay: (Specify Cognitive Area; attention, decision making, etc.)
☐ Hypothermia
☐ Hyperthermia
☐ Knowledge Deficit (Specify)
☐ Sensory-Perceptual Alteration: Input Excess or Sensory Overload
☐ Sensory-Perceptual Alteration: Input Deficit or Sensory Deprivation
☐ Thermoregulation, Ineffective
☐ Thought Processes, Altered
☐ Unilateral Neglect

Self-perception/self-concept

☐ Anxiety
☐ Body Image Disturbance
☐ Fear
☐ Hopelessness
☐ Personal Identity Confusion
☐ Powerlessness (Severe, Low, Moderate)
☐ Self-Esteem Disturbance

Role relationship

☐ Communication, Impaired Verbal
☐ Developmental Delay: Communication Skills
☐ Developmental Delay: Social Skills
☐ Family Processes, Altered
☐ Grieving, Anticipatory
☐ Grieving, Dysfunctional
☐ Parenting, Altered: Actual or Potential

☐ Role Performance, Disturbance in
☐ Social Interactions, Impaired
☐ Social Isolation (Rejection)

Sexuality/reproductive

☐ Rape-Trauma Syndrome: Compounded
☐ Rape-Trauma Syndrome: Silent Reaction
☐ Sexual Dysfunction
☐ Sexuality Patterns, Altered

Coping/stress tolerance

☐ Adjustment, Impaired
☐ Coping, Ineffective Individual
☐ Coping, Ineffective Family: Compromised
☐ Coping, Ineffective Family: Disabling
☐ Coping, Family: Potential for Growth
☐ Developmental Delay (Specify area)
☐ Post-Trauma Response
☐ Violence, Potential for (Self-Directed or Directed at Others)

Value/belief

☐ Spiritual Distress (Distress of Human Spirit)

You are now ready to develop a nursing care plan for this client. Use the following blank pages to do so. Then refer to the author's formulation, diagnostic summary, care plan, and summary.

NURSING CARE PLAN

Complete the chart below to develop a nursing care plan for this client.

Discharge outcomes/long-term goals	

Nursing diagnosis	Nursing intervention	

	Predicted outcomes/short-term goals (include time frame)	**Date/signature**

Return to Formulation, page 256

and denied any auditory or visual hallucinations. Although she was preoccupied with body image, weight loss, and consumption of food, this preoccupation was not of a delusional quality. She denied any experiences of depersonalization or any fears of panic proportions, except as relating to excessive weight gain.

Jana denied homicidal ideation, but admitted several past suicide attempts. These attempts, all of which occurred while she was intoxicated, involved cutting her wrists until she began to feel pain and see blood. (This information pointed to the possibility that Jana may experience some degree of depersonalization under stress that causes her to act impulsively and destructively.) The latest attempt represented the first time she had ever ingested a large quantity of pills with alcohol. When questioned about her intention, Jana reported a strong desire to be dead, explaining that she could no longer live with the anxiety and depression she had been experiencing. She admitted that her binging and purging were out of control and felt she no longer could get meaningful help to assist her with her impulsive, destructive behaviors.

Reader may now complete Recording the Data, Assigning Nursing Diagnoses, and Nursing Care Plan.

FORMULATION

Jana's adaptation to chronic distorted self-concept involved a long-term depression and development of a severe eating disorder. A decline in her general functioning over a 7-year period paralleled the progression of her eating disorder. She clearly revealed this on admission when describing her gradually increasing social isolation. Even her sustained interactions, such as with people at work or with a few friends, were characterized by a limited degree of involvement. In contrast, her early history—before the eating disorder worsened—revealed some ability to be social, date, and even have a relationship that involved a healthy sexual exchange. A differential diagnosis would determine any deficit in her personality structure. The psychiatric evaluation process would include an assessment of her personality and ego functioning and the degree to which they contribute to the severity of the disease process. This assessment, besides providing insight into the nature of the disorder, would also help define certain approaches in dealing with the individual at risk (Wilson and Mintz, 1985).

Another sign of life-interruption was her developing anhedonia, a symptom of depression. Gradually, she lost all interest in her usual leisure activities of tennis and rug weaving. She had become apathetic to her work situation and was indifferent to seeking a change.

But a more significant factor interrupting her life functioning—one that was becoming life-threatening—was her growing impulsivity. This was evidenced by the exacerbation of her binging and vomiting, which resulted in decreased potassium levels that endangered her cardiac function, as well as by problems in other body systems: esophageal irritation with infrequent bleeding upon vomiting, erosion of tooth enamel, and bowel disturbances. Her actual weight of 117 pounds was established as appropriate for her height of 5'7".

Jana also exhibited possible personality disintegration in the form of dissociative episodes, which increased the potential for other forms of unpredictable, impulsive behavior. While the actual occurrence of dissociation was unclear, she clearly had become increasingly impulsive with her self-mutilating behaviors over the past 6 months, culminating in a serious lethal attempt and also in increased alcohol consumption.

Jana described herself as being in much turmoil and psychic pain. She readily identified her maladaptive behavior: binging and vomiting out of control, with a progressive increase in anxiety prior to binging and guilt and shame afterwards. Vomiting brought progressively less relief from these feelings. According to Johnson (1984), the binge-purge cycle initially takes an adaptive, integrating function for the individual in the relief of tension but eventually begins to fail, leading to a resumption of the original state of low self-esteem with feelings of worthlessness, despair, and accompanying dysphoria. Jana was able to demonstrate some insight into the process of her anxiety and her response by identifying certain provoking precipitants to binging and vomiting: difficult family interactions, particularly as relating to eating habits; extremely high anxiety when in a large social group; and times of intense self-negation. But in terms of identifying specific thoughts and feelings that activated her binge-purge behavior, she remained confused and unclear.

One critical variable to Jana's impulsivity was her rigid way of thinking and reacting in response to stress. Generally, in response to increased stress, she lost her ability to problem-solve and essentially coped very poorly. For instance, when a client or coworker became irritated or demanding, she would respond by internalizing and personalizing the incident, seeing herself as accountable and responsible for almost everything that happened in the office. She also reported the inability to cope with any form of criticism or constructive feedback at work; in response to such incidents, she would experience overwhelming anxiety and frequently would need to rush to the bathroom to vomit. Clearly, she was not able to differentiate and define her boundaries at these times.

Continued on page 277

DIAGNOSTIC SUMMARY FOR JANA

Data	Functional health pattern	Nursing diagnosis
—Presents with hypovolemia, hypokalemia, dehydration, muscle cramping, chronic fatigue, weight loss of 10 lbs. in 2 weeks, tooth enamel erosion, and past history of cardiopathy hypotension	Health Perception/ Health Management	Potential complications of hypovolemia, negative nitrogen balance, hypokalemia, and esophageal bleeding (collaborative diagnosis) Potential for injury related to fatigue and vertigo secondary to orthostatic hypotension
—Has a past history of esophageal bleeding	Nutritional/ Metabolic	Altered oral mucous membrane related to chronic vomiting secondary to bulimia
—Sleeps poorly (3 hours per night for the past year) —Is unable to fall asleep and remain asleep	Sleep/Rest	Sleep pattern disturbance related to anxiety and fear secondary to depressive symptoms and bulimia
—Complains of chronic constipation —Admits laxative abuse	Elimination	Altered bowel elimination: constipation, related to depression, chronic eating disorder, and laxative abuse
—Displays impulse dyscontrol, as manifested by binging and purging, self-mutilation, and suicide attempts —Experiences dissociative episodes	Self-Perception/ Self-Control	Fear and anxiety related to depression and chronic distorted self-image secondary to disease process
—Engages in binging and vomiting episodes, self-mutilation, and suicide attempts —Admits to social isolation and alcohol abuse —Has an inability to ask for help —Experiences increased anxiety in evening hours	Coping/Stress Tolerance	Ineffective individual coping related to depression secondary to bulimia Potential for self-harm related to past history and effects of depression

Data	Functional health pattern	Nursing diagnosis
—Expresses gross body image disturbances; views herself as always being too large —Experiences overwhelming feelings of worthlessness, extreme self-negation, and self-derogatory ideation —Has an increased dependency on others to meet her needs and an inability to make decisions on her own —Has a poor ability to express herself, especially when angry, and to identify various feeling states, particularly anger —Complains of anhedonia, apathy, and chronic dysphoria	Self-Perception/ Self-Concept	Altered self-esteem related to distorted perceptions of self and depression secondary to bulimia
—Holds a delusion of inhaling oxygen from rommate —Displays a rigid, inflexible thinking process with increased referential thinking —Experiences periodic dissociative episodes	Cognitive/Perceptual	Altered thought processes related to negative cognitive set secondary to disease process

NURSING CARE PLAN

Complete the chart below to develop a nursing care plan for this client.

Discharge outcome/long-term goals			
1. Jana will be restored to homeostasis with all bodily functions intact by discharge. 2. She will return to an optimal level of functioning in her personal,		social, and work life by discharge. 3. She will be prepared to maintain her physical and emotional life with an improved self-concept, better self-control, and effective coping mechanisms by discharge.	

Nursing diagnosis	Nursing intervention	Predicted outcome/short-term goals (include time frame)	Date/signature
Potential complications of hypovolemia, negative nitrogen balance, hypokalemia, and esophageal bleeding (collaborative diagnosis)	—Take orthostatic vital signs as ordered and when Jana complains of vertigo. Instruct her to get up from a sitting position slowly to minimize symptoms —Ensure that Jana remains under nursing supervision for 1 hour after each dose of potassium via day-room restriction —Monitor compliance with prescribed fluid intake (according to her physician's orders it should be 180 cc every 2 hours)	—Jana will not fall or be injured due to syncopal episodes during hospital stay —Her potassium levels will be maintained within normal limits within 3 days —Dehydration will resolve itself within 5 days —Her blood pressure will rise and stabilize within 5 days —She will not lose any more weight during hospitalization —She will not experience cardiac decompensation during hospitalization	2/5 JE
Potential for injury related to fatigue and vertigo secondary to orthostatic hypotension	—Take her weight weekly, in the morning after voiding but before breakfast, with her dressed in a patient gown —See intervention for weight maintenance under nursing diagnosis: individual coping —Observe her for any changes in vital signs or complaints of chest pain		2/5 JE
Altered oral mucous membrane related to chronic vomiting secondary to bulimia	—If Jana complains of abdominal pain or vomits any blood, take her vital signs and call the physician	—Jana will not experience any further esophageal bleeding (starting immediately)	2/5 JE
Altered bowel elimination: constipation related to depression, chronic	—Ensure increased hydration (2 liters per day) —Monitor effectiveness of milk of magnesia as ordered —Teach Jana about	—Within 3 weeks, regular patterns in bowel movements will be established	2/5 JE

Nursing diagnosis	Nursing intervention	Predicted outcome/short-term goals (include time frame)	Date/signature
EATING DISORDER AND LAXATIVE ABUSE	BOWEL FUNCTIONING AND THE EFFECTS OF CHRONIC LAXATIVE ABUSE —ENCOURAGE HER TO EAT FOODS HIGH IN FIBER: FRESH FRUITS, BRAN, FRUIT JUICES		
SLEEP PATTERN DISTURBANCE RELATED TO ANXIETY AND FEAR SECOND-ARY TO DE-PRESSIVE SYMPTOMS AND BULIMIA	—ENCOURAGE JANA TO USE RELAXATION TAPES BEFORE HOUR OF SLEEP TO DECELERATE —ARRANGE A BRIEF (10-MINUTE) MEETING BETWEEN JANA AND ASSIGNED NIGHT STAFF TO DISCUSS ANY CON-CERNS THAT MAY BE PREVENTING SLEEP —OFFER HER WARM MILK OR A HOT BATH/SHOWER BEFORE MEDICATION —MEDICATE AS ORDERED AND EVALUATE EFFEC-TIVENESS, IF ITEMS ABOVE PROVE INEFFEC-TIVE	—WITHIN 1 MONTH, JANA WILL SLEEP 5 TO 8 HOURS PER NIGHT UNINTERRUPTED	2/5 JE
FEAR AND ANX-IETY RELATED TO DEPRESSION AND CHRONIC DISTORTED SELF-IMAGE SECONDARY TO DISEASE PROCESS	—USE BEHAVIOR MODI-FICATION TECHNIQUES TO INCREASE JANA'S RESPONSIBILITY FOR SELF-CONTROL ·TEACH JANA TO USE A SUBJECTIVE ANXIETY RATING SCALE (A SCALE OF 1 TO 10, WITH 1 BEING THE LEAST SEVERE AND 10 BEING THE MOST SEVERE) AND TO RATE HERSELF EVERY TIME SHE RECOGNIZES ANY SIGNS OF INCREAS-ING ANXIETY; i.e., RACING PULSE, RAPID BREATHING, COLD, CLAMMY SKIN ·EXPLAIN THE INTER-VENTIONS YOU PLAN TO EMPLOY FOR EACH RAT-ING CATEGORY. A RATING OF 1 TO 3 WILL EARN HER REGULAR STATUS ON THE UNIT, AD LIB USE OF HER ROOM, THE	—HER VOMITING EPISODES WILL BE REDUCED FROM 2 TIMES A DAY TO 2 TIMES A WEEK —SHE WILL DEMONSTRATE IN-CREASED IMPULSE CONTROL OF ANXIETY AND FEAR IN CRITICAL SITUATIONS THAT PRECIPITATE SELF-MUTI-LATION AND SUICIDE AT-TEMPTS AND EPISODES OF BINGING AND VOMITING. THIS WILL BE EVIDENCED BY HER ABILITY TO IDENTIFY ANXIOUS FEELINGS AND TO EXERT SOME LEVEL OF CON-TROL USING LEARNED COPING SKILLS. SHE WILL INITIALLY REQUIRE STAFF HELP FOR 3 WEEKS; WITHIN 5 WEEKS, SHE WILL BE ABLE TO FOLLOW-THROUGH ON APPROPRIATE MEASURES WITHOUT STAFF SUPERVISION	2/5 JE

Continued

Nursing Care Plan *continued*

Nursing diagnosis	Nursing intervention	Predicted outcome/short-term goals (include time frame)	Date/signature
	PRIVILEGE TO LEAVE THE UNIT FOR ACTIVITIES AND GROUP WALKS, ETC. •A RATING OF 4 TO 7 WILL REQUIRE THE IMPLEMENTATION OF 15-MINUTE SELF-CHECKS FOR A PERIOD OF 3 HOURS. DURING THIS PERIOD, SHE MAY HAVE USE OF HER ROOM, BUT WILL NOT BE ALLOWED TO LEAVE THE UNIT		
	•A RATING OF 7 TO 10 WILL REQUIRE THE IMPLEMENTATION OF DAYROOM RESTRICTION, WITH ACCOMPANYING 15-MINUTE SELF-CHECKS FOR A PERIOD OF 3 HOURS. LIFT THIS RESTRICTION ONLY AFTER HER RATING DROPS TO 6 OR BELOW; SHE CAN THEN RETURN TO REGULAR STATUS OF ROOM		
	PRIVILEGES, BUT MUST PERFORM 15-MINUTE SELF-CHECKS FOR 3 HOURS FOLLOWED BY 30-MINUTE SELF-CHECKS FOR 2 MORE HOURS. LIFT THESE RESTRICTIONS ONLY FOR A RATING OF 3 OR LOWER •INSTRUCT JANA TO CONTACT THE STAFF IF SHE RATES AN EPISODE OF ANXIETY BETWEEN 4 AND 10 ON THE SCALE. EXPLAIN THAT THE STAFF WILL TALK WITH HER BRIEFLY AND ASSIST HER IN IDENTIFYING POSSIBLE SOURCES OF ANXIETY •INSTRUCT HER TO RATE ANXIETY DURING ANY EPISODES OF BINGING AND VOMITING AND TO RECORD THESE RATINGS IN HER EATING JOURNAL CHART		

Nursing diagnosis	Nursing intervention	Predicted outcome/short-term goals (include time frame)	Date/signature
	(SEE PAGE 274 FOR SAMPLE OF SUCH A JOURNAL) ALSO HAVE HER RATE HER ANXIETY AFTER EACH MEAL EATEN AND IF HER LEVEL IS BETWEEN 4 AND 7, TO REMAIN ON DAYROOM RESTRICTION WITH 15-MINUTE SELF-CHECKS FOR 1 HOUR. EXPLAIN THAT SHE IS TO REMAIN IN HER ROOM UNTIL SHE RATES A 3 OR LOWER TO ENSURE THAT NO VOMITING WILL OCCUR. INSTRUCT HER TO IMPLEMENT COPING STRATEGIES (SEE COPING SECTION, PAGE 264) IMMEDIATELY AFTER ALL MEALS REGARDLESS OF HER ANXIETY RATING, AND TO PERFORM SUCH COPING STRATEGIES FOR NOT LESS THAN 45 MINUTES · WHEN SHE IS ABLE TO FOLLOW THROUGH AND CONTACT STAFF FOR THOUGHTS OF SELF-HARM, STRONGLY ENCOURAGE HER TO VENTILATE HER FEELINGS OF FEAR AND ANGER AND TO EXTERNALIZE THE ANGER THROUGH PREPLANNED COPING STRATEGIES. STRESS THAT SHE SHOULD NOT ISOLATE IN HER ROOM IF HER ANXIETY LEVEL IS BETWEEN 4 AND 10 — PROVIDE DIRECT INTERVENTION FOR ANY SELF-MUTILATION ATTEMPTS · IF SHE DOES ACTUAL HARM TO HERSELF, PLACE HER ON DAYROOM RESTRICTION FOR ONE 8-HOUR PERIOD WITH 15-MINUTE SELF-CHECKS WHILE AWAKE.		

Continued

Nursing Care Plan *continued*

Nursing diagnosis	Nursing intervention	Predicted outcome/short-term goals (include time frame)	Date/signature
	AFTERWARDS, IMPLE-MENT THE INTERVEN-TIONS FOR AN ANXIETY RATING OF 7 TO 10 (SEE PAGE 262) TO EN-SURE CONTROL OF IM-PULSIVE BEHAVIOR		
	·IF SHE IS OBSERVED TO BE IN OBVIOUS DIS-TRESS AND HAS NOT COMMUNICATED TO THE STAFF, IMPLEMENT THE INTERVENTIONS		
	APPROPRIATE FOR AN ANXIETY RATING OF 4 TO 7		
	·IF SHE REVEALS THAT SHE'S EXPERIENCED SELF-DESTRUCTIVE THOUGHTS WITH A DEFINITE PLAN AND THAT SHE DID NOT CONTACT STAFF AT THE TIME OF ONSET OF THE IDEATION,		
	EVALUATE HER IMPULSIVITY BY ASSESSING HER ABILITY TO CONTRACT TO NOT HARM HERSELF AND HER SELF-RATING, AND IMPLEMENT THE APPRO-PRIATE INTERVENTIONS (SEE "POTENTIAL FOR SELF-HARM", PAGE 267)		
	−IF JANA EXPERIENCES ANY EPISODES OF DIS-SOCIATION, PLACE HER ON IMMEDIATE CLOSE OBSERVATION, EITHER IN THE DAYROOM OR ON ONE-TO-ONE STATUS, AND ASSESS HER NEED FOR MEDICATION	−JANA WILL REPORT ANY DISSOCIATIVE EXPERIENCES TO PRIMARY NURSE WITHIN 3 WEEKS	
INEFFECTIVE INDIVIDUAL COP-ING RELATED TO DEPRESSION SECONDARY TO BULIMIA	−TEACH JANA IMPROVED COPING SKILLS TO ASSIST HER IN CONTROLLING HER FEAR AND ANXIETY IN CRITICAL SITUATIONS ·FOCUS ON INCREASING HER KNOWLEDGE OF THE DISEASE PROCESS AND ON DEVELOPING EFFECTIVE METHODS TO COPE WITH LONE-LINESS AND UNSTRUC-TURED TIME PERIODS	−WITHIN 5 WEEKS, JANA WILL DEMONSTRATE AN ABILITY TO IMPLEMENT COPING BEHAVIORS (OUTLINED ON PAGE 264) IN AN EFFORT TO REDUCE THE RISK OF BINGING AND VOMITING WITHOUT STAFF REINFORCEMENT −WITHIN 5 WEEKS, HER EATING HABITS WILL BEGIN TO NORMALIZE −SHE WILL BE ABLE TO USE ANXIETY RATING SCALE AND	2/5 JE

Nursing diagnosis	Nursing intervention	Predicted outcome/short-term goals (include time frame)	Date/signature
	—FOR HER BINGING AND VOMITING: ·TEACH HER TO MAKE DAILY ENTRIES ON A DAILY INTAKE SHEET (PAGE 276). EXPLAIN THAT SHE IS TO MAKE AN ENTRY BEFORE EACH MEAL AND IS TO EAT REGARDLESS OF HER LEVEL OF ANXIETY. INSTRUCT HER TO CONTACT STAFF SHOULD HER ANXIETY LEVEL BE BETWEEN 4 AND 7 · INSTRUCT HER TO SELF-RATE HER ANXIETY AFTER EVERY MEAL OR SNACK AND RECORD IMMEDIATELY THE EX- PERIENCE OF EATING: ANXIETY LEVEL BEFORE EATING, WHAT SHE CONSUMED, ANXIETY LEVEL AFTER EATING, ANY THOUGHTS OF VOMITING (SEE PAGE 274 FOR A SAMPLE EATING JOURNAL CHART). IF SHE VOMITS EVEN AFTER THE HOUR RE- STRICTION IN THE DAY- ROOM, SHE IS TO ALSO RECORD THAT EPISODE WITH ACCOMPANYING FEELINGS, THOUGHTS, AND ANY OTHER COPING SHE MAY HAVE EMPLOYED. SHE IS TO MAKE THESE ENTRIES AFTER EACH MEAL AND HAND IN A COM- PLETED CHART AT THE END OF EACH DAY ·ENSURE THAT STAFF MEETS WITH JANA AT THE END OF EACH SHIFT TO REVIEW HER DAILY INTAKE SHEET. THIS REVIEW SHOULD INCLUDE AN EVALUATION OF ITS COMPLETENESS (WITH A	IMPLEMENT A PLAN TO CONTROL IMPULSES FOR SELF-HARM, WITHIN 2 WEEKS	

Continued

Nursing Care Plan *continued*

Nursing diagnosis	Nursing intervention	Predicted outcome/short-term goals (include time frame)	Date/signature
	DISCUSSION OF ANY IN-COMPLETENESS AND OF THE REASONS BEHIND IT); A REVIEW OF ALL MEAL TIMES; POSITIVE REINFORCEMENT FOR EATING APPROPRIATE AMOUNTS AS PRESCRIBED BY THE DIETICIAN; POSITIVE REINFORCE-MENT OF HER ATTEMPTS AT IDENTIFYING LEVELS OF ANXIETY AND EM-PLOYING APPROPRIATE COPING STRATEGIES;		
	AND AN EXPLORATION OF ANY BINGING AND VOMITING OR VOMITING AFTER EATING REGULAR AMOUNTS OF FOOD, FO-CUSING ON POSSIBLE PRECIPITANTS TO OVER-WHELMING ANXIETY AND REASONS FOR HER FAILURE TO IMPLE-MENT COPING STRATE-GIES		
	·REINFORCE THE DIETI-CIAN'S TEACHING ON NUTRITIONAL NEEDS AND CALORIC REQUIREMENTS AND EVALUATE HER LEVEL OF LEARNING. (JANA HAS CONTRACTED TO EAT A TOTAL OF 2500 CALORIES A DAY, APPROXIMATELY 840 CALORIES A MEAL. EACH MEAL IS PREARRANGED AND ITS CALORIES ARE RECORDED ON A PAPER FOR HER TO SEE AT EACH MEAL TIME) ·WEIGH HER EVERY OTHER DAY IN THE MORN-ING AFTER VOIDING AND BEFORE BREAKFAST AND DRESSED IN THE SAME CLOTHING. HAVE HER RECORD HER WEIGHT AND HER CALORIC RECORD ON TWO GRAPHS OPENLY DISPLAYED ON HER DESK OR BULLETIN BOARD THIS WILL HELP	JANA WILL CONSUME 840 CALORIES PER MEAL, 2,500 CALORIES PER DAY	

Nursing diagnosis	Nursing intervention	Predicted outcome/short-term goals (include time frame)	Date/signature
	HER VISUALIZE HER PRO-GRESS, WHICH IN TURN WILL REINFORCE APPRO-PRIATE CONTROLS OF NORMAL EATING AND MAINTENANCE OF AP-PROPRIATE WEIGHT ·REVIEW THE PATHO-PHYSIOLOGICAL AND PSYCHOLOGICAL EFFECTS OF CHRONIC BINGING, VOMITING, AND LAXA-TIVE AND DIURETIC A-BUSE, GASTRIC DILATION, ESOPHAGEAL BLEEDING, TOOTH EROSION, SEVERE METABOLIC DISTUR-BANCES OVERWHELMING ANXIETY, PANIC, LOSS OF CONTROL, AND SEVERE SELF-INCRIMINATION ·EMPHASIZE OTHER APPROPRIATE METHODS OF WEIGHT CONTROL, SUCH AS EXERCISE. EN-COURAGE HER TO DEVEL-OP AN EXERCISE PLAN IN COORDINATION WITH THE RECREATION THERAPIST		
POTENTIAL FOR SELF-HARM RELATED TO PAST HISTORY AND EFFECTS OF DEPRESSION	—FOR SELF-MUTILATION AND SUICIDE ATTEMPTS: ·OBTAIN HER AGREE-MENT TO FOLLOW THROUGH ON THE PLAN FOR IMPULSE CONTROL AND TO NOT HARM HER-SELF WHILE IN THE HOSPITAL ·IF SHE EXPRESSES THOUGHTS OF SELF-HARM, STRONGLY ENCOURAGE HER TO VENTILATE FEEL-INGS OF FEAR, ANGER, AND ANXIETY. HELP HER EXTERNALIZE THESE FEELINGS THROUGH VER-BALIZATION AND TO USE COPING MEASURES TO GIVE HER DISTANCE AND TO INTERRUPT THE POTENTIAL FOR SELF-HARM. EMPHA-SIZE STRONGLY THAT	—JANA WILL NOT HARM SELF WHILE IN HOSPITAL	2/5 JE

Continued

Nursing Care Plan *continued*

Nursing diagnosis	Nursing intervention	Predicted outcome/short-term goals (include time frame)	Date/signature
	SHE SHOULD NOT ISO-LATE HERSELF IN HER ROOM, AS THAT ONLY SERVES TO INCREASE POTENTIAL FOR UNPRE-DICTABILITY. FINALLY, INSTRUCT HER TO RATE HER ANXIETY LEVEL WHEN SHE HAS THOUGHTS OF SELF-HARM, AND TO FOLLOW THROUGH ON THE APPROPRIATE INTERVEN-TION FOR HER RATING		
	—FOR SOCIAL ISOLATION: ·STRONGLY ENCOURAGE HER TO PARTICIPATE IN ALL SCHEDULED ACTIV-ITIES	—SHE WILL BECOME MORE SPONTANEOUS IN INITIATING ACTIVITIES WITH PEERS AND OTHER CLIENTS IN 3 WEEKS	
	·OBSERVE HER FOR PARTICIPATION AND THE QUALITY OF ENGAGE-MENT WITH OTHERS. IF SHE PERSISTS IN WITH-DRAWING, PROMPT HER TO BECOME MORE IN-VOLVED. BRIEFLY EX-PLORE ANY RESISTANCE/RELUCTANCE TO PARTI-CIPATION		
	·OBSERVE WHETHER SHE INITIATES ANY CONVERSATIONS OR AC-TIVITIES WITH PEERS. WHEN SHE INITIATES, GIVE MUCH POSITIVE REINFORCEMENT		
	—FOR ALCOHOL ABUSE: ·CONFRONT AND EXPLORE HER ALCOHOL ABUSE IN SESSIONS. STRESS THE PART THAT ALCOHOL PLAYS IN HER LACK OF CONTROL OVER BINGING AND VOMITING AND ALSO, MORE IMPORTANT-LY, IN HER LETHALITY. DISCUSS THE CONTROL SHE CAN EXERT OVER HER DESIRE TO DRINK BY PARTICIPATION IN ALCOHOLICS ANONY-MOUS (AA), BY RECOG-NIZING AND DEALING WITH THE ANXIETY THAT PRECIPITATES	—WITHIN 5 WEEKS, JANA WILL BE MORE OPEN TO TALKING ABOUT ALCOHOL ABUSE AND WILL ATTEND AN AA MEETING	

Nursing diagnosis	Nursing intervention	Predicted outcome/short-term goals (include time frame)	Date/signature
	HER DRINKING, AND BY USING THE COPING STRATEGIES SHE HAS LEARNED		
	·TO ENSURE HER EX- POSURE TO AA, GRANT HER UNSUPERVISED TIME OFF THE UNIT TO ATTEND DAILY AA MEETINGS		
	—FOR HER INABILITY TO ASK FOR HELP:		
	·WHEN SHE DOES FOL- LOW THROUGH ON PLAN FOR IMPULSE CONTROL AND SEEKS STAFF AS- SISTANCE, CONTINUE		
	TO PROVIDE MUCH POS- ITIVE REINFORCEMENT		
	·HOWEVER, CONFRONT SUCH PASSIVE BEHAVIOR AND EXPLORE ITS POS- SIBLE MEANING (e.g., "COULD YOU POSSIBLY BE ANGRY AT THE STAFF, AND THIS IS A WAY FOR YOU TO GAIN ATTENTION?")		
	—FOR UNSTRUCTURED TIME, HELP HER DEVEL- OP AND INITIATE A PLAN OF ACTIVITIES FOR HER EVENING HOURS. INSTRUCT HER TO USE THE ANXIETY RATING SCALE EVERY HOUR FROM 4 P.M. TO BED- TIME, AND TO RECORD THE RESULTS IN HER JOURNAL. ALSO ENCOUR- AGE HER TO BEGIN DE- VELOPING A PLAN FOR HER UNSTRUCTURED TIME OUTSIDE THE HOSPITAL IN PREPAR- ATION FOR DISCHARGE		
	—ENCOURAGE JANA TO USE THE FOLLOWING COPING ACTIVITIES (WHICH SHE SELECTED), AS INDICATED BY HER LEVEL OF ANXIETY:		
	·RELAXATION AND CLASSICAL MUSIC TAPES		
	·TABLE GAMES		
	·STATIONARY BICYCLE		

Continued

Nursing Care Plan *continued*

Nursing diagnosis	Nursing intervention	Predicted outcome/short-term goals (include time frame)	Date/signature
	· RUG HOOKING · READING · OCCUPATIONAL THER- APY PROJECTS · COLLAGE WITH USE OF MAGAZINE PICTURES · TIME OFF THE UNIT TO RUN AT THE TRACK		
ALTERED SELF-ESTEEM RE-LATED TO DIS-TORTED PER-CEPTIONS OF HERSELF AND DEPRESSION SECONDARY TO BULIMIA	— HELP JANA DEVELOP AN IMPROVED SELF-CON-CEPT THROUGH CONFRON-TATION OF DISTORTED THINKING, ENCOURAGE-MENT OF INDEPENDENT BEHAVIORS, STRUCTUR-ING OF CORRECTIVE EMOTIONAL EXPERI-ENCES, AND ASSERTIVE-NESS TRAINING — DEAL WITH HER VER-BALIZATION OF DIS-TORTED BODY IMAGE IN A SUPPORTIVE AND NONTHREATENING MANNER. EXPLORE FEARS THAT GIVE BIRTH TO THE DISTOR-TIONS, THEN TEST THE REALITY OF HER PER-CEPTIONS; i.e., THAT SHE IS NOT OBESE AND ACTUALLY IS AT AN APPROPRIATE WEIGHT. FOCUS PRIMARILY ON FEELINGS AND IDEAS OF SELF AND HOW SHE IS CONSUMED WITH WEIGHT AS PART OF HER SELF-ESTEEM. — FOR ANY VERBALIZA-TION OF SELF-IN-CRIMINATING IDEAS, INTERVENE IN THE SAME WAY. FOCUS ON HER FEELINGS OF IN-ADEQUACY; ENCOURAGE HER TO IDENTIFY HER POSITIVE BEHAVIORS THAT CONTRIBUTE TO HER WELL-BEING AND COMFORT. COLLABORATE WITH OTHER STAFF TO PROVIDE CORRECTIVE EXPERIENCES THAT AL-	— WITHIN 1 MONTH, JANA WILL BEGIN TO PERCEIVE HER PRESENT BODY WEIGHT AS NORMAL — WITHIN 1 MONTH, SHE WILL DEMONSTRATE LESS SELF-NEGATION AND BEGIN TO DEMONSTRATE SIGNS OF A MORE POSITIVE SELF-IMAGE BY VERBALIZING HER POSI-TIVE ACTIONS — SHE WILL DEMONSTRATE THE ABILITY TO ARRIVE AT OTHER WAYS OF PERCEIVING A POTENTIALLY THREATENING SITUATION WITHIN 1 MONTH — SHE WILL SEEK LESS STAFF APPROVAL AND DIRECT GUID-ANCE AND BE ABLE TO SET REALISTIC GOALS ON HER OWN IN 3 WEEKS — SHE WILL BEGIN TO DEMON-STRATE THE ABILITY TO UNDERSTAND ANGER AND EX-PRESS HERSELF ASSERTIVELY IN 1 MONTH — WITHIN 1 MONTH, SHE WILL SHOW MORE INTEREST IN PREVIOUSLY ENJOYED LEISURE ACTIVITIES AS EVIDENCED BY PARTICIPATING IN ONE PROJECT PER WEEK — HER MOOD AND ENERGY LEVEL WILL IMPROVE WITHIN 3 WEEKS AS EVIDENCED BY MORE SPONTANEOUS COMMUNICATION AND LESS ISOLATION	2/5 JE

Nursing diagnosis	Nursing intervention	Predicted outcome/short-term goals (include time frame)	Date/signature
	LOW HER TO SUCCEED AND GAIN A SENSE OF SATISFACTION AND PLEASURE		
	— INSTRUCT HER THAT EX-CEPT FOR SEEKING STAFF HELP WHEN FEELING IM-PULSIVE, AT ALL OTHER TIMES SHE IS TO PROBLEM-SOLVE AND MAKE DE-CISIONS ON HER OWN. SHE SHOULD INVOLVE		
	STAFF ONLY AFTER SHE HAS ARRIVED AT A SATISFACTORY CONCLU-SION FOR HER PROBLEMS OR GOALS. STAFF WILL LISTEN ONLY, AND WILL NOT BECOME A PART OF THE PROBLEM-SOLVING PROCESS BUT RATHER WILL ENCOUR-AGE HER OWN THINKING, AND REINFORCE HER FEELINGS OF SATISFAC-TION WHEN SHE DOES SO SUCCESSFULLY		
	— HOLD DAILY 20-MIN-UTE SESSIONS TO DEAL WITH FEELINGS, ESPECIALLY ANGER. REFLECT UPON AND DISCUSS HER RESPONSES TO ANXIETY AND SUB-SEQUENT MALADAP-TIVE COPING. ENCOUR-AGE HER TO IDENTIFY SITUATIONS THAT CAUSE INCREASED ANX-IETY AND ANGRY FEEL-INGS THAT RESULT FROM UNRESOLVED SITUATIONS. POINT OUT HOW ANGER IS MAIN-TAINED IF NOT EX-PRESSED IN AN AP-PROPRIATE, EXTERNAL MANNER AND THE SENSE OF POWERLESS-NESS THAT ALSO EN-SUES. MAKE THE CON-NECTION BETWEEN IN-WARDLY TURNED AN-GER AND HER BINGING, VOMITING, AND SELF-		

Continued

Nursing Care Plan *continued*

Nursing diagnosis	Nursing intervention	Predicted outcome/short-term goals (include time frame)	Date/signature
	MUTILATION. TEACH HER MORE EFFECTIVE METHODS OF HANDL-ING ANGER THROUGH ROLE-MODELING AND THE USE OF ASSER-TIVENESS TRAINING TECHNIQUES		
	- STRONGLY ENCOURAGE HER TO PARTICIPATE IN PREVIOUSLY ENJOYED ACTIVITIES WHILE IN THE HOSPITAL. RE-ASSURE HER THAT AS HER MOOD IMPROVES AND ENERGY INCREASES, SHE WILL DEVELOP MORE SPONTANEOUS INTEREST IN THESE ACTIVITIES		
ALTERED THOUGHT PRO-CESSES RELATED TO NEGATIVE COGNITIVE SET SECONDARY TO DISEASE PROCESS	- PERFORM REALITY-TEST-ING WHEN JANA BEGINS TO EXPERIENCE AND VERBALIZE DELUSIONS. ENCOURAGE HER TO START PRACTICING SIMI-LAR TESTING ON HER OWN AND REPORT THE RESULTS TO STAFF. CON-STANTLY EDUCATE HER ON REALITY AND CON-TRAST IT WITH UNREAL-ITY OF WHAT SHE IS EX-PERIENCING. ASSESS FOR IMPULSIVITY AND INTER-VENE ACCORDINGLY, AS PREVIOUSLY OUTLINED - IN AND OUTSIDE OF SESSIONS, STRONGLY ENCOURAGE HER TO EX-AMINE OTHER PERCEP-TIONS OF A VULNERABLE SITUATION, AND PROB-LEM-SOLVE FOR OTHER POSSIBLE ALTERNATE WAYS OF THINKING AND REACTING. PROVIDE FREQUENT POSITIVE REINFORCEMENT. ENCOURAGE HER SELF-ASSESSMENT RELATED TO BEHAVIOR WITH OTHERS IN THE MILIEU - DO REALITY TESTING	- JANA WILL BE ABLE TO RECOGNIZE DELUSIONS VS. REALITY WITHIN 3 WEEKS - HER REFERENTIAL THINKING WILL DECREASE IN 3 WEEKS - WITHIN 3 WEEKS, HER CAPA-BILITY FOR EXPANSIVE THINKING WILL INCREASE AS EVIDENCED BY PROBLEM-SOLVING AT LEAST ONE HYPOTHETICAL SITUATION	2/5 JE

Nursing diagnosis	Nursing intervention	Predicted outcome/short-term goals (include time frame)	Date/signature
	WHEN SHE REPORTS IN-CREASED REFERENTIAL THINKING		
	-ASSESS JANA FOR IMPUL-SIVITY WHEN SHE'S EXPER-IENCING DISSOCIATIVE EPISODES; INTERVENE ACCORDINGLY, AS PREVI-OUSLY DESCRIBED. DURING THESE EPISODES, OBSERVE CAREFULLY AND EMPLOY PRECAUTIONS FOR SELF-MUTILATIVE BEHAVIOR		

EATING JOURNAL CHART

Date & Time	What was happening before the binge	Binge foods eaten and quantity	Where eaten

Others present	Consequences: feelings & thoughts after binging	Amount of time after binge to vomit	Consequences: thoughts & feelings after vomiting

DAILY INTAKE SHEET

Date: _____

a. Breakfast _____   Calories _____   oz _____
_____   _____   _____
_____   _____   _____

*Fluids _____   _____   _____
b. Snack (midmorn) _____   _____   _____
_____   _____   _____

*Fluids _____   _____   _____
c. Lunch _____   _____   _____
_____   _____   _____
_____   _____   _____

*Fluids _____   _____   _____
d. Snack (afternoon) _____   _____   _____
_____   _____   _____

e. Dinner _____   _____   _____
_____   _____   _____
_____   _____   _____
_____   _____   _____

*Fluids _____   _____   _____
f. Snack (evening) _____   _____   _____
_____   _____   _____

*Fluids _____   _____   _____
Additional foods _____   _____   _____
_____   _____   _____
_____   _____   _____

*Additional fluids _____   _____   _____
_____   _____   _____
_____   _____   _____

     Total _____   Total _____

Comments/Questions _____
_____
_____

        Primary Nurse's Initials _____
Please turn in on completion   Physician's Initials _____

*Note—If help is required with fluid calculation, contact assigned nursing staff.

Jana admitted that her suicidal attempt was serious and her behavior was out of control. She had difficulty recognizing the contribution of alcohol use to her depression and denied that she was an alcoholic.

SUMMARY

Over Jana's 10-week course of hospitalization, her mood and affect improved markedly, and her health problems—hypovolemia and hypokalemia, muscle cramping, cardiopathy, dehydration, vertigo, and chronic fatigue—diminished significantly. Nursing interventions focused on monitoring vital signs, educating her on the importance of adequate hydration, and preventing her from vomiting after potassium administration. Jana seemed to do well with self-checks around the hydration schedule, which provided her with some responsibility for her own care. Her sleep improved moderately, increasing from 3 hours to 5 hours per night. She acknowledged deriving some benefit from use of the relaxation tapes in falling asleep.

Jana required intensive intervention in the areas of impulse control, coping, and her distorted self-image. The proposed and implemented behavioral interventions for these problems necessitated continuous reinforcement from the nursing staff.

Regarding Jana's dysfunction in fear, anxiety, and coping, she initially was unable or unwilling to follow through on utilizing the anxiety rating scale, contacting staff, and implementing preplanned coping strategies in an effort to decrease the potential for impulsive actions. Consequently, the primary and associate nurses concentrated their efforts towards establishing a strong therapeutic and supportive relationship with her in order to engage her in the attempt to follow-through on proposed interventions designed to interrupt the vicious cycle of impulsive, destructive behavior. Other staff members caring for Jana needed to be apprised of all aspects of care so that consistency and clarity could be maintained in the absence of the primary and associate nurses.

During the course of her care, Jana experienced three panic attacks in immediate response to an explosive family meeting, a case conference, and the anticipation of a preplanned home visit with her mother. Twice, she had scratched her wrists with a paper clip and reported the incidents after the fact instead of contacting staff before acting upon her feelings. At these times, she was assessed as being in a dissociative state and possibly in need of antianxiety or neuroleptic medication. Staff repeatedly reinforced the fact that she need only to come immediately to them when she felt out of control, and that by not doing so, she was putting herself at risk for self-injury and demonstrating to the staff that she was not learning how to successfully interrupt the self-destructive process. In another incident, she had revealed to staff a plan to ingest insecticide while on a pass to visit her mother. She did not carry out this plan but once again had not sought help when the increased anxiety and self-incriminating ideation first appeared. These two incidents of self-destructive behavior required implementation of direct supervision in day-room restriction, followed by the self-monitoring as outlined in the nursing care plan. During the remainder of her stay, Jana would admit to daily thoughts of being "gone" but did not act-out with any further self-mutilation.

The anxiety rating scale proved very helpful in improving Jana's coping skills. Whenever she appeared anxious or verbalized anxiety, and even often when she seemed calm, the primary and associate nurses would inquire as to her self-rating of anxiety. This encouraged her constant awareness of feeling states and supported the implementation of preplanned coping strategies. While this strategy may be seen to foster dependency, in reality it served to give a strong message to Jana as to the importance of interrupting the cycle of impulsive acting-out. The continuous use of reinforcement is a sound behavioral concept utilized when first establishing newly learned behaviors. This is usually followed by use of intermittent reinforcement, which fosters generalization of the new behaviors. Jana openly stated liking the anxiety rating scale; it helped her reduce her fears of feeling anxious.

Regarding her impulsive behavior of vomiting, Jana experienced extreme difficulty in following through on contacting staff. Initially, she claimed she was not vomiting and stated that she "absolutely" would not allow herself to do so. This again demonstrated her "all-or-nothing" mode of thinking and reacting. After initiation of once-a-week intensive family meetings and her dietary plan, her vomiting commenced, occurring once or twice a day. This continued for 2½ weeks, even with the hourly restriction after mealtimes. In essence, Jana was refusing to follow through with contacting staff. After being confronted about this behavior and the meaning behind it (which staff interpreted as ambivalence in changing her maladaptive behavior), she was able to engage in exploration of her ambivalence and, with much prompting and support, express some feelings. During the remainder of her hospitalization, she vomited only three times.

For most bulimics, the vomiting behavior is an old and ingrained way of coping and the most difficult to give up. After discharge, vomiting typically resumes to a frequency equal to that before admission. This behavior, often interpreted as a response to discharge anxiety, must be examined during discharge planning to stress and reinforce the implementation of new coping skills.

With regard to her alcohol abuse, Jana would not admit to alcoholism. She viewed the wine she drank at night as her "friend" and would not concur with the idea that drinking only served to increase her impulsivity. She was encouraged to attend Alcoholic Anonymous (AA) meetings, but refused. Because of this overt denial, she was not granted any pass time by herself; she was told of the reason for this action.

In addition to the coping strategies for containment of impulsivity described above, other coping mechanisms were introduced to Jana in an effort to increase her sense of power and control. Particular emphasis was placed on learning appropriate dietary measures with regard to her weight. Although weight gain was not an issue with Jana, she needed to learn ways to control her weight other than vomiting and food restriction. A number of appropriate methods of controlling weight were identified and explored. While she implemented some of them (such as increasing exercise during recreational therapy, asking staff for permission to go out for walks, and using a stationary bicycle), her actual level of internalization of these strategies was in question.

The most difficult area to deal with was Jana's altered self-esteem. She presented with a gross body image disturbance, extreme self-incrimination, and a poor ability to identify and express her feelings, particularly anger. But as therapy continued, she expressed an increasing desire to meet with staff to talk about her fears. These meetings provided the staff with an excellent opportunity to encourage her to verbalize her distorted thoughts and subsequently to identify accompanying feelings of fear and anxiety. Consequently, staff was able to develop interventions to confront her distortions in a supportive way so as not to arouse defensiveness. Interventions included self-reality testing, introduced in an effort to provide her with a new perspective. Of course, the more complex issues of body image and weight concerns necessitate long-term therapeutic effort. She did appear to handle anxious situations better toward the end of hospitalization.

The remaining problem area involved her thought processes. Her "all-or-nothing" thinking was assessed to be a definite contributor to her impulsivity. In one-to-one sessions, when presented with a situation to which she reacted in a singular, inflexible way, staff attempted to get her to examine other possible ways of thinking and then reacting. But although she was amenable to discussing this problem and the proposed alternative behaviors, she infrequently practiced what was proposed. She was, however, able to report her ambivalence with implementation to staff, thus leaving open the opportunity to continue exploring her problem and supporting any progress.

In terms of accomplishing discharge goals, by discharge the staff felt that Jana had progressed in self-control and coping so as to reduce her impulsivity, which decreased the threat to her life. But more importantly, they felt that she was finally beginning to learn different ways of thinking about herself and to assume more appropriate control over her feelings.

REFERENCES

Johnson, C. "Family Characteristics of Bulimic and Normal Women: A Comparative Study," Unpublished data, 1984.

Wilson, C.P., and Mintz, I. "Anorexia and Bulimia in Anorexia Nervosa. A Study of Psycho-Social Functioning and Associated Psychiatric Symptomatology," *British Journal of Psychiatry* 146:648-52, 1985.

SELECTED BIBLIOGRAPHY

American Psychiatric Association. *Diagnostic and Statistical Manual,* 3rd ed. Washington, D.C.: American Psychiatric Association, 1980.

Bardwick, J. *Psychology of Women: A Study of Biocultural Conflicts.* New York: Harper & Row Publishers, 1971.

Bruch, H. "Anorexia Nervosa: Therapy and Theory," *American Journal of Psychiatry* 139(12):1531-38, 1982.

Casper, R.C. "Hypothalmic Dysfunction and Symptoms of Anorexia Nervosa," *Psychiatric Clinics of North America* 201-204, June, 1984.

Garfinkel, P.E., et al. "The Heterogeneity of Anorexia Nervosa: Bulimia as a Distinct Subgroup," *Archives of General Psychiatry* 3:1030-39, 1980.

Garner, D.M., et al. "Clinical Comparison Between Bulimia in Anorexia and Bulimia in Normal-Weight Women," *Report of the Fourth Ross Conference on Medical Research,* 6-11, 1983.

Gwirtsman, H.E., et al. "Constructing an Inpatient Treatment Program for Bulimia," Study at National Institutes of Mental Health, Bethesda, Md., 1985.

Hubert, J.L. "Bulimic Syndrome at Normal Body Weight: Reflection on Pathogenesis and Clinical Features," *International Journal of Eating Disorders* 2:59-66, 1982-1983.

Johnson, C.L. Bulimia: "A Descriptive Survey of 316 Cases," *International Journal of Eating Disorders* 2:3-16, 1982.

Johnson, C.L., and Hagman, J. "The Syndrome of Bulimia: Review and Synthesis," *Psychiatric Clinics of North America* 7(2):247-70, 1984.

Keltner, N.L. "Bulimia: Controlling Compulsive Eating," *Journal of Psycho-Social Nursing* 22(8):24-29, 1984.

Lehmann, A. "Emancipation by Emaciation," *The Canadian Nurse* 78(10):31-33, 1982.

Marks, R.G. "Anorexia and Bulimia: Eating Habits That Can Kill," *RN* 44-47, January 1984.

Mars, D., et al. "Anorexia Nervosa: A Disorder with Severe Acid-Base Derangements," *Southern Medical Journal* 1038-1042, September 1982.

Potts, N.L. "Eating Disorders: The Secret Pattern of Binge and Purge," *American Journal of Nursing* 32-34, January 1984.

Russel, G. "Bulimia Nervosa," *Psychological Medicine* 9:429-48, 1979.

Savage, M.S. "Bulimia Nervosa," *Nursing Times,* 43-45, August 1984.

Visselman, J.O., and Roig, M. "Depression and Suicidality in Eating Disorders," *Journal of Clinical Psychiatry* 46(4):118-22, 1985.

Wilson, C.P., and Mintz, I. "Abstaining and Bulimic Anorexics: Two Sides of the Same Coin," *Primary Care* 9:517-30, 1982.

Martin:
Substance Abuse

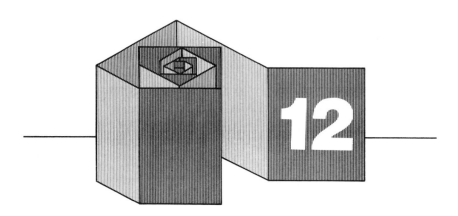

Deidre O'Connor Rea, MSN, RN

As this case study illustrates, the client with a substance abuse problem invariably demonstrates maladaptive coping styles. Many times, depression or feelings of inadequacy underlie the primary substance abuse disorder. When caring for such a client, the nurse must work carefully to uncover the source of and encourage the expression of inadequate, hopeless, and helpless feelings and to introduce new, more effective coping strategies. With the help of interested and supportive family members, the client is usually able to reenter society with adequate therapeutic follow-up, such as individual therapy in conjunction with attendance of support groups such as Alcoholics Anonymous, Narcotics Anonymous, and Alanon.

CASE STUDY

This was the second psychiatric hospitalization for Martin, a 28-year-old married, white, Protestant male of English and German descent. Martin had a G.E.D. and worked as a machinist at a local factory. He lived with his wife of 7 years, Patricia, a high school graduate and a secretary.

During his admission interview, Martin dated the onset of his current difficulties to approximately 2 months prior to hospitalization, when he began having increasing conflicts with his wife concerning his drug use. At that time, he had decided to try to sell heroin and cocaine to earn extra money. But far from making money, he found he was using most of the drugs himself. He estimated his daily substance use at approximately $150 worth of cocaine, $100 worth of heroine, varying amounts of marijuana, and two six-packs of beer, with an occasional dose of diazepam (Valium) to "take the edge off the crash." He also smoked two to three packs of cigarettes per day. In general, his standard method of drug use involved intravenous injection of a heroin and cocaine mixture (known as a "speedball"), although he also often engaged in "freebasing" (smoking refined cocaine) to energize himself.

During the course of the previous 2 months, Martin had used up the couple's entire savings on drug purchases and then began stopping at his company's credit union to extract small loans that he spent on drugs. As his drug use increased, his work functioning deteriorated; he was often late for work, missed days due to drug intoxication, and made an increasing number of mistakes due to being "high" while operating the machinery. Patricia finally became aware of the extent of Martin's drug use only after attempting to make a bank withdrawal and finding their savings account empty. At first extremely angry, she then became frightened and worried after Martin fell asleep at the stove while cooking. Martin's work supervisor also initially expressed concern for Martin's changing behavior but eventually threatened to fire him if he did not seek help.

Martin continued to deny that he had a drug problem until he was stopped by the police for erratic driving. Found with cocaine in his car, he was charged with driving while intoxicated (DWI) and with possession of a controlled substance. Upon learning of the arrest, Patricia threatened to leave Martin unless he sought treatment for his addiction. Martin finally agreed to attend a drug program, but only if Patricia did the work to find him one. After visiting several hospitals, he chose the program he thought would be the fastest and easiest to complete.

Martin had a previous history of psychiatric treatment. His first contact occurred at age 7, when he was taken to a psychiatrist for evaluation of his hyperactive behavior. He was begun on methylphenidate (Ritalin) at an unknown dosage and maintained on this medication for approximately 3 years with good effect. Previously distractable and unable to sit still, he ultimately was able to focus on schoolwork and eventually to transfer out of his special education classes.

Martin started using street drugs at age 12; his use escalated steadily until he required hospitalization at age 19. He was admitted to a 28-day program for detoxification from glutethimide (Doriden) and codeine and completed the treatment program. He did not take the program seriously, however, and returned to drug use the day after discharge. Not wishing to be drug-free, he was noncompliant with all aspects of his aftercare.

Martin's developmental history contained numerous medical, behavioral, and substance abuse problems. He was the product of an unwanted pregnancy that his mother attempted to end by taking "morning after" pills of unknown type and dosage. His mother took Valium and drank alcohol throughout much of her pregnancy, fell twice, and ultimately became toxemic. Her labor with Martin lasted 22 hours, and delivery was finally achieved with the use of high and low forceps.

As a neonate, Martin had both crying and eating difficulties and was overly responsive to both light and sound. Because he was "hyperactive" as a toddler, his mother would often put opium tincture (Paregoric) in his bottle to "slow him down." He contracted all the usual childhood illnesses and also developed croup at age 3. Although he developed a 104° F. fever with associated febrile convulsions, he was not hospitalized for croup. He denied any hospitalizations for medical purposes, except for a tonsillectomy at age 7. He was highly accident-prone as a child and sustained numerous head injuries with concussions. He actually lost consciousness on two occasions—once as the result of an automobile accident sustained while "high" and again from a blow on the head with a lead pipe received while attempting a drug sale.

At age 12, Martin began using dextroamphetamine (Dexedrine), which was prescribed by his doctor for weight control. He continued to take this medication for 5 years, and began abusing it by age 14. By age 14, he had also begun using marijuana; by age 19, he had used amyl nitrate, volatile solvents, hallucinogens, oral and injectable opioids, methaqualone (Quaaludes), and other barbiturates/sedative-hypnotics. His alcohol use included a minimum of a case of beer and up to a fifth of bourbon per weekend. Although he often had blackouts, he never experienced delirium tremens. At the time of admission, he presented with a skin abscess in the left antecubital space secondary to use of an unsterilized needle for drug injection.

Martin reached most developmental milestones on time with the exception of speech, which was delayed until age 3. A hyperkinetic child, he was difficult to care for as he required constant observation and attention. His childhood was marked by abnormal behaviors: destroying his clothes and toys; displaying fidgety, distractible behavior with poor attention and concentration; engaging in frequent temper tantrums and fights; and remaining unresponsive to discipline. He was enuretic until age 8 and also set many fires, including one at his school for which he was expelled. He loved animals and was never cruel to them. (During his interview, he actually related that he preferred animals to people.)

Martin began kindergarten at age 5. While school staff recommended he be held back a year because of his immaturity, his mother enrolled him anyway in order to allow herself a break from his behavior at home. In his early grammar school years, he rapidly developed into a highly disruptive "class clown." During one of their many parent-teacher conferences in the second grade, Martin's teacher recommended to Martin's mother that Martin see a psychiatrist to obtain treatment for hyperkinesis. Following through on this recommendation, Martin was begun on Ritalin. The effect of the medication was positive, allowing him several uneventful years during which he was able to achieve As and Bs in his schoolwork.

By age 11, Martin had gained a considerable amount of weight. With both his parents drinking heavily, many household responsibilities—including cooking meals—fell to him. He never felt as if he had a relationship with his parents, as he never saw them sober. At night, alone in his room, he would hear them arguing about finances and the children and occasionally engaging in physical abuse. Food became an easy solace, and Martin ate almost constantly. This led to obesity, for which he received his first prescription for Dexedrine.

Junior high school was a turning point for Martin in terms of his general attitudes. Angry at his life situation, he no longer cared about responsibility. At every opportunity, he engaged in behaviors that were "fun" without considering or caring about the consequences. After being expelled in the eighth grade for setting the classroom on fire, Martin transferred schools. At his new school, he quickly connected socially with people much like himself. He began getting into fights with other students and expanding his drug repertoire, and became increasingly truant from school. By age 15, he had been incarcerated in detention centers three times for vandalism, destruction of public property, and breaking and entering. With his schoolwork having deteriorated to constant Fs, he dropped out of school in the tenth grade on his 16th birthday.

In order to make money to buy drugs, Martin began making street sales for major drug distributors in his area. His criminal activity progressed from misdemeanors to felonies, including two counts of grand larceny for car theft and for stealing a diamond necklace from a jewelry store window. Set up by his friends, Martin was caught by the police and sent to jail where he remained for 8 months. Feeling badly about the charges only because he was caught, Martin nonetheless decided to take advantage of his incarceration. He obtained his G.E.D. and trained in the use of a variety of machines, which provided him with valuable skills. Upon his release, Martin returned almost immediately to drug use. However, his parole officer, recognizing Martin's returning behavioral pattern, was influential in having him admitted to a treatment program for detoxification and rehabilitation. Martin completed the program, but again resumed drug use immediately after discharge.

Martin met Patricia in a bar when he was 20 and she was 18. Their initial contact centered around a drug sale, with Patricia attempting to buy marijuana from him. They began dating and sharing their drug use and married 1 year later, after Patricia believed she might be pregnant. After the marriage, Patricia stopped all her drug use (even though she was not pregnant) and tried to persuade Martin to do the same. But although he greatly reduced his use, he did not stop completely and eventually began lying about the amount and frequency of his use.

At this point, Martin attempted to "settle down" by pursuing a conventional job. His father helped him get a construction job, which he held for 3 years. During this period he was seen as a responsible and reliable employee, and his drug use did not interfere with his job performance. He eventually transferred to another, better-paying job in which he could utilize the specialty skills he had developed in jail. During his interview, Martin stated that he and Patricia could have been financially stable were it not for all the money he spent on drugs. However, he also admitted that, because Patricia's income met their monthly expenses, he felt no need to save his own money.

In terms of the couple's relationship, Martin believed it was stable despite his two extramarital affairs and Patricia's threats to leave him. His own expressed wish was to remain married and improve communication with Patricia so as not to replicate his own parents' relationship.

Martin's family history contained many clues to the origin of his current problems. Martin was born the older of two siblings to a lower-middle class family of English and German extraction. Although his parents divorced, they both lived in the same town as Martin. His father, a vocational school graduate, worked in construction. His mother had an eleventh-grade education and was unemployed. His 26-year-old sister graduated from college, married, and moved across the country. She had one child and was the owner of a small boutique.

Martin's mother, Mrs. Tyson, was an alcoholic who abused Valium for many years. At one point, she was hospitalized for a 5-month treatment program; since that time, she had remained sober and drug-free for the ensuing 9 years. One maternal aunt had a history of Valium abuse, and two maternal cousins had spent time in jail on drug charges. Martin's father was an untreated alcoholic and a diabetic. His paternal grandfather also abused alcohol and died of medical complications of alcoholism. One paternal uncle died of leukemia, and family history was also positive for brain cancer and epilepsy.

During Martin's early years, his family relationships were chaotic and a poor example of what family life should be. Martin often took care of not only his sister, but also his parents. Looking back, Martin's mother admitted that it took Martin's prison term to convince her of the need to seek treatment. After her successful course of treatment, she had spent the last 9 years trying to repair the damage done to herself and her children.

Mrs. Tyson stated that she became pregnant with Martin out of wedlock and tried to end the pregnancy rather than marry Mr. Tyson. When this proved unsuccessful, the couple was married. But the marriage was not a happy one; each partner carried much resentment because of the circumstances surrounding the wedding. After 19 years of disharmony and almost constant intoxication, Mrs. Tyson finally realized that she could not live with her husband and his drinking, and so instituted divorce proceedings. Since the divorce, Martin had gravitated more towards his father, while her daughter became closer to her. Mrs. Tyson remained highly supportive of Martin's treatment, however, and hoped to provide him with a positive example of how a person's life can change for the better.

On formal mental status examination, Martin presented as a casually dressed white male appearing somewhat older than his stated age of 28. He seemed tense, restless, and irritable. He made almost no eye contact throughout the entire interview, and provided only basic factual information in generally underproductive speech. He made several sarcastic comments and expressed annoyance at having to engage in the interview. As the interview progressed, he became progressively more agitated; finally the interview was interrupted so that he could obtain medication for withdrawal symptoms. When the interview resumed, he appeared calmer and was more cooperative; however, he was still fairly guarded and hostile in his presentation. His facial expression was bland, and although his affect was appropriate to the content of the discussion, his range of affect seemed quite constricted. His thinking, while logical, was generally concrete; he denied any hallucinations, delusions, or first-rank Schneiderian criteria (1971). He further denied ever feeling depressed or having any suicidal or homicidal ideation.

Formal cognitive testing revealed that Martin was oriented in four spheres with recent and remote memory essentially intact. His recall was two out of three objects at 5 minutes and was related to his difficulty concentrating and focusing on the task at hand. He performed serial sevens slowly, with multiple mistakes. His digit span was six forward and three backward, and his fund of knowledge was above-average for his educational level. While his similarity responses were fairly abstract, his proverbs were markedly concrete. His responses to social judgment questions indicated an understanding of appropriate social norms, but his initial responses were remarkable for their antisocial tendencies. (For instance, when asked what he would do if he smelled smoke in a crowded movie theatre, Martin responded with a laugh, "I'd go to the nearest exit so I'd be the first one out, then yell 'fire' at the top of my lungs.")

Continued on page 294

RECORDING THE DATA

After you have read the case, cluster significant data into functional health patterns.

Health management/health perception ⸻⸻⸻⸻⸻

⸻⸻⸻⸻⸻⸻⸻⸻

⸻⸻⸻⸻⸻⸻⸻⸻

⸻⸻⸻⸻⸻⸻⸻⸻

⸻⸻⸻⸻⸻⸻⸻⸻

Nutritional/metabolic ⸻⸻⸻⸻⸻⸻

⸻⸻⸻⸻⸻⸻⸻⸻

⸻⸻⸻⸻⸻⸻⸻⸻

⸻⸻⸻⸻⸻⸻⸻⸻

Elimination ⸻⸻⸻⸻⸻⸻⸻

⸻⸻⸻⸻⸻⸻⸻⸻

⸻⸻⸻⸻⸻⸻⸻⸻

⸻⸻⸻⸻⸻⸻⸻⸻

Activity/exercise ⸻⸻⸻⸻⸻⸻⸻

⸻⸻⸻⸻⸻⸻⸻⸻

⸻⸻⸻⸻⸻⸻⸻⸻

⸻⸻⸻⸻⸻⸻⸻⸻

Cognitive/perceptual ⸻⸻⸻⸻⸻⸻

⸻⸻⸻⸻⸻⸻⸻⸻

⸻⸻⸻⸻⸻⸻⸻⸻

⸻⸻⸻⸻⸻⸻⸻⸻

Sleep/rest _____

_____

_____

_____

Self-perception/self-concept _____

_____

_____

_____

Role relationship _____

_____

_____

_____

Sexuality/reproductive _____

_____

_____

_____

Coping/stress tolerance _____

_____

_____

_____

Value/belief _____

_____

_____

_____

ASSIGNING NURSING DIAGNOSES

Use your clustered data to select appropriate nursing diagnoses.

Health perception/health management

- [ ] Growth and Development, Altered (see Developmental Delay)
- [ ] Health Maintenance, Altered
- [ ] Infection, Potential for
- [ ] Injury (Trauma): Potential for
- [ ] Noncompliance (Specify)
- [ ] Poisoning: Potential for
- [ ] Suffocation: Potential for

Nutritional/metabolic

- [ ] Body Temperature, Potential Alteration in
- [ ] Developmental Delay: Physical Growth and Development
- [ ] Fluid Volume, Altered: Excess or Excess Fluid Volume
- [ ] Fluid Volume Deficit, Actual
- [ ] Fluid Volume Deficit, Potential
- [ ] Nutrition, Altered: Less Than Body Requirements or Nutritional Deficit (Specify)
- [ ] Nutrition, Altered: More Than Body Requirements or Exogenous Obesity
- [ ] Nutrition, Altered: Potential for More Than Body Requirements or Potential for Obesity
- [ ] Oral Mucous Membrane, Altered
- [ ] Skin Integrity, Impaired or Skin Breakdown
- [ ] Skin Integrity, Impaired or Potential Skin Breakdown
- [ ] Swallowing, Impaired or Uncompensated Swallowing Impairment
- [ ] Tissue Integrity, Impaired

Elimination

- [ ] Bowel Elimination, Altered: Constipation
- [ ] Bowel Elimination, Altered: Diarrhea
- [ ] Bowel Elimination, Altered: Incontinence

- [ ] Developmental Delay: Bowel/ Bladder Control
- [ ] Incontinence: Functional
- [ ] Incontinence: Reflex
- [ ] Incontinence: Stress
- [ ] Incontinence: Total
- [ ] Incontinence: Urge
- [ ] Urinary Elimination, Altered Patterns of
- [ ] Urinary Retention

Activity/exercise

- [ ] Activity Intolerance
- [ ] Activity Intolerance, Potential
- [ ] Airway Clearance, Ineffective
- [ ] Breathing Pattern, Ineffective
- [ ] Cardiac Output, Altered: Decreased
- [ ] Developmental Delay: Mobility
- [ ] Developmental Delay: Self-Care Skills
- [ ] Diversional Activity Deficit
- [ ] Gas Exchange, Impaired
- [ ] Home Maintenance Management, Impaired (Mild, Moderate, Severe, Potential, Chronic)
- [ ] Mobility, Impaired Physical
- [ ] Self-Care Deficit: Feeding
- [ ] Self-Care Deficit: Bathing/ Hygiene
- [ ] Self-Care Deficit: Dressing/ Grooming
- [ ] Self-Care Deficit: Toileting
- [ ] Self-Care Deficit: Total
- [ ] Tissue Perfusion, Altered: (Specify)

Sleep/rest

- [ ] Sleep Pattern Disturbance

Cognitive/perceptual

- [ ] Comfort, Altered: Pain
- [ ] Comfort, Altered: Chronic Pain

☐ Developmental Delay: (Specify Cognitive Area; attention, decision making, etc.)
☐ Hypothermia
☐ Hyperthermia
☐ Knowledge Deficit (Specify)
☐ Sensory-Perceptual Alteration: Input Excess or Sensory Overload
☐ Sensory-Perceptual Alteration: Input Deficit or Sensory Deprivation
☐ Thermoregulation, Ineffective
☐ Thought Processes, Altered
☐ Unilateral Neglect

Self-perception/self-concept

☐ Anxiety
☐ Body Image Disturbance
☐ Fear
☐ Hopelessness
☐ Personal Identity Confusion
☐ Powerlessness (Severe, Low, Moderate)
☐ Self-Esteem Disturbance

Role relationship

☐ Communication, Impaired Verbal
☐ Developmental Delay: Communication Skills
☐ Developmental Delay: Social Skills
☐ Family Processes, Altered
☐ Grieving, Anticipatory
☐ Grieving, Dysfunctional
☐ Parenting, Altered: Actual or Potential

☐ Role Performance, Disturbance in
☐ Social Interactions, Impaired
☐ Social Isolation (Rejection)

Sexuality/reproductive

☐ Rape-Trauma Syndrome: Compounded
☐ Rape-Trauma Syndrome: Silent Reaction
☐ Sexual Dysfunction
☐ Sexuality Patterns, Altered

Coping/stress tolerance

☐ Adjustment, Impaired
☐ Coping, Ineffective Individual
☐ Coping, Ineffective Family: Compromised
☐ Coping, Ineffective Family: Disabling
☐ Coping, Family: Potential for Growth
☐ Developmental Delay (Specify area)
☐ Post-Trauma Response
☐ Violence, Potential for (Self-Directed or Directed at Others)

Value/belief

☐ Spiritual Distress (Distress of Human Spirit)

You are now ready to develop a nursing care plan for this client. Use the following blank pages to do so. Then refer to the author's formulation, diagnostic summary, care plan, and summary.

NURSING CARE PLAN

Complete the chart below to develop a nursing care plan for this client.

Discharge outcomes/long-term goals	

Nursing diagnosis	Nursing intervention	

	Predicted outcomes/short-term goals (include time frame)	Date/signature

Return to Formulation, page 294

His judgment responses were consistent with the judgment he had used in his own life, and his overall level of insight was limited. At this point, Martin's goals for treatment were unclear but appeared to center around avoiding the consequences for his actions prior to admission.

Reader may now complete Recording the Data, Assigning Nursing Diagnoses, and Nursing Care Plan.

FORMULATION

Martin Tyson presented with a history and symptoms most notable for their chaotic, uncontrolled nature. In terms of his addiction, Martin's substance abuse, for all intents and purposes, extended back to the date of his conception. With a strong genetic loading for substance abuse and an addictive mother who continued to abuse a variety of substances throughout her pregnancy, Martin was born with a predisposition to drug use beyond his control. Through the course of his childhood years, he was maintained on sedatives, followed by Ritalin and then appetite suppressants—lending full support to his growing perception that he needed to rely on external objects to control his inner feelings and drives.

However, while in some ways a learned method of coping, Martin's notion that he needed medication may not have been totally erroneous. Prenatal difficulties and his mother's drug use during the pregnancy, compounded by a difficult forceps delivery, may have produced some cognitive damage by the time of Martin's birth. Further neurological insults in the form of his head injuries, high fevers, seizures, and loss of consciousness could only have served to worsen the situation, possibly resulting in the hyperkinetic behavior and attention deficit disorder apparent in his history. As such, his abilities to focus, attend, problem-solve, and delay gratification were impaired, and he probably *was* in need of medication, albeit of a more appropriate type.

In examining a person's rationale and response to hospitalization, Childress (1970) suggests looking foremost to the person's motivation to change his life. Martin appeared at best ambivalent and at worst frightened of truly facing an addictive life-style. In reviewing his early experiences, illicit drugs provided Martin with the only available mechanism of escape from the feelings aroused by his chaotic family situation, perceived rejection, and his own recognition of his inadequacies. Without drugs, Martin would have to face the many issues he had long been repressing. Because these issues touched the very core of his identity, Martin was necessarily ambivalent about treatment. To overcome this ambivalence, he needed much support, encouragement, and confrontation. Toward this end, the inclusion of the drug-free members of his family on the "treatment team" was an important aspect of his care. Through involvement

Continued on page 302

DIAGNOSTIC SUMMARY FOR MARTIN

Data	Functional health pattern	Nursing diagnosis
—Experiencing discomfort: muscle cramps, restlessness, increased perspiration, chills, and vital sign fluctuations	Cognitive/Perceptual	Altered comfort: pain related to effects of opiate withdrawal secondary to drug abuse
—Complains of difficulty falling asleep, early awakening in morning, awakening during night, restless sleep, and increased irritability	Sleep/Rest	Sleep pattern disturbance related to opiate and cocaine withdrawal secondary to addition
—Exhibits an interruption in skin integrity (abcess), with reddened and inflamed skin surrounding an open, oozing wound	Health Perception/ Health Management	Potential for infection related to possible contagious agents secondary to use of street injectable drugs and presence of abscess
—Expresses a desire to leave treatment quickly —Has failed to make progress in previous therapy —Denies illness —Has a history of noncompliant behavior —Perceives recommended treatment as ineffective	Health Perception/ Health Management	Noncompliance related to failure to adhere to medical regime secondary to denial of disease process
—Denies substance use as a problem —Minimizes use of drugs —Manipulates others to meet needs —Engages in only superficial interactions and relationships —Attempts to gain power and control in treatment setting —Bargains with and splits staff —Lacks adequate coping skills for dealing with stress	Coping/Stress Tolerance	Ineffective individual coping for dependent and manipulative behaviors to meet needs secondary to addictive personality traits
—Expresses growing family conflict due to his drug use —Divorce secondary to substance use of parents —With spouse, engages in inappropriate shared activities	Coping/Stress Tolerance	Ineffective family coping: compromised related to effects and interference of substance use on all family relationships secondary to disease process
—Reports boredom, identifies few interests or skills —Uses drugs for social/ interpersonal and individual leisure pursuits —Displays a need for appropriate leisure-time pursuits postdischarge	Activity/Exercise	Diversional activity deficit related to use of substances as only form of leisure time activity/pursuit secondary to ineffective coping

NURSING CARE PLAN

Complete the chart below to develop a nursing care plan for this client.

Discharge outcome/long-term goals	
1. MARTIN WILL VERBALIZE ABSENCE OF DRUG WITHDRAWAL SYMPTOMS. 2. MARTIN WILL REGULARLY SLEEP 8 HOURS PER NIGHT WITH NO DISTURBANCES.	

Nursing diagnosis	Nursing intervention	Predicted outcome/short-term goals (include time frame)	Date/signature
ALTERED COMFORT: PAIN RELATED TO EFFECTS OF OPIATE WITHDRAWAL SECONDARY TO DRUG ABUSE	–DOCUMENT SIGNS AND SYMPTOMS OF WITHDRAWAL –MONITOR VITAL SIGNS EVERY 4 HOURS –ADMINISTER MEDICATIONS FOR DETOXIFICATION –RESPECT MARTIN'S SUBJECTIVE EXPERIENCE OF DISCOMFORT; DO NOT DEVALUE OR JUDGE HIM –TEACH MARTIN TO CONTROL HIS DISCOMFORT THROUGH RELAXATION TECHNIQUES –SUGGEST COMFORT MEASURES, SUCH AS WARM SHOWERS, HOT CHOCOLATE, REST PERIODS, ETC. –PROVIDE BLANKETS TO KEEP MARTIN WARM –MONITOR MARTIN'S BOWEL AND BLADDER FUNCTION	–WITHIN 1 WEEK, CLIENT WILL VERBALIZE ONSET OF WITHDRAWAL SYMPTOMS AND REQUEST THE NURSE'S ASSISTANCE (i.e., MEDICATION, COMFORT MEASURES) –WITHIN 1 WEEK, MARTIN WILL INITIATE RELAXATION EXERCISES WHEN WITHDRAWAL SYMPTOMS BECOME APPARENT	8/28 dn
SLEEP PATTERN DISTURBANCE RELATED TO OPIATE AND COCAINE WITHDRAWAL SECONDARY TO ADDICTION	–ENCOURAGE MARTIN TO VERBALIZE AND EXPRESS HIS CONCERNS AND FEARS RELATED TO BOTH SLEEP DISTURBANCES AND DRUG WITHDRAWAL –ENCOURAGE HIS PARTICIPATION IN RELAXATION EXERCISES –LIMIT INCREASED PHYSICAL ACTIVITY PRIOR TO BEDTIME (RAISES THE NOREPINEPHRINE LEVEL) –ESTABLISH A BEDTIME ROUTINE; e.g., A WARM BATH, A GLASS OF WARM MILK, ADEQUATE BLANKETS, PILLOWS, AND QUIET TO PROVIDE COMFORT –ADMINISTER MEDICATIONS IF OTHER MEASURES INEFFECTIVE	–WITHIN 2 WEEKS, MARTIN WILL FALL ASLEEP WITHIN 10 MINUTES AFTER GOING TO BED, AND WILL REPORT FEELING RESTED UPON AWAKENING IN THE MORNING	8/28 dn

Discharge outcome/long-term goals			
1. MARTIN'S NEEDLE ABSCESS WILL HEAL COMPLETELY WITHOUT COMPLICATIONS.			

Nursing diagnosis	Nursing intervention	Predicted outcome/short-term goals (include time frame)	Date/signature
POTENTIAL FOR INFECTION RELATED TO POSSIBLE CONTAGIOUS AGENTS SECONDARY TO USE OF STREET INJECTABLE DRUGS AND PRESENCE OF ABSCESS	—ASSESS FOR SIGNS OF INFLAMMATION AND INFECTION —CULTURE WOUND AS ORDERED BY PHYSICIAN AND REPORT RESULTS —REPORT TO INFECTION CONTROL NURSE IF ORGANISMS GROWN FROM CULTURES ARE PATHOGENIC —CHANGE DRESSING DAILY, AND APPLY TOPICAL MEDICATION AS ORDERED BY PHYSICIAN —DOCUMENT WOUND APPEARANCE DAILY —TEACH MARTIN PROPER CARE OF WOUND TO PREVENT INFECTION —PRACTICE MEDICAL ASEPSIS IN WOUND CARE, ESPECIALLY HANDWASHING —OBSERVE FOR SIGNS OF HEPATITIS AND, IF PRESENT, PLACE ON HEPATITIS AND NEEDLE PRECAUTIONS —TO AVOID CONTAMINATION, OBSERVE STRICT STERILE TECHNIQUE WHEN PERFORMING INTRUSIVE PROCEDURES, SUCH AS VENIPUNCTURE —TEACH MARTIN HOW TO PREVENT SPREAD OF INFECTION THROUGH APPROPRIATE PLACEMENT OF DRESSINGS, BED LINEN, AND CLOTHING; HANDWASHING AND AVOIDANCE OF SHARING FOOD, CIGARETTES, ETC.. HAVE MARTIN REPEAT PROCEDURES TO DETERMINE DEGREE OF LEARNING	—MARTIN WILL DEVELOP GRANULATION TISSUE WITHIN 2½ WEEKS —MARTIN WILL LIST THREE WAYS TO PREVENT INFECTION WITHIN 1 WEEK	8/28 dm

Continued

Nursing Care Plan *continued*

Discharge outcome/long-term goals	
I. MARTIN WILL VERBALIZE A COMMIT-MENT TO CONTINUED OUTPATIENT TREATMENT/FOLLOW-UP POSTDIS-CHARGE.	

Nursing diagnosis	Nursing intervention	Predicted outcome/short-term goals (include time frame)	Date/signature
NONCOMPLIANCE RELATED TO FAILURE TO ADHERE TO MED-ICAL REGIME SECONDARY TO DENIAL	—ASSESS MARTIN'S LEVEL OF KNOWLEDGE AND PERCEPTIONS REGARD-ING HIS ILLNESS AND ITS MANIFESTATIONS —HELP HIM IDENTIFY WHAT BEING "WELL" AND "HEALTHY" MEAN TO HIM —IDENTIFY DEFENSE MECHANISMS HE USES TO DEFEND AGAINST COMPLIANCE—DENIAL, MINIMIZING, RATIONAL-IZATION —ASSIST MARTIN IN EX-PLORING WAYS OF MAIN-TAINING CONTROL OF HIS LIFE WHILE STILL COM-PLYING WITH TREAT-MENT	—MARTIN WILL VERBALIZE THREE POTENTIAL POSITIVE ASPECTS OF REMAINING IN TREATMENT WITHIN 2 WEEKS	8/28 drc

Discharge outcome/long-term goals			
1. MARTIN WILL IDENTIFY THREE APPROPRIATE ALTERNATE METHODS OF DEALING WITH STRESS OTHER THAN SUBSTANCES AND WILL VERBALIZE A COMMITMENT TO A SUBSTANCE-FREE LIFE.			
Nursing diagnosis	**Nursing intervention**	**Predicted outcome/short-term goals (include time frame)**	**Date/signature**
INEFFECTIVE INDIVIDUAL COPING RELATED TO DEPENDENT AND MANIPULATIVE BEHAVIORS TO MEET NEEDS SECONDARY TO ADDICTIVE PERSONALITY TRAITS	—ENCOURAGE MARTIN TO IDENTIFY HIS BEHAVIORS WHICH HAVE CAUSED HIM PROBLEMS IN THE PAST —CONFRONT AND REDIRECT HIM WHEN HE ATTEMPTS TO BLAME HIS PROBLEMS ON OTHERS —CONSISTENTLY DIRECT MARTIN'S FOCUS TO HIS RESPONSIBILITY FOR HIS PROBLEMS AND TO THE CONTROL HE HAS OVER CHANGING THEM —ASSIST MARTIN IN IDENTIFYING THE CHANGES IN HIS LIFE HE NEEDS TO MAKE —TEACH HIM PROBLEM-SOLVING SKILLS AND PROVIDE ASSERTIVENESS TRAINING —SET LIMITS WITH HIM AROUND MANIPULATIONS AND BE CONSISTENT —POINT OUT MANIPULATIVE BEHAVIORS AND RELATE TO HOW THEY MANIFEST THEMSELVES IN PROBLEMS OUTSIDE THE HOSPITAL —ASSIST CLIENT IN IDENTIFICATION OF APPROPRIATE BEHAVIORS AND REINFORCE THEIR USE —ROLE-PLAY DIFFERENT SITUATIONS	—MARTIN WILL IDENTIFY THREE NEGATIVE CONSEQUENCES OF DRUG ABUSE WITHIN 2½ WEEKS —HE WILL REQUEST A ONE-TO-ONE WITH A STAFF MEMBER INSTEAD OF MEDICATION WITHIN 3 WEEKS	8/28 _dn_

Continued

Nursing Care Plan *continued*

Discharge outcome/long-term goals	
1. MARTIN AND HIS WIFE WILL CLARIFY THEIR RELATIONSHIP AND MAKE A DECISION WHETHER TO END OR CONTINUE THE MARRIAGE.	

Nursing diagnosis	Nursing intervention	Predicted outcome/short-term goals (include time frame)	Date/signature
INEFFECTIVE FAMILY COPING COMPROMISED RELATED TO EFFECTS AND INTERFERENCE OF SUBSTANCE USE ON ALL FAMILY RELATIONSHIPS SECONDARY TO DISEASE PROCESS	—ROLE-MODEL CLEAR, EFFECTIVE COMMUNICATIONS BY POINTING OUT INEFFECTIVE FAMILY COMMUNICATIONS AND SUGGESTING ALTERNATIVE MEANS OF RELATING —POINT OUT PROBLEMS IN COMMUNICATION (e.g., INTERRUPTING, SPEAKING FOR ANOTHER, CRITICIZING) AND ASSIST FAMILY IN CHANGING THEIR APPROACH/ STYLE OF RELATING — REFER THE FAMILY TO ALANON —INCLUDE FAMILY MEMBERS IN BEHAVIORAL CONTACT; e.g., MARTIN'S WIFE WILL NOT "RESCUE" HIM BY PAYING HIS DRUG DEBTS —ENCOURAGE MARTIN TO SEEK OUT STAFF IF COMMUNICATION BECOMES BLOCKED DURING A VISIT	—WITHIN 4 WEEKS, MARTIN AND FAMILY WILL REPORT THAT NO ARGUMENTS OCCURRED ON THREE VISITS IN A ROW —HE AND HIS WIFE WILL IDENTIFY THREE AREAS IN NEED OF CHANGE IN THEIR RELATIONSHIP WITHIN 4 WEEKS	8/28 dn

Discharge outcome/long-term goals			
1. MARTIN WILL EXPLORE AND BEGIN PARTICIPATION IN ONE VOLUNTEER POSITION AND ONE DIVERSIONAL ACTIVITY PRIOR TO AND AFTER DISCHARGE.			
Nursing diagnosis	Nursing intervention	Predicted outcome/short-term goals (include time frame)	Date/signature
DIVERSIONAL ACTIVITY, DEFICIT RELATED TO USE OF SUBSTANCES AS ONLY FORM OF LEISURE-TIME ACTIVITY/ PURSUIT SECONDARY TO INEFFECTIVE COPING	—IDENTIFY MARTIN'S PAST INTERESTS AND POSSIBLE TALENTS AND APTITUDES—MUSICAL, ATHLETIC, ARTISTIC, ETC.	—MARTIN WILL IDENTIFY TWO POTENTIAL AREAS OF INTEREST WITHIN 4 WEEKS	8/28 dwr
	—ASSIST MARTIN IN EXPLORING WAYS OF REUTILIZING SKILLS AND APTITUDES	—HE WILL REQUEST READING MATERIAL TO EXPLORE INTERESTS WITHIN 5 WEEKS	
	—ASSIST MARTIN IN IDENTIFYING HOW PAST ACTIVITIES WERE PLEASURABLE		
	—REFER HIM FOR OCCUPATIONAL/RECREATION ASSESSMENT OF SKILLS (MOTOR CONTROL, SOCIAL SKILLS, ETC.)		
	—PROVIDE HIM WITH NEWSPAPER AND OTHER SOURCES TO LOCATE ACTIVITIES AND GROUPS IN THE COMMUNITY THAT INTEREST HIM		

and alliance, Martin's family thus formed the supportive framework for his aftercare plans.

SUMMARY

Approximately halfway through the detoxification program, Martin became extremely uncomfortable and frightened at the prospect of becoming drug-free. Consequently, he signed himself out of the hospital, only to be readmitted 3 days later in an intoxicated state. Later, after recognizing that a continued life of drug use was in fact undesirable, he became aware of the extent of assistance he would need to change his life attitudes, goals, and expectations.

Both his wife and his mother were involved in the treatment program. This created the need for some changes in the care plan as family issues brought out much buried anger and guilt. However, once Martin's motivation was activated, he responded to therapeutic intervention with few setbacks. As part of therapy, Martin was begun on a low-dose tricyclic antidepressant, which proved highly effective in helping him increase his concentration and focus his attention on the therapy (much like Ritalin had helped him as a child).

In terms of discharge plans, Martin was referred to Narcotics Anonymous to complete 90 meetings in 90 days. He was also referred to continued treatment in couples' therapy and to a follow-up psychiatrist for individual therapy and medication maintenance.

REFERENCES

Childress, G. "The Role of the Nurse with the Drug Abuser and Addict," *Journal of Psychiatric Nursing and Mental Health Services* 2:21-26, 1970.

Schneider, K. *Klinische Psychopathologie*, 9th ed. Stuttgart, W. Germany: Thieme, 1971.

SELECTED BIBLIOGRAPHY

Ewan, C.E., and Whaite, A. "Training Health Professionals in Substance Abuse: A Review," *The International Journal of the Addictions* 17:1211-29, 1982.

Field, K.L. "Helping the Patient Off the Not-So-Merry-Go-Round," *Nursing84*, 14:79-80, 1984.

Kosten, T.R., et al. "*DSM-III* Personality Disorders in Opiate Addicts," *Comprehensive Psychiatry* 23:572-81, 1982.

Stevenson, R.C.K. "Dealing with Drug Abusers," *RN* 48:37-39, 1985.

Paul:
Schizoaffective Disorder

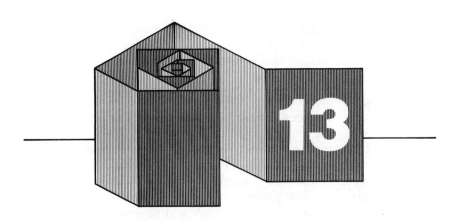

Deidre O'Connor Rea, MSN, RN

Acute inpatient hospitalization of the client with schizoaffective disorder has as its major goals the stabilization of maladaptive behavior and disposition to the home, extended care facility, and/or community. Various treatments may be employed to achieve these goals, including but not limited to individual and family psychotherapy, medication therapy, and nursing care focused on ongoing monitoring and modification of behavior. As demonstrated in this case study, the client who denies illness presents a particular challenge; the greater the denial, the greater the resistance to the staff's therapeutic efforts. A client responds only when *ready*. In the meantime, nursing care focuses on maintaining a supportive, positive hospital experience for the duration of treatment.

CASE STUDY

This was the third psychiatric hospitalization for Paul, a 24-year-old, single, white, Catholic male of Irish and Italian extraction. A high school graduate, Paul was employed as a stockroom clerk at a local hospital and lived in a nearby suburban area with his parents at the time of admission.

During his admission interview, Paul dated the onset of his current difficulties as 2 days prior to admission. However, when interviewed, his work supervisor noted a behavioral change approximately 4 months previously, when Paul reportedly burst into a hospital operating room yelling bizarre statements about God and Jesus Christ. When asked about that incident, Paul stated that God had been calling him to the ministry for some time, but he had refused to acknowledge this calling because he had been "a sinner." However, on that day, he had decided that his time to preach had come and that interrupting the operation was the best way for him to begin. Paul also reported that he "may be Jesus Christ" and that the devil was attempting to control him and plant evil thoughts in his head against his will.

Although his parents had noted no overt change, Paul's occupational functioning had in fact been deteriorating for 8 months prior to admission. Sleeping only 4 hours per night, Paul was spending most of his nocturnal hours composing songs and poetry and engaging in philosophical and religious discussions with himself. Consistently arriving late to work, he would then sleep on the job. Coworkers reported an increase in inappropriate sexual comments towards females, along with verbalization of suspicious thoughts regarding both friends and superiors. Paul's supervisor referred him to a physician, Dr. Brown, for an outpatient evaluation of his psychiatric symptoms. At that point he was diagnosed as paranoid schizophrenic and given a prescription for the neuroleptic medication chlorpromazine (Thorazine) 200 mg q.i.d. However, Paul was noncompliant with the medication regimen and soon discontinued it completely. He complained of the medication "not making him feel right."

About a month prior to this admission, Paul had begun to absorb himself in religion. He often left work during the day to attend church meetings, and started to feel more energized with a decreased need for sleep. He began to form the belief that he was "on a mission from God." He also experienced an increase in appetite and libido and asked a variety of female coworkers to engage in sexual relations. His mood was irritable, however, and he presented with increasingly bizarre and paranoid thoughts, illogical thinking, flight of ideas, and clang associations. He was admitted to the crisis unit at the county mental health center, but was noncompliant with treatment and signed out against medical advice after 3 days. As a result of Paul's outburst in the operating room and out of fear for his, staff's, and clients' safety, Paul's supervisor brought him directly to the hospital, where he was subsequently admitted.

This was not Paul's first psychiatric contact; that had occurred almost 4 years previously, several weeks after he began working at the hospital. At that time, he was seen in outpatient treatment by a Dr. Smith for medication maintenance. Paul's first hospitalization occurred approximately 4 months later, after he was found directing traffic in the middle of a busy street. On admission, he stated that his brother was trying to kill him and accused his brother of being "the devil." Paul was hospitalized for 1 month; during the hospitalization, he was treated with a variety of medications, none of which had much effect on his symptoms. A brief series of electroconvulsive therapy was utilized with some effect, but his symptoms reemerged shortly after his release.

Following discharge from this first hospitalization, Paul continued in outpatient treatment with Dr. Smith for approximately 8 months. Feeling that Paul's major problem was depression, Dr. Smith instituted medication trials of doxepin (Sinequan), amitriptyline (Elavil), protriptyline (Vivactil), trifluoperazine (Stelazine), and desipramine (Norpramin). Each of the 1- to 2-month trials proved ineffective, as Paul continued to feel depressed and to sleep constantly. The only medication that produced a positive effect was Stelazine; however, because the drug made him feel that he was better, Paul discontinued it and remained medication-free until his contact with Dr. Brown.

Paul's medical history was mostly unremarkable. He was the product of a normal full-term pregnancy and a planned cesarean delivery. He contracted all the normal childhood illnesses, as well as several ear infections. During the interview, he denied ever having any high or prolonged fevers or seizures and stated that his occasional headaches are relieved by aspirin. Although he also denied any major head injuries or loss of consciousness, he may have sustained minor trauma secondary to his headbanging behaviors as a child. His only medical hospitalization was for hernia repair surgery at age 4. According to his mother, he had major difficulties with the separation and was highly fearful during his entire stay. Paul denied any allergies and stated he had never smoked cigarettes. His alcohol consumption consisted of up to three cans of beer per weekend, with drug use limited to an occasional marijuana cigarette.

According to Paul's mother, Paul reached all developmental milestones early and displayed no overt behavioral problems as a child. He had no history of enuresis, fire-setting, or cruelty to animals. He did, however, exhibit a significant degree of separation anxiety upon his hospitalization at age 4 and again when he entered kindergarten. Fearful of leaving his mother, he reportedly would hide under his bed in an effort to avoid school.

When discussing his history, Paul stated that many of his difficulties began at age 5, when he was forced to perform fellatio on a neighbor (an incident he kept to himself until his first hospitalization). He did fairly well in school until the fourth grade, but then his family moved to a different part of the county where the school was more advanced; consequently, he was forced to repeat fourth grade. This situation occurred again in the sixth grade, when the family moved to their current home in a different state. Again, the new school was more advanced than the former, and Paul had to repeat the sixth grade. Although he was having increasingly pronounced difficulties with math, he was never formally tested for an actual learning disability and remained in regular classes, where he did poorly.

Paul related that he had much difficulty adjusting to each move and found making friends difficult. His retention in each grade further separated him from his peers and became the source for much social rejection. His poor grades were a constant irritation to his father and often served as the cause for a beating, restriction of what little social contact he had, and confinement to his room. Although Paul attempted to be outgoing, he had few friends and no close relationships.

On his entry into high school, Paul became active in various sports, including the wrestling team, and began writing songs. His grades averaged in the B to C range, and he appeared better adjusted. According to his mother, however, he continued to have difficulty with friends and girlfriends and generally remained quiet, isolated, and centered on his home life. He always tried to spend time with his father and help him with jobs around the house, but was invariably disappointed as his father tended only to recognize his faults and criticize him.

During his last year of high school, Paul enrolled in a work-study program in which he attended school half-time and worked in a fast-food restaurant the rest of the day. At this time, he reportedly became preoccupied with "the communists" and fearful that people were after him. Consequently, his mother withdrew him from school and arranged for private tutoring at home until he was deemed ready for graduation following a Child Study Evaluation. Although given the option to participate in the high school graduation exercises, Paul did not attend and received his diploma in absentia.

Paul obtained his job at the hospital shortly after graduation. While his job functioning was only marginal, his supervisors kept him on because they found him quite likeable. Even after this latest admission, they continued to express a willingness to keep him on staff.

In terms of relationships, Paul admitted engaging in sexual relations with a prostitute on two occasions but denied ever having a relationship beyond a casual encounter. He admitted to wanting a girlfriend and identified his mother, whom he believed to be perfect, as the general model against which he would judge a girlfriend.

Paul's family provided many clues to the origins of his illness. Paul was born the youngest of four siblings to a middle-class family of Italian and Irish descent. His brother, age 29, and two sisters, ages 27 and 26, were all high school graduates; one of the sisters completed junior college. All were married, lived outside the home, and held full-time employment.

The family history included several psychologic and medical disorders. Paul's mother had been hospitalized briefly on two occasions for paranoid thoughts and bizarre behavior. She had been stable for the past 8 years while maintained on Stelazine. Paul's maternal grandfather was institutionalized in a state psychiatric hospital when in his 30s and had died there 2 years before Paul's hospitalization. (The exact nature of his illness and cause of death were unknown.) The paternal side of the family was marked by alcohol abuse in Paul's father, grandfather, and several uncles. Despite behavioral problems associated with the alcohol use and some evidence of depression, none had ever sought treatment. The family history was also notable for cardiovascular disease and diabetes.

In terms of family function, Paul's mother stated that Paul was unplanned and that her husband was angry about the pregnancy. Unemployed at the time and drinking heavily, he reportedly focused much of his anger on his unborn child. After Paul's birth, his father rarely acknowledged his existence other than to occasionally physically abuse him for small infractions. He also periodically beat Paul's mother who had become overly protective of Paul.

Paul's siblings adopted their father's attitudes towards Paul; according to his mother, they generally teased and ostracized him from their groups and activities. Even after the abuse stopped, Paul's mother remained his protector and "best friend" and admittedly discouraged him from attempting to move out on his own. Her relationship with her husband continued to be poor, but while they often considered the possibility of divorce, they always decided to remain together while there were still children in the family home.

On formal mental status examination, Paul presented as a well-nourished but unkempt white male appearing his stated age of 24. His speech was rapid and pressured, and he exhibited normal psychomotor activity. He made little to no eye contact throughout the entire interview, but voiced a variety of inappropriate statements, such as requests for kisses and sexual innuendos about women on the unit. In general, he appeared to be an unreliable historian; his thoughts were illogical and disconnected and he contradicted himself quite frequently. He exhibited marked perseveration on issues of a sexual and religious nature and displayed evidence of flight of ideas with occasional loose and clang associations, thought broadcasting, paranoid delusions, and referential thinking. Believing he may be Jesus Christ, Paul stated that he had ESP, received messages from the radio and television, had thought insertion, and believed that God and Satan were fighting to gain control over him. He denied any current hallucinations but admitted to having heard voices in the past.

Although Paul reported feeling depressed at the time of the interview, his general presentation vacillated between angry and irritable to

Continued on page 314

RECORDING THE DATA

After you have read the case, cluster significant data into functional health patterns.

Health management/health perception _____

_____

_____

_____

_____

Nutritional/metabolic _____

_____

_____

_____

Elimination _____

_____

_____

_____

Activity/exercise _____

_____

_____

_____

Cognitive/perceptual _____

_____

_____

_____

Sleep/rest _____

_____

_____

_____

Self-perception/self-concept _____

_____

_____

_____

Role relationship _____

_____

_____

_____

Sexuality/reproductive _____

_____

_____

_____

Coping/stress tolerance _____

_____

_____

_____

Value/belief _____

_____

_____

_____

ASSIGNING NURSING DIAGNOSES

Use your clustered data to select appropriate nursing diagnoses.

Health perception/health management

☐ Growth and Development, Altered (see Developmental Delay)
☐ Health Maintenance, Altered
☐ Infection, Potential for
☐ Injury (Trauma): Potential for
☐ Noncompliance (Specify)
☐ Poisoning: Potential for
☐ Suffocation: Potential for

Nutritional/metabolic

☐ Body Temperature, Potential Alteration in
☐ Developmental Delay: Physical Growth and Development
☐ Fluid Volume, Altered: Excess or Excess Fluid Volume
☐ Fluid Volume Deficit, Actual
☐ Fluid Volume Deficit, Potential
☐ Nutrition, Altered: Less Than Body Requirements or Nutritional Deficit (Specify)
☐ Nutrition, Altered: More Than Body Requirements or Exogenous Obesity
☐ Nutrition, Altered: Potential for More Than Body Requirements or Potential for Obesity
☐ Oral Mucous Membrane, Altered
☐ Skin Integrity, Impaired or Skin Breakdown
☐ Skin Integrity, Impaired or Potential Skin Breakdown
☐ Swallowing, Impaired or Uncompensated Swallowing Impairment
☐ Tissue Integrity, Impaired

Elimination

☐ Bowel Elimination, Altered: Constipation
☐ Bowel Elimination, Altered: Diarrhea
☐ Bowel Elimination, Altered: Incontinence

☐ Developmental Delay: Bowel/Bladder Control
☐ Incontinence: Functional
☐ Incontinence: Reflex
☐ Incontinence: Stress
☐ Incontinence: Total
☐ Incontinence: Urge
☐ Urinary Elimination, Altered Patterns of
☐ Urinary Retention

Activity/exercise

☐ Activity Intolerance
☐ Activity Intolerance, Potential
☐ Airway Clearance, Ineffective
☐ Breathing Pattern, Ineffective
☐ Cardiac Output, Altered: Decreased
☐ Developmental Delay: Mobility
☐ Developmental Delay: Self-Care Skills
☐ Diversional Activity Deficit
☐ Gas Exchange, Impaired
☐ Home Maintenance Management, Impaired (Mild, Moderate, Severe, Potential, Chronic)
☐ Mobility, Impaired Physical
☐ Self-Care Deficit: Feeding
☐ Self-Care Deficit: Bathing/Hygiene
☐ Self-Care Deficit: Dressing/Grooming
☐ Self-Care Deficit: Toileting
☐ Self-Care Deficit: Total
☐ Tissue Perfusion, Altered: (Specify)

Sleep/rest

☐ Sleep Pattern Disturbance

Cognitive/perceptual

☐ Comfort, Altered: Pain
☐ Comfort, Altered: Chronic Pain

- [ ] Developmental Delay: (Specify Cognitive Area; attention, decision making, etc.)
- [ ] Hypothermia
- [ ] Hyperthermia
- [ ] Knowledge Deficit (Specify)
- [ ] Sensory-Perceptual Alteration: Input Excess or Sensory Overload
- [ ] Sensory-Perceptual Alteration: Input Deficit or Sensory Deprivation
- [ ] Thermoregulation, Ineffective
- [ ] Thought Processes, Altered
- [ ] Unilateral Neglect

Self-perception/self-concept

- [ ] Anxiety
- [ ] Body Image Disturbance
- [ ] Fear
- [ ] Hopelessness
- [ ] Personal Identity Confusion
- [ ] Powerlessness (Severe, Low, Moderate)
- [ ] Self-Esteem Disturbance

Role relationship

- [ ] Communication, Impaired Verbal
- [ ] Developmental Delay: Communication Skills
- [ ] Developmental Delay: Social Skills
- [ ] Family Processes, Altered
- [ ] Grieving, Anticipatory
- [ ] Grieving, Dysfunctional
- [ ] Parenting, Altered: Actual or Potential

- [ ] Role Performance, Disturbance in
- [ ] Social Interactions, Impaired
- [ ] Social Isolation (Rejection)

Sexuality/reproductive

- [ ] Rape-Trauma Syndrome: Compounded
- [ ] Rape-Trauma Syndrome: Silent Reaction
- [ ] Sexual Dysfunction
- [ ] Sexuality Patterns, Altered

Coping/stress tolerance

- [ ] Adjustment, Impaired
- [ ] Coping, Ineffective Individual
- [ ] Coping, Ineffective Family: Compromised
- [ ] Coping, Ineffective Family: Disabling
- [ ] Coping, Family: Potential for Growth
- [ ] Developmental Delay (Specify area)
- [ ] Post-Trauma Response
- [ ] Violence, Potential for (Self-Directed or Directed at Others)

Value/belief

- [ ] Spiritual Distress (Distress of Human Spirit)

You are now ready to develop a nursing care plan for this client. Use the following blank pages to do so. Then refer to the author's formulation, diagnostic summary, care plan, and summary.

NURSING CARE PLAN

Complete the chart below to develop a nursing care plan for this client.

Discharge outcomes/long-term goals	

Nursing diagnosis	Nursing intervention	

	Predicted outcomes/short-term goals (include time frame)	**Date/signature**

Return to Formulation, page 314

silly and euphoric. He also exhibited an inappropriate affect that was incongruent to his stated mood and the content of the discussion. He denied any current suicidal or homicidal ideas but admitted to having had suicidal thoughts during his hospitalization 5 years before. (During that hospitalization, he was found attempting to jump from a window while nude, stating that he would be brought closer to God.) Paul denied any episodes of depersonalization but admitted to derealization, *jamais vu,* and *deja vu*—believing these were all episodes from past lives.

On formal cognitive testing, Paul was oriented in four spheres with recent and remote memory seemingly impaired. (However, his paranoid thought content may have prevented his giving an accurate history.) His recall was one out of three objects at 5 minutes; his serial sevens were done slowly with three mistakes; and his digit span was five forward and three in reverse. His fund of knowledge was generally below-average for his educational level. Paul's responses to similarities were primarily concrete, and his proverb interpretations were comprised of cliches, quotes, and lines and titles of popular songs (e.g., to "Every cloud has a silver lining," he responded " 'Joy Inside My Tears' by Stevie Wonder"). His responses to social judgment questions showed evidence of impairment and a limited level of insight. In 5 years' time, he expected to be a brain surgeon, to have published a Pulitzer Prize–winning book, to be preaching and possibly a chaplain, and to be happily married to the woman of his choice. (He did, however, firmly believe that his wife would die a widow, as "people [were] out to kill [him].")

Reader may now complete Recording the Data, Assigning Nursing Diagnoses, and Nursing Care Plan.

FORMULATION

Paul presented with a symptom constellation of a mixed nature, with evidence of both psychotic and affective components. He had been diagnosed previously as schizophrenic based on the disordered thinking, delusions, and Schneiderian criteria (1971), so that the grandiose nature of his delusions, increased energy, neurovegetative changes, and negative/nihilistic overtones could not be ignored. Previous attempts at treatment appeared to have been medication-oriented and aimed primarily at the presenting symptomatology, either depressive or psychotic. While these treatments were essentially appropriate, few addressed both symptoms in conjunction or the underlying dynamics and Paul's seeming need to sabotage his treatment regimens with noncompliance.

Davidhizar (1982) notes that, when addressing noncompliance, the clinician must consider the client's general attitudes regarding self, illness,

Continued on page 321

DIAGNOSTIC SUMMARY FOR PAUL

Data	Functional health pattern	Nursing diagnosis
—Expresses persistent belief that people are attempting to harm him —Verbalizes grandiose ideas of inflated self-worth (e.g., believes he's Jesus Christ) —Exhibits perseveration on false beliefs, loose associations, and illogical thinking —Expresses grandiose, inflated beliefs —Is easily distractible —Displays increased energy, flight of ideas, and poor judgment and impulse control —Decreased sleep —Too busy to eat —Displays hypergraphia—writing poems and music—and hypersexuality	Cognitive/Perceptual	Altered thought processes related to psychosis secondary to schizoaffective illness
—Has a lack of interest and initiative in bathing himself —Exhibits an inappropriate appearance, with improper dressing and overall poor personal hygiene	Activity/Exercise	Self-care deficit: bathing/hygiene and dressing/grooming related to preoccupation with delusional thoughts secondary to schizoaffective disorder
—Denies illness —Has a history of noncompliance with medication regimens and therapy appointments —Perceives his problem to be of limited risk	Health Perception/Health Management	Noncompliance related to lack of follow-through with prescribed medical regime secondary to denial of illness
—Has demonstrated failure to follow through with previous recommendations and medication regimens —Verbalizes an inadequate understanding of his illness and the side effects of medications —Had inadequate performance on test of knowledge re: medications	Cognitive/Perceptual	Knowledge deficit related to his illness and lack of insight regarding the need for medication
—Needs family support —Experiences negative sibling relationships —Has overly close relationship with mother and distant, conflictual relationship with father —Family in transitional stages of development (empty nest)	Coping/Stress Tolerance	Ineffective family coping: compromised related to longstanding conflict between all family members and client secondary to multigenerational substance abuse history

NURSING CARE PLAN

Complete the chart below to develop a nursing care plan for this client.

Discharge outcome/long-term goals	
1. PAUL WILL NOT VERBALIZE BELIEFS THAT CANNOT BE CONSENSUALLY VALIDATED.	
2. PAUL'S MOOD WILL BE EUTHYMIC, WITH AN ABSENCE OF OMNIPOTENT BELIEFS.	

Nursing diagnosis	Nursing intervention	Predicted outcome/short-term goals (include time frame)	Date/signature
ALTERED THOUGHT PROCESSES RELATED TO PSYCHOSIS SECONDARY TO SCHIZOAFFECTIVE ILLNESS	—MEDICATE PAUL WITH NEUROLEPTICS ACCORDING TO PHYSICIAN'S ORDERS; ADMINISTER OTHER MEDICATIONS AS ORDERED	—WITHIN 14 DAYS, PAUL WILL BE ABLE TO INTERACT WITH A STAFF MEMBER FOR 15 MINUTES WITHOUT DISCUSSING DELUSIONAL MATERIAL	4/1 *dn*
	—ASSESS HIS REALITY ORIENTATION TO PERSON, PLACE, TIME, AND SITUATION EVERY SHIFT		
	—OBSERVE HIM FOR EXTRAPYRAMIDAL SYMPTOMS (EPS) AND MEDICATE AS APPROPRIATE		
	—FOCUS ON REALITY-BASED IDEAS		
	—ENCOURAGE PAUL TO EXPRESS ANY DOUBTS ABOUT HIS FALSE BELIEFS		
	—HELP HIM TO IDENTIFY HOW SUCH FALSE BELIEFS INTERFERE WITH HIS DAILY FUNCTIONING		
	—RESPOND TO THE THEMES OF DELUSIONAL CONTENT; e.g., THE NEED FOR IMPORTANCE, ACCEPTANCE, AND RESPECT		
	—ASSESS FOR LITHIUM TOXICITY; MONITOR INPUT, OUTPUT, AND LITHIUM LEVELS	—PAUL WILL SLEEP FOR 6 TO 8 HOURS PER NIGHT WITHIN 2 WEEKS	
	—ADMINISTER LITHIUM ACCORDING TO PHYSICIANS ORDERS	—HE WILL MAKE NO SEXUALLY PROVOCATIVE STATEMENTS IN 3 WEEKS	
	—USE A CALM BUT FIRM APPROACH WITH HIM		
	—USE DISTRACTION AND REFOCUSING TECHNIQUES TO REDIRECT HIM TO APPROPRIATE THOUGHTS AND ACTIVITIES		
	—LIMIT HIS NUMBER OF VISITORS, TIME IN GROUPS, AND OTHER STIMULATION UNTIL HE GAINS MORE CONTROL OVER HIS MOOD AND BEHAVIOR		

Nursing diagnosis	Nursing intervention	Predicted outcome/short-term goals (include time frame)	Date/signature
	—PROVIDE QUIET TIMES TO DECREASE STIMULATION		
	—MONITOR FOOD/FLUID INTAKE AND SLEEP PATTERNS AND WEIGHT WEEKLY		
	—PROVIDE POSITIVE FEEDBACK TO REINFORCE APPROPRIATE BEHAVIOR		
	—SET FIRM LIMITS ON INAPPROPRIATE SEXUAL STATEMENTS		
	—PROTECT HIM FROM OTHERS' RIDICULE DUE TO INAPPROPRIATE BEHAVIOR	—WITHIN 7 DAYS, PAUL WILL BE ABLE TO CONTROL HIS BEHAVIOR DURING A MILIEU ACTIVITY FOR ½ HOUR	
	—PROVIDE HIM WITH A STRUCTURED ROUTINE TO MINIMIZE BEHAVIORAL ESCALATION. GIVE A COPY OF THIS SCHEDULE TO PAUL AND KEEP ANOTHER COPY POSTED AT THE NURSING STATION		

Continued

Nursing Care Plan *continued*

Discharge outcome/long-term goals	
1. PAUL WILL REGULARLY EXHIBIT PROPER HYGIENE AND APPEARANCE WITHOUT BEING REMINDED OR SUPERVISED. 2. PAUL WILL VERBALIZE A COMMIT-MENT TO CONTINUED MEDICATION AND	THERAPY POST DISCHARGE.

Nursing diagnosis	Nursing intervention	Predicted outcome/short-term goals (include time frame)	Date/signature
SELF-CARE DEFICIT: BATH-ING/HYGIENE, DRESSING/GROOMING RE-LATED TO PRE-OCCUPATION WITH DELUSION-AL THOUGHTS SECONDARY TO SCHIZOAFFEC-TIVE DISORDER	—EXPLAIN TASKS, SUCH AS GROOMING, IN SHORT, SIMPLE SEN-TENCES —GIVE PAUL ADEQUATE TIME TO COMPLETE TASKS —ENCOURAGE HIM TO MAKE CHOICES ON TIME OF DAY FOR BATHING, DRESSING, ETC. —ASSIST HIM, WHEN NECESSARY, IN PROVID-ING APPROPRIATE FEED-BACK REGARDING HY-GIENE AND DECISIONS —REDIRECT HIM WHEN NECESSARY TO HELP HIM COMPLETE A TASK	—IN 1 WEEK, PAUL WILL TAKE A SHOWER AND BRUSH HIS TEETH, SHAVE, AND COMB HIS HAIR —HE WILL DRESS APPROPRIATELY FOR UNIT ACTIVITIES WITHIN 3 WEEKS	
NONCOMPLIANCE RELATED TO LACK OF FOL-LOW-THROUGH WITH PRESCRIB-ED MEDICAL REGIME SEC-ONDARY TO DENIAL OF ILLNESS	—ASSESS PAUL'S OVER-ALL UNDERSTANDING AND ACCEPTANCE OF HIS ILLNESS AND ITS MANIFESTATIONS —ASSIST HIM IN UNDER-STANDING THE RELA-TIONSHIP BETWEEN TAKING MEDICATIONS AND HEALTH/PRODUC-TIVE FUNCTIONING —ASSESS HIS LEVEL OF ANGER OR GUILT RE-GARDING CHRONIC ILL-NESS/IMPAIRMENT —ACTIVATE SUPPORT SYSTEMS IN ENCOUR-AGING FOLLOW-UP TREATMENT —ASSIST HIM IN PLAN-NING THE SIMPLEST AND LEAST DISRUPTIVE SCHEDULE FOR TAKING MEDICATIONS OUTSIDE THE HOSPITAL	—PAUL WILL SWALLOW ALL MEDICATIONS WHEN ADMIN-ISTERED THROUGHOUT THE HOSPITALIZATION —HE WILL IDENTIFY THREE POSITIVE EFFECTS OF MEDI-CATIONS WITHIN 3 WEEKS	4/1 dcr

Discharge outcome/long-term goals			
1. PAUL WILL BE ABLE TO STATE TWO CONDITIONS THAT NECESSITATE CALLING HIS PHYSICIAN WHILE ON NEUROLEPTIC MEDICATION AND LITHIUM POSTDISCHARGE.			

Nursing diagnosis	Nursing intervention	Predicted outcome/short-term goals (include time frame)	Date/signature
KNOWLEDGE DEFICIT RELATED TO HIS ILLNESS AND LACK OF INSIGHT RE: NEED FOR MEDICATION	—ASSESS PAUL'S READINESS AND ABILITY TO LEARN INFORMATION	—IN 2 WEEKS, PAUL WILL BE ABLE TO STATE EFFECTS AND SIDE EFFECTS OF EACH MEDICATION	4/1 ᴅᴍ
	—ASSESS HIS LEVEL OF KNOWLEDGE REGARDING BOTH MEDICATIONS AND ILLNESS AND CORRECT MISPERCEPTIONS WHERE NECESSARY	—IN 3 TO 4 WEEKS, HE WILL BE ABLE TO DESCRIBE OVERALL NATURE OF ILLNESS AND BEHAVIORS THAT SIGNIFY RESURGENCE OF SYMPTOMS	
	—RESPOND TO HIS QUESTIONS CLEARLY, CONCISELY, AND IN LANGUAGE HE CAN UNDERSTAND		
	—IDENTIFY WHAT HE WANTS TO KNOW, AND BUILD ON KNOWLEDGE HE ALREADY HAS		
	—ASSOCIATE NEW INFORMATION WITH ASPECTS OF HIS SYMPTOMS AND BEHAVIORS TO INCREASE THE POTENTIAL FOR RECALL AND COMPLIANCE		
	—DEMONSTRATE, IF POSSIBLE, AS YOU GIVE INSTRUCTIONS		
	—INVOLVE FAMILY MEMBERS IN TEACHING WHEN POSSIBLE		
	—PROVIDE WRITTEN MATERIAL THAT HE CAN SAVE AND REFER TO AT LATER POINTS IN TIME		
	—TEST PAUL 1 TO 2 WEEKS FOLLOWING TEACHING TO ASCERTAIN HIS DEGREE OF LEARNING		
	—REINFORCE LEARNING WITH PRAISE THROUGHOUT LENGTH OF STAY		
	—REVIEW MATERIAL HE HAS NOT LEARNED ON A WEEKLY BASIS		

Continued

Nursing Care Plan *continued*

Discharge outcome/long-term goals	
1. PAUL WILL BE ABLE TO SPEND 8 HOURS WITH HIS PARENTS ON A PASS WITHOUT ANY ARGUMENTS.	

Nursing diagnosis	Nursing intervention	Predicted outcome/short-term goals (include time frame)	Date/signature
INEFFECTIVE FAMILY COP- ING: COMPROM- ISED RELATED TO LONG- STANDING CON- FLICT BETWEEN ALL FAMILY MEMBERS AND PAUL SEC- ONDARY TO MULTI-GEN- ERATION SUB- STANCE ABUSE HISTORY	—DEVELOP A THERA- PEUTIC RELATIONSHIP WITH PAUL'S FAMILY —USE THE FAMILY'S LANGUAGE WHEN IN- TERVENING (AVOID MEDICAL JARGON) —ROLE-MODEL CLEAR, EFFECTIVE COMMUNI- CATION BY POINTING OUT INEFFECTIVE WAYS OF COMMUNI- CATING AND SUGGEST- ING ALTERNATIVES —ENCOURAGE EACH FAMILY MEMBER TO IDENTIFY WHAT HE/ SHE PERCEIVES AS "THE PROBLEM" —DO NOT TAKE SIDES WITH FAMILY MEM- BERS —IDENTIFY MOTIVATION AND WILLINGNESS OF FAMILY MEMBERS TO CHANGE —CONTRACT WITH FAMILY MEMBERS FOR ASSISTANCE IN MEETING TREATMENT GOALS	—PAUL WILL LIMIT HIS PHONE CALLS HOME TO TWO PER DAY WITHIN 14 DAYS —PAUL AND HIS FATHER WILL IDENTIFY TWO AREAS OF COMMON INTEREST WITHIN 2 WEEKS —PARENTS WILL ENSURE PAUL'S COOPERATION AND COMPLIANCE IN OUT-PATIENT FOLLOW-UP CARE	4/1 *dn*

and wellness. Moreover, as treatment and/or the course of the illness progresses, so might the client's attitudes change. As a result, ongoing assessment of Paul's changing beliefs was deemed an important part of his treatment, with interventions—especially teaching—geared towards his current state and his availability and readiness to learn.

A second major area of consideration was Paul's family situation. Essentially rejected by his father and siblings, Paul had bonded closely with his mother. Fueled by the family's lack of acceptance of mental illness, their attachment had been strengthened by the shared similarities of their symptoms. Superimposed was the intersection of Paul's mother's own unresolved issues with Paul's attempts at mastering the developmental tasks of his age. According to Critchley (1982), successful treatment of a child demands dealing with the parents' issues that unconsciously foster and encourage their child's pathology. As such, concentration needed to be placed on addressing the parental discord and the role Paul played in maintaining the marriage by focusing attention on his symptoms and away from his parents' difficulties.

Of final concern was Paul's prognosis and the identification of realistic expectations for hospitalization. Given his past history and the probability of symptom exacerbation, the goals for this admission were aimed at stabilization with a rapid return to the community. Target symptoms for medication included not only those of the formal thought disorder, but also those of mania and depression. A regimen of teaching, medication, and psychotherapy in conjunction with the establishment of a solid, supportive outpatient network, was implemented in an attempt to maintain his functioning at an adaptive level on an outpatient basis.

SUMMARY

The course of Paul's hospitalization proved erratic; it included one episode of agitation that required restraints for 2 hours. An emergency plan of care was devised that included monitoring of intake and output, range-of-motion, skin integrity, sensory deprivation/stimulation, agitation, and disordered thinking. To assist in stabilization, Paul was begun on lithium and fluphenazine (Prolixin), with plans to convert him to fluphenazine decanoate (Prolixin Decanoate) just prior to discharge. As his lithium level approached the therapeutic range, his symptoms gradually decreased to a level that allowed him to begin obtaining passes from the unit to return to work.

Unfortunately, Paul's family situation did not stabilize, but rather appeared to deteriorate when basic dynamics were addressed. Recognizing that Paul would decompensate on return to the family home, plans were geared toward placing him in a halfway house. Further referral was established with the community mental health center, where Paul could receive group support and individual contact to oversee his progress. In the health center, continued lithium levels would be obtained and regular medication teaching updates given to ensure compliance. Paul's work passes from the hospital seemed to smooth his overall transition back to the community, and he appeared to handle discharge well.

REFERENCES

Critchley, D.L. "Interventions with Disorganized Parents of Disturbed Children," *Issues in Mental Health Nursing* 4:199-215, 1982.

Davidhizar, R.E. "Tool Development for Profiling the Attitude of Clients with Schizophrenia Toward Their Medication, Using Fishbein's Expectancy-Value Model," *Issues in Mental Health Nursing* 4:343-57, 1982.

Schneider, K. *Klinische Psychopathologie*, 9th ed. Stuttgart, W. Germany: Thieme, 1971.

SELECTED BIBLIOGRAPHY

Bernstein, L.R. "Patterns of Dysfunctional Reality Orientation," in *Comprehensive Psychiatric Nursing,* 3rd ed. Edited by Haber, J., et al. New York: McGraw-Hill Book Co., 1987.

Buckwalter, K.C. "Emergency Department Nursing of the Manic Patient," *Journal of Emergency Nursing* 8:239-42, 1982.

Buckwalter, K.C. "Psychiatric Disorders in the Work Setting: Identification and Management of the Manic Individual," *Occupational Health Nursing* 30:17-19, 1982.

Fletcher, A. "Schizoaffective Disorder," *Nursing Times* 79:29-32, 1983.

George, L., and Neufeld, R.W.J. "Cognition and Symptomatology in Schizophrenia," *Schizophrenia Bulletin* 11(2):264-82, 1985.

Grossman, L.S., et al. "The Longitudinal Course of Schizoaffective Disorders," *Journal of Nervous and Mental Disease* 172:104-49, 1984.

Scheflin, A.E. *Levels of Schizophrenia.* New York: Brunner-Mazel, 1981.

A.J.:
Sexual Acting-Out and Aggression in a Boy

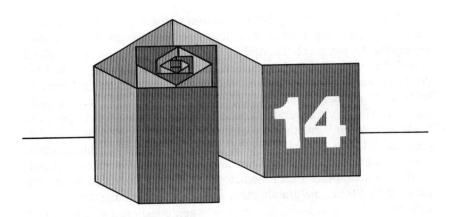

Dessye-Dee Clark, MSN, RN

Representatives from governmental, congressional, and health professional groups have brought us a heightened awareness of child abuse in the 1980s. The McMartin case in California, where day care center administrators were accused of sexually abusing young students, heightened public awareness of the problem of physical and sexual child abuse in our homes and schools.

Using this new awareness, nurses have begun to gain familiarity with the phenomena associated with trauma syndromes resulting from rape or other forms of abuse. Various interventions strategically designed to meet the needs of this young, vulnerable population, such as play therapy techniques and parent training, are incorporated into the treatment regimen. The involvement of parental figures is key, as abusers as well as victims require the special skills of an understanding, empathic professional nurse. The following case exemplifies the work of a nurse with an 8-year-old child who has a history of sexual abuse. The child's self-destructive behavior pointed to this abuse and became the initial focus of nursing care.

CASE STUDY

The subject of this case study, A.J., was an 8-year-old black boy who resided in an inner-city shelter with his 28-year-old mother and 6-month-old half-brother. He was enrolled in a regular second-grade class in a racially integrated school.

This was the first psychiatric admission for A.J. However, he had been seen as an outpatient on an emergency basis the previous day after attempting to jump off the roof of the shelter. After he was "talked down" from the roof by his mother, he expressed sad feelings and the desire to hurt himself and others. When questioned about the incident, he told his mother "I want to kill myself"; "I'm bad, I should go to jail." He also made several violent comments such as "I hate you, I'm going to stab you," and then revealed that he had witnessed his stepfather rape and kill two women 4 months earlier. In addition to this incident, 2 weeks previously, during a 3-day family visit to A.J.'s maternal grandmother in his mother's rural hometown, A.J. had attempted to set four fires. At that time, the grandmother insisted that her daughter get some help for A.J. According to his mother, when questioned about the fires A.J. stated that "My stepfather told me to burn the house down"; "The other side of me wants to do this"; and "I can't forget the feeling to burn things."

A.J. reportedly had set a fire 4 years prior to the latest incident; this act prompted no psychiatric evaluation, however. He had one psychiatric evaluation at age 5, at which time he was diagnosed as hyperactive; however, no psychopharmacological treatments were recommended.

A.J. had been in relatively good health, except for numerous cases of otitis media during his toddler years. At age 3, tubes were placed in his ears that helped decrease infections and seemed to improve his hearing. He is the result of an unexpected, uncomplicated pregnancy and a normal spontaneous vaginal delivery. His mother did acknowledge using alcohol and occasionally marijuana throughout the pregnancy. Mother and infant had contact within the first 3 hours of birth, and were able to leave the hospital after 24 hours of observation. A.J. always displayed a good appetite—in fact, he was preoccupied with eating—and reportedly often gorged his favorite meals to the point of vomiting. Upon physical examination by the pediatrician, A.J. was found to be overweight, within the 97th percentile rating on the growth chart for overall height/weight indices. He had not been exposed to any recent illnesses, had no known allergies, and had up-to-date immunizations. His VDRL lab value was negative. He exhibited no evidence of penile discharge, sexually transmitted disease, or genital trauma. However, his anus was reddened and enlarged, with flaccid sphincter muscles. A.J.

was extremely anxious throughout the physical examination and defecated in his pants at its conclusion.

A.J.'s early feeding history was unremarkable; he was bottle-fed at his mother's preference and convenience. His motor and language milestones were within developmental norms. His first social smile was noticed between 4 to 6 weeks, and he never demonstrated any stranger anxiety. He began talking at age 13 months, and began simple two-word conversations by age 2.6 years. By age 3, he was aware that he was a boy and selected typical male-typed play objects. But also at age 3, he was observed to undress a big doll and then himself and lay on top of the doll.

Although A.J. had achieved full bowel and bladder control by age 4 and had been "dry" since his 5th birthday, recently he had been enuretic three to four times a week. In addition Mrs. Composa, A.J.'s mother, reported some settling problems. A.J. did not settle until 2 to 3 hours after going to bed, stood confused in his room, remade the bedclothing, refused to undress, insisted the light be left on, and refused to let others enter his room. A.J.'s mother also noted that A.J. "seems to like kissing people's feet" and "plays in the bath, I can't get him out of the water." Over the 2 months prior to admission, A.J. had experienced several violent nightmares and reported recurrent, intrusive visions of the incident when his stepfather stabbed two women. He visualized the blood in these dreams.

A.J. began school at age 5. Teachers reported he had "dyslexia" and "wrote his letters backward," "couldn't sit still for class," and often was caught lying about minor things. One teacher described him as "likeable; he responds well to praise, but forgets easily." A.J. was achieving D level performance in his schoolwork, yet school testing showed him to be of average intelligence. A.J. had few friends in school, often fought, and acted as the "class clown" to gain attention. Recently, he began to withdraw from peers, choosing inappropriate sex and age toys, such as dolls, and pretending to kill or stab them. In the school bathrooms, he was found on at least two occasions with male peers in the same toilet stall with their pants down. The observing teacher saw A.J. attempting to put his penis up against the other boy's buttocks. When questioned by a male teacher, A.J. bit the teacher's hand.

A.J. had no history of truancy or cruelty to animals. He had been known to steal money from his mother's purse and often did not mind her. He had frequent, severe temper-tantrums, and was easily frustrated. His mother denied ever hitting him; for discipline, she sent him to his room. According to Mrs. Composa, her aunt, who lived in town, was very supportive, and her own mother was supportive but often critical and also "lets A.J. eat anything he wants to."

Mrs. Composa reported that A.J.'s stepfather was physically and sexually abusive to her and the children. He made verbal threats to kill A.J. and the rest of the family. She admitted knowing that the stepfather gave A.J. marijuana to smoke. She also reported that he once took A.J. into a back room, and as A.J. told her, "put his bone on me." Actual anal penetration was probable. Mrs. Composa was afraid to report this incident, as the stepfather often told A.J. to "burn the house down if mother tried to leave." The Department of Social Services (DPSS) investigated these events several months before, but the case was closed after the stepfather's incarceration.

A.J.'s parents never married but lived together for the first 6 months of A.J.'s life, then off-and-on for 4 years prior to the father's arrest on robbery and murder charges. He was incarcerated at the time of A.J.'s admission. Although never hospitalized himself, he had frequent "mood swings" and a "violent temper," and "ran with the wrong crowd," according to Mrs. Composa. A.J. remembered having "many daddies" in the house, not being able to go outside, and being put in a closet for asking for more food to eat. The family's neighborhood was the scene of frequent assaults and robberies. The family changed apartments often during A.J.'s early years because of burglary attempts, harrassment from landlords, and financial problems.

Mrs. Composa married A.J.'s stepfather when A.J. was age 6. Her current husband had been jailed recently on charges of rape and murder, but prior to this incarceration had been living with the family for the previous 2 years. During the time that A.J.'s stepfather was living in the home, A.J. witnessed frequent marital violence and intoxication from his stepfather.

A.J.'s paternal grandparents resided in a nearby city but had no contact with the family. Although neither of A.J.'s parents expressed a religious preference, A.J.'s maternal grandmother was a devout Baptist and Mrs. Composa had been raised with strong fundamentalist beliefs. Mrs. Composa's father, who had been deceased for the past 20 years, reportedly had "learning problems" and also "drank some."

A.J.'s mother was also physically and sexually abused as a child by her stepfather. Nevertheless, she denied any history of psychiatric disorder or suicide on her side of the family. She had been working as an electronic parts assembler for 2 years, after training with an urban job support program. Three months ago, Mrs. Composa took the family into the shelter, as A.J.'s stepfather had threatened to kill them.

During his formal mental status examination, A.J. appeared well-developed, mildly overweight, and physically hyperactive, moving from seat to seat and crawling under desks. He was dressed in clothes that appeared one size too small, with the middle shirt button missing. He displayed poor eye contact. Initially, he refused to talk to the therapist and exhibited much immature behavior, such as "baby talk," crawling and rolling on the floor, and sticking his fingers into his mouth while talking. Later, he sought physical attention by holding hands and making inappropriate physical contact with the therapist (rubbing up against her front, licking her hand, and pointing at her breasts with jabbing movements). During the interview, A.J. was noncompliant with many requests and appeared impulsive and easily distracted. He required constant reassurance and redirection. He displayed clear evidence of thought disorder, but made frequent jokes that made it hard to discern between his fantasy life and his real world comprehension. He related that he was "in jail" at the hospital because "I tried to burn things, because I'm bad like my dad." His recent and remote memory were judged to be good.

While in the play room, A.J. grabbed a doll and exhibited violent gestures by pretending to kill or stab the doll with an object. He stated mechanically that he was going to "put a neighbor girl on the bed or the floor" and then showed a humping movement of his body to indicate what he would do. Given the probability of sexual abuse, A.J. was presented with anatomically correct dolls to provide an opportunity for him to visually describe what had happened. Without hesitation, he undressed the dolls, then grinned upon discovering the exposed genitals and asked the therapist to touch them. At one point during the interview, A.J. became somewhat frenzied, getting down on his hands and knees, rocking back and forth, and groaning while attempting to perform fellatio on the male doll. At the end of the admission session, he urinated into the anus of the male doll.

Reader may now complete Recording the Data, Assigning Nursing Diagnoses, and Nursing Care Plan.

FORMULATION

A.J. was diagnosed by the therapist as having both attention deficit disorder with hyperactivity (ADDH) and post-traumatic stress disorder (PTSD) due to the mother's reports of the stepfather's abuse and the doll interview findings. The therapist also made a rule-out diagnosis of learning disability at the time of admission.

A.J. presented as an 8-year-old black boy with average intelligence but poor school achievement skills, marked emotional regression and depressive symptoms, and serious maladaptive behaviors that posed a danger to himself and others. His history included target behaviors of fire setting, aggression toward others, suicidal ideation, severe and fre-

Continued on page 334

RECORDING THE DATA

After you have read the case, cluster significant data into functional health patterns.

Health management/health perception _____

_____

_____

_____

_____

Nutritional/metabolic _____

_____

_____

_____

Elimination _____

_____

_____

_____

Activity/exercise _____

_____

_____

_____

Cognitive/perceptual _____

_____

_____

_____

Sleep/rest _____

_____

_____

_____

Self-perception/self-concept _____

_____

_____

_____

Role relationship _____

_____

_____

_____

Sexuality/reproductive _____

_____

_____

_____

Coping/stress tolerance _____

_____

_____

_____

Value/belief _____

_____

_____

_____

ASSIGNING NURSING DIAGNOSES

Use your clustered data to select appropriate nursing diagnoses.

Health perception/health management

- ☐ Growth and Development, Altered (see Developmental Delay)
- ☐ Health Maintenance, Altered
- ☐ Infection, Potential for
- ☐ Injury (Trauma): Potential for
- ☐ Noncompliance (Specify)
- ☐ Poisoning: Potential for
- ☐ Suffocation: Potential for

Nutritional/metabolic

- ☐ Body Temperature, Potential Alteration in
- ☐ Developmental Delay: Physical Growth and Development
- ☐ Fluid Volume, Altered: Excess or Excess Fluid Volume
- ☐ Fluid Volume Deficit, Actual
- ☐ Fluid Volume Deficit, Potential
- ☐ Nutrition, Altered: Less Than Body Requirements or Nutritional Deficit (Specify)
- ☐ Nutrition, Altered: More Than Body Requirements or Exogenous Obesity
- ☐ Nutrition, Altered: Potential for More Than Body Requirements or Potential for Obesity
- ☐ Oral Mucous Membrane, Altered
- ☐ Skin Integrity, Impaired or Skin Breakdown
- ☐ Skin Integrity, Impaired or Potential Skin Breakdown
- ☐ Swallowing, Impaired or Uncompensated Swallowing Impairment
- ☐ Tissue Integrity, Impaired

Elimination

- ☐ Bowel Elimination, Altered: Constipation
- ☐ Bowel Elimination, Altered: Diarrhea
- ☐ Bowel Elimination, Altered: Incontinence

- ☐ Developmental Delay: Bowel/ Bladder Control
- ☐ Incontinence: Functional
- ☐ Incontinence: Reflex
- ☐ Incontinence: Stress
- ☐ Incontinence: Total
- ☐ Incontinence: Urge
- ☐ Urinary Elimination, Altered Patterns of
- ☐ Urinary Retention

Activity/exercise

- ☐ Activity Intolerance
- ☐ Activity Intolerance, Potential
- ☐ Airway Clearance, Ineffective
- ☐ Breathing Pattern, Ineffective
- ☐ Cardiac Output, Altered: Decreased
- ☐ Developmental Delay: Mobility
- ☐ Developmental Delay: Self-Care Skills
- ☐ Diversional Activity Deficit
- ☐ Gas Exchange, Impaired
- ☐ Home Maintenance Management, Impaired (Mild, Moderate, Severe, Potential, Chronic)
- ☐ Mobility, Impaired Physical
- ☐ Self-Care Deficit: Feeding
- ☐ Self-Care Deficit: Bathing/ Hygiene
- ☐ Self-Care Deficit: Dressing/ Grooming
- ☐ Self-Care Deficit: Toileting
- ☐ Self-Care Deficit: Total
- ☐ Tissue Perfusion, Altered: (Specify)

Sleep/rest

- ☐ Sleep Pattern Disturbance

Cognitive/perceptual

- ☐ Comfort, Altered: Pain
- ☐ Comfort, Altered: Chronic Pain

☐ Developmental Delay: (Specify Cognitive Area; attention, decision making, etc.)
☐ Hypothermia
☐ Hyperthermia
☐ Knowledge Deficit (Specify)
☐ Sensory-Perceptual Alteration: Input Excess or Sensory Overload
☐ Sensory-Perceptual Alteration: Input Deficit or Sensory Deprivation
☐ Thermoregulation, Ineffective
☐ Thought Processes, Altered
☐ Unilateral Neglect

Self-perception/self-concept

☐ Anxiety
☐ Body Image Disturbance
☐ Fear
☐ Hopelessness
☐ Personal Identity Confusion
☐ Powerlessness (Severe, Low, Moderate)
☐ Self-Esteem Disturbance

Role relationship

☐ Communication, Impaired Verbal
☐ Developmental Delay: Communication Skills
☐ Developmental Delay: Social Skills
☐ Family Processes, Altered
☐ Grieving, Anticipatory
☐ Grieving, Dysfunctional
☐ Parenting, Altered: Actual or Potential

☐ Role Performance, Disturbance in
☐ Social Interactions, Impaired
☐ Social Isolation (Rejection)

Sexuality/reproductive

☐ Rape-Trauma Syndrome: Compounded
☐ Rape-Trauma Syndrome: Silent Reaction
☐ Sexual Dysfunction
☐ Sexuality Patterns, Altered

Coping/stress tolerance

☐ Adjustment, Impaired
☐ Coping, Ineffective Individual
☐ Coping, Ineffective Family: Compromised
☐ Coping, Ineffective Family: Disabling
☐ Coping, Family: Potential for Growth
☐ Developmental Delay (Specify area)
☐ Post-Trauma Response
☐ Violence, Potential for (Self-Directed or Directed at Others)

Value/belief

☐ Spiritual Distress (Distress of Human Spirit)

You are now ready to develop a nursing care plan for this client. Use the following blank pages to do so. Then refer to the author's formulation, diagnostic summary, care plan, and summary.

NURSING CARE PLAN

Complete the chart below to develop a nursing care plan for this client.

Discharge outcomes/long-term goals	

Nursing diagnosis	Nursing intervention	

	Predicted outcomes/short-term goals (include time frame)	**Date/signature**

Return to Formulation, page 327

quent temper tantrums, difficulty in getting along with peers, noncompliance with adult demands, lying, enuresis, settling difficulties, overeating, and compulsive sexual acting-out. A.J.'s reports of witnessing severe violence and rape and of being molested by his stepfather were corroborated by his mother; physical examination findings reinforced the report of sexual molestation.

From A.J.'s perspective, he felt "bad," "mad," and "sad." He was able to connect these dysphoric feelings with his stepfather and believed that his behavior (fire-setting) had gotten him punished (put in the hospital). A.J. also wanted to punish himself and felt "split" by having multiple feelings at the same time. He suffered from poor self-esteem and was suspicious of his environment. Ambivalent toward both mother and stepfather, A.J. was confused and anxious about getting his needs met.

Although A.J. made no reference to his younger half-brother, his recurring infantile behavior may have represented some underlying feelings of sibling rivalry and emotional deprivation. He was aware of the reason for his stepfather's absence (jail), but did not express any sense of loss or separation. He was unaware of the maladaptive aspects of his sexual acting-out, and associated sexual behaviors with violence toward others.

Developmentally, A.J. was not yet capable of abstract reasoning and had been culturally "trained" by early life experience into precocious sexual activity. He experienced internal distress and a sense of deprivation and thus could not perceive his own abilities for success. He displayed no evidence of formal thought disorder, but exhibited some signs of a learning disability, with attentional difficulties and a high level of motor activity possibly suggestive of some mild underlying neurological disorder. This may have served to exacerbate symptoms by contributing to his frustration with school and to his poor task mastery.

Although A.J. had expressed a wish to kill himself and others prior to admission, his ideation was impulsive and lacked a definite plan, and he was easily "talked down" by his mother. Suicidal and homicidal risks were thus judged to be moderate, given the protective environment of the inpatient unit, but with possible lethal potential if he did not receive immediate treatment. Looking back, A.J.'s suicidal attempt can be seen as an urgent request for help and a belief that he must be punished for wrong-doing. A.J. demonstrated a growing identification with his stepfather as a powerful and violent person, and began to have considerable trouble controlling his aggressive impulses. In response to his own victimization, A.J. identified with his aggressor by imitating his stepfather's violence. His predominant moods consisted of sadness and anger. He

Continued on page 345

DIAGNOSTIC SUMMARY FOR A.J.

Data	Functional health pattern	Nursing diagnosis
—Experiences enuresis three to four times a week (had been dry since age 5) —Exhibits sleep disorder: settles poorly 2 to 3 hours after bedtime; stands in confused state in room; perseverates at remaking his bedclothes; will not undress into pajamas; insists the light be left on; refuses to have male staff in room; and reports violent nightmares —Engages in compulsive sex-play: masturbates in public and attempts to disrobe and display body, kiss other's feet, urinate on peer's bed and doll's anus, direct sex-play with peers, and touch staff's breasts; will assume sexual postures and make grunting, snorting, farting sounds with giggling and a starry-eyed, glazed look	Sexuality/ Reproductive	Rape-Trauma Syndrome: compound reaction, related to witnessing rape and violence and experiencing sexual abuse by stepfather
—Displays violent behavior: hits peers and bites adults; while in play room, grabbed a doll and exhibited violent gestures by holding an object in his hands and pretending to kill or stab the doll —Has made one suicide attempt —Expresses homicidal and suicidal ideation —Has engaged in fire-setting —Shows regressive "babyish" behaviors (crawling, whining) —Exhibits constant hyperactivity and anxiety —Engages in excessive water play and bathing with masturbation —Demonstrates blurred distinctions between his fantasy life and real world comprehension	Coping/Stress Tolerance	Potential violence to self and others, related to verbal threats and witnessing of violent act 4 months ago Ineffective individual coping related to maladaptive compulsive sex play with self and peers secondary to Rape-Trauma Syndrome

NURSING CARE PLAN

Complete the chart below to develop a nursing care plan for this client.

Discharge outcome/long-term goals	
I. BY DISCHARGE, A.J. WILL SHOW IMPROVED POSTTRAUMATIC ADJUSTMENT, DEMONSTRATED BY: ABSENCE OF HYPERSEXUAL BEHAVIOR (INAPPROPRIATE TOUCHING/SEX-PLAY); ABSENCE OF AGGRESSIVE	BEHAVIOR TOWARDS SELF AND OTHERS (HITTING, BITING, SUICIDAL GESTURES); AND AN INCREASE IN SELF-ESTEEM, DEMONSTRATED BY ATTEMPTS TO SOCIALIZE AND TRY NEW ACTIVITIES AND BY VERBALIZED COMMENTS OF PERCEIVED

Nursing diagnosis	Nursing intervention	Predicted outcome/short-term goals (include time frame)	Date/signature
RAPE-TRAUMA SYNDROME, COMPOUND REACTION RELATED TO WITNESSING RAPE AND VIOLENCE AND EXPERIENCING SEXUAL ABUSE BY STEPFATHER	—HELP A.J. ADJUST TO THE UNIT, WORKING TO IMPROVE HIS RESPONSE TO STAFF BY CREATING A FAMILIAR ROUTINE, AND CONSISTENTLY NURTURING ENVIRONMENT —ASSIST A.J. IN FEELING ACCEPTED BY SHOWING HIM ATTENTION AND AFFECTION WHILE NOT REINFORCING HIS MALADAPTIVE BEHAVIORS; i.e., "CATCH HIM BEING GOOD" —ENSURE THAT A.J. HAS 20 MINUTES OF UNINTERRUPTED TIME WITH HIS PRIMARY AND/OR ASSOCIATE NURSE EACH SHIFT —INTRODUCE A.J. TO UNIT ROUTINES AND SHOW HIM UNIT CALENDAR OF DAILY ACTIVITIES (SCHOOL, SWIMMING, THERAPY TIMES, ETC.) —AVOID EXPRESSIVE PITY OR RESPONDING TO A.J.'S REQUESTS MADE IN BABY-TALK; VERBALLY PROMPT A.J. TO ASK FOR THINGS LIKE A "BIG BOY" AND ACTIVELY IGNORE WHINING OR CRAWLING TO AVOID REINFORCING REGRESSIVE DEPENDENT BEHAVIORS —IMMEDIATELY RESPOND TO A.J. AS SOON AS HE BEGINS TO DEMONSTRATE ANY "BIG BOY" TYPE BEHAVIORS (e.g., REMOVES HIS FINGERS FROM HIS MOUTH WHEN SPEAKING, STOPS WHINING, ASKS DIRECTLY FOR SOMETHING OR STANDS UP AFTER CRAWLING) PRAISE THIS BEHAVIOR —AVOID ASKING QUESTIONS RE: DETAILS OF TRAUMA	—BY END OF FIRST WEEK, A.J. WILL ADJUST TO THE UNIT AS DEMONSTRATED BY: DECREASED USE OF REGRESSIVE, "BABYISH" BEHAVIORS (CRAWLING, PUTTING FINGERS IN MOUTH, ETC.); AVOIDANCE OF GORGING HIMSELF AT MEALS; COMPLIANCE WITH UNIT PROCEDURES AND "RULES"; e.g., TAKING TIME-OUT WHEN NONCOMPLIANT WITH STAFF'S REQUESTS FOR SAFE PLAY; AGGRESSIVE WITHOUT PHYSICAL STRUGGLE; RAPPORT WITH STAFF, SHOWN BY SPONTANEOUSLY SEEKING OUT HIS PRIMARY NURSE; ABILITY TO STATE REASONS FOR HIS HOSPITALIZATION; USE OF STARS TO BUY TOYS AT TOKEN STORE OR TO EARN SPECIAL TIME WITH STAFF FOR ADLs; AND SAFELY USE TIMER HIMSELF 5 OUT OF 7 DAYS PER WEEK (BOTH MORNING AND AFTERNOON)	5/2 DDC

Discharge outcome/long-term goals	
INNER CONTROL OF SELF.	

Nursing diagnosis	Nursing intervention	Predicted outcome/short-term goals (include time frame)	Date/signature
	—DO NOT CRITICIZE A.J.'s STEPFATHER		
	—GIVE A.J. CHOICES; ALLOW HIM TO SAY "NO" WHEN FEASIBLE		
	—REWARD A.J. WITH A STAR FOR COMPLETING SELF-CARE ADLs IN THE MORNING (ONE STAR EACH FOR: GETTING UP, MAKING HIS OWN BED, DRESSING HIMSELF IN LESS THAN 20 MINUTES, WASHING HIS FACE, AND BRUSHING HIS TEETH) AND AT BEDTIME (BRUSHING HIS TEETH, PUTTING HIS DIRTY CLOTHES IN HAMPER, TAKING A BATH IN LESS THAN 20 MINUTES, DRESSING IN PAJAMAS, AND STAYING IN BED QUIETLY AFTER "LIGHTS OUT"		
	—PRAISE A.J. LAVISHLY AND COMMENT ON HIS PROGRESS WHEN PLACING STARS ON CHART. ALLOW HIM TO PLACE STARS ON CHART HIMSELF IF HE DESIRES		
	—USE TIMER FOR FUN AND CHALLENGE, TO PLAY "BEAT THE CLOCK" AND PROVIDE MULTISENSORY REINFORCEMENT. A.J. MAY SET THE TIMER HIMSELF WITH STAFF SUPERVISION, IF HE DEMONSTRATES SAFE USE OF IT		
	—REWARD EACH SAFE USE OF TIMER AND COMPLETION OF ADLs BY LAVISH PRAISE: "A.J., YOU SURE ARE BEING VERY SAFE AND RESPONSIBLE WITH THE TIMER," "GREAT! YOU BEAT THE CLOCK AGAIN!		

Continued

Nursing Care Plan *continued*

Nursing diagnosis	Nursing intervention	Predicted outcome/short-term goals (include time frame)	Date/signature
	YOU EARN ANOTHER STAR!"		
	—ALLOW A.J. TO EARN UP		
	TO A TOTAL OF FIVE STARS		
	PER SHIFT (TEN STARS =		
	ONE FULL STAR CHART,		
	WHICH HE MAY CASH IN		
	THE NEXT DAY AT "TOKEN		
	STORE" FOR TOYS OR SPE-		
	CIAL TIME WITH STAFF)		
	—REINFORCE THE CONCEPT		
	THAT "EVERY DAY IS A		
	NEW OPPORTUNITY"		
POTENTIAL VIO-	—DISCUSS "SAFE PLAY"	—BY THE END OF THE FIRST	5/2
LENCE TO SELF	CONCEPTS WITH A.J. AT	WEEK, A.J. WILL HAVE EARNED	DOC
AND OTHERS, RE-	BEGINNING OF EACH MI-	AT LEAST FIVE POINTS FOR	
LATED TO VER-	LIEU GROUP. WHENEVER	"SAFE PLAY" WITH PEERS IN	
BAL THREATS	POSSIBLE, "CATCH HIM BE-	MILIEU GROUPS (BASELINE —	
AND WITNESSING	ING GOOD" BY PROVIDING	A.J. CANNOT PLAY SAFELY	
OF A VIOLENT	IMMEDIATE VERBAL PRAISE	WITH PEER IN ANY MILIEU	
ACT 4 MONTHS	OF ALL POSITIVE PEER CON-	GROUP FOR THE ENTIRE 45-	
AGO (RAPE AND	TACTS AND EXAMPLES OF	MINUTE PERIOD)	
MURDER)	ANY SPONTANEOUS SAFE		
	CARE OF SELF AND OTHERS		
	(e.g., KEEPING SHOE LACES		
	TIED, HOLDING DOOR OPEN		
	FOR OTHERS, HOLDING A		
	YOUNGER CHILD'S HAND IN		
	TRANSIT TO SCHOOL AS A		
	"SAFETY HELPER"		
	—REWARD A.J. WITH ONE		
	POINT FOR EACH MILIEU		
	GROUP IN WHICH HE IS ABLE		
	TO DO "SAFE PLAY" WITH		
	PEERS (i.e., NO TIME-OUTS		
	FOR AGGRESSION OR		
	UNSAFE PLAY)		
	—USE EXAMPLES OF PHYS-		
	ICAL DANGER AND CON-		
	CEPT OF BODILY SAFETY		
	AS A METAPHOR FOR		
	SAFETY OF PSYCHOLOGICAL		
	SELF AND PERSONAL IN-		
	TEGRITY		
	—IDENTIFY AVAILABLE		
	SUPPORT SYSTEMS (TIMES,		
	PEOPLE, RESOURCES)		
	DAILY		
	—PROVIDE SHORT, CONCISE		
	WARNINGS ABOUT PO-		
	TENTIALLY DANGEROUS		
	BEHAVIOR, REMOVE ANY		
	DANGEROUS OBJECTS AND		
	KEEP NOISE AND VISUAL		
	STIMULI LOW		

Nursing diagnosis	Nursing intervention	Predicted outcome/short-term goals (include time frame)	Date/signature
	—PROVIDE A.J. WITH A CALENDAR OF VISITS AND APPOINTMENTS	—BY THE END OF THE FIRST WEEK, A.J. WILL HAVE DE-CREASED HIS NEED FOR TIME-OUTS FROM NINE TO ONLY TWO PER SHIFT	
	—ENCOURAGE A.J. TO TALK RATHER THAN ACT OUT PHYSICALLY. ROLE-MODEL TURN-TAKING, SHARING, ETC.		
	—ROLE-MODEL SOCIAL CONVERSATION SKILLS (BE CALM, QUIET, INTER-ESTED IN OTHERS WITH FULL EYE CONTACT; DIS-CUSS IMPORTANCE OF CARING ABOUT SELF AND OTHERS)		
	—REINFORCE REALITY AND SOCIAL BOUNDARIES (i.e., TIME, PLACE, PERSON, GOALS) AT BEGINNING OF EACH MILIEU GROUP TO PROMPT SAFE PLAY BEHAVIOR		
	—IF A.J. EXHIBITS UN-SAFE PLAY (e.g., CLIMB-ING ON FURNITURE, TIP-PING CHAIR), ACTS AG-GRESSIVELY TOWARD OTHERS, OR DOES NOT COMPLY WITH STAFF RE-QUESTS TO ADHERE TO SOCIAL RULES OF UNIT (e.g., STAYING WITH GROUP ON WALKS) GIVE ONE VERBAL WARNING AND WAIT 5 SECONDS CALMLY. AFTER THIS, IF HE'S STILL NONCOM-PLIANT, IMMEDIATELY ESCORT HIM TO A COR-NER OF THE ROOM FOR A 2-MINUTE "TIME OUT" MAKE NO DIRECT EYE CONTACT WHILE HE'S IN THE CORNER; STAND NEARBY WITH YOUR FACE AND BODY TURNED PAR-TIALLY AWAY. IN THE CASE OF AGGRESSION, IF A.J. IS STILL AGITAT-ED IN THE CORNER, IN-CREASE THE TIME TO 5 MINUTES, WITH THE LAST MINUTE SPENT		

Continued

Nursing Care Plan *continued*

Nursing diagnosis	Nursing intervention	Predicted outcome/short-term goals (include time frame)	Date/signature
	IN SILENCE. TELL HIM THAT "WHEN YOU ARE SITTING QUIETLY AND FEEL CALM YOU CAN COME OUT OF CORNER AND BACK TO OUR PLAY GROUP". IF HE BECOMES EXTREMELY AGITATED PLACE HIM IN A SECLU- SION ROOM ON AN EMERGENCY BASIS. NO- TIFY PHYSICIAN OF CHANGE IN A.J.'s CON- DITION. FOLLOW THE SECLUSION/RESTRAINT PROTOCOL OUTLINED IN YOUR HOSPITALS POLICY MANUAL		
	—RESTRICT A.J. FROM ROOF-TOP DECK ACTIVITIES ON UNIT — ALLOW A.J. TO TALK ABOUT RESTRICTIONS ON ACTIVITY — DON'T THREATEN A.J.'s SELF-ESTEEM OR SENSE OF CONTROL; e.g., DON'T CONFRONT HIM IN A PUNITIVE MANNER WITH SUCH THREATS AS "IF YOU DON'T STOP ____, I'LL PUT YOU IN THE CORNER." INSTEAD, WHEN- EVER POSSIBLE ALLOW A.J. TO MAKE A DECISION ABOUT HIS OWN BEHAV- IOR AND PHRASE LIMITS IN A POSITIVE LIGHT ("YOU HAD A GOOD START TO THIS GROUP, A.J.. NOW, YOU CAN TRY TO KEEP YOURSELF AND OTHERS SAFE FOR THE REST OF THE PERIOD OR YOU CAN SIT IN THE CORNER UNTIL YOU CALM DOWN") — MAINTAIN A.J. ON STEP-DOWN FROM STRICT SO (SUICIDAL OBSERVATION) STATUS, DUE TO SUICIDAL IDEATION AND RECENT ROOF JUMP ATTEMPT (NOTE: HIS CURRENT SUI- CIDAL LETHALITY IS AS- SESSED AS MODERATE,		

Nursing diagnosis	Nursing intervention	Predicted outcome/short-term goals (include time frame)	Date/signature
	DUE TO THE STRUCTURED MILIEU, HIS RESPONSIVENESS TO POSITIVE SOCIAL REINFORCERS, HIS LACK OF AN IDENTIFIED PLAN, AND THE ABSENCE OF OVERT SUICIDAL IDEATION SINCE HOSPITALIZATION) THUS, DURING NORMAL WAKING HOURS, MAINTAIN A.J. ON CE (CONSTANT EYESIGHT) STATUS TO ALLOW HIM OPPORTUNITIES TO JOIN PEERS IN MILIEU WITHOUT SPECIAL		
	ONE TO ONE ASSIGNMENT, WHICH MIGHT INADVERTENTLY GIVE MORE ATTENTION TO SUICIDAL IDEATION AND REINFORCE MALADAPTIVE DEPENDENCY BEHAVIORS. AT NIGHT, MAINTAIN HIM ON CLOSE OBSERVATION, WITH CHECKS EVERY 15 MINUTES — TO HELP A.J. EXPRESS HIS FEELINGS, PROVIDE HIM WITH FEELINGS CHARTS THAT SHOW A VARIETY OF FACIAL EXPRESSIONS — HAPPINESS, SORROW, ANGER, FEAR, ETC.		
INEFFECTIVE INDIVIDUAL COPING RELATED TO MALADAPTIVE COMPULSIVE SEX-PLAY WITH SELF AND PEERS SECONDARY TO RAPE-TRAUMA SYNDROME	— VERBALLY INTERRUPT ALL OF A.J.'s COMPULSIVE SEX-PLAY ACTIVITIES TOWARD SELF AND OTHERS, USING NONPUNITIVE REDIRECTING STATEMENTS SUCH AS "WE DON'T PLAY TOUCH/SHOW GAMES HERE; IF YOU LIKE, YOU MAY TOUCH YOURSELF UNDER THE COVERS ALONE AT NIGHT AFTER LIGHTS-OUT" — REDIRECT A.J. INTO ALTERNATIVE ADAPTIVE MODES OF RELATING USING PROMPTS SUCH AS "A.J. REMEMBER TO KEEP HANDS TO	— BY THE END OF WEEK 1, A.J. WILL BE ABLE TO ENGAGE IN SAFE PLAY WITH PEERS IN AT LEAST TWO MILIEU GROUPS PER DAY WITHOUT ANY SEXUAL ACTING-OUT	5/2 PDC

Continued

Nursing Care Plan *continued*

Nursing diagnosis	Nursing intervention	Predicted outcome/short-term goals (include time frame)	Date/signature
	YOURSELF; LET'S PLAY _____." OR "A.J., WHEN YOU WANT TO TALK WITH ME, CALL MY NAME. I DON'T WANT YOU TO TOUCH ME THERE"		
	—VISUALLY DEMONSTRATE THE NORMAL PHYSICAL BOUNDARIES BETWEEN PEOPLE BY STEPPING BACK AWAY FROM HIM, OFFERING A HANDSHAKE TO MAINTAIN SOCIAL CONNECTEDNESS, AND PERHAPS DRAWING AN IMAGINARY CIRCLE A-ROUND YOURSELF, THEN HIM. EXPLAIN THAT YOU ARE IN CHARGE OF YOUR BODY AND HE IS IN CHARGE OF HIS		
	—REMIND HIM THAT HE IS A SPECIAL "SAFETY KID" WITH HIS OWN "MAGIC CIRCLE" OF PRO-TECTION AROUND HIS BODY THAT PUTS HIM IN CHARGE AND GIVES HIM THE RIGHT TO SAY "NO" IF SOMEONE TRESPASSES INTO IT		
	—EXPLAIN THESE LIMIT-SETTING GAMES TO A.J. IN A CALM, SUPPORTIVE, NONJUDGMENTAL BUT FIRM MANNER THAT SHOWS CLEARLY THAT HE IS O.K., BUT HIS IN-TRUSIVE, UNASKED-FOR TOUCHING BEHAVIOR IS NOT		
	—RECORD THE FREQUEN-CY OF A.J.'s SEX-PLAY ATTEMPTS TOWARD SELF AND OTHERS/OBJECTS	—BY THE END OF WEEK 1, A.J. WILL EARN "SMELLY STICKERS" FOR AT LEAST ONE MILIEU GROUP PER DAY (BASELINE = 15 MINUTES OF ONE 45-MIN-UTE GROUP WITHOUT COM-PULSIVELY TOUCHING HIMSELF OR OTHERS OR MAKING SEX-UAL GESTURES/NOISES	
	—GIVE A.J. A "SMELLY STICKER" FOR EACH MILIEU GROUP SESSION HE IS ABLE TO COM-PLETE WITH "KEEPING HIS HANDS TO HIMSELF"		
	—INCLUDE A.J. AS A MEMBER OF THE "SAFE-TY KIDS CLUB" TWICE A	—BY COMPLETION OF TWO SESSIONS IN THE "SAFETY KIDS CLUB, A.J. WILL SPON-TANEOUSLY SHARE AT LEAST ONE PERSONAL SAFETY CON-	

Nursing diagnosis	Nursing intervention	Predicted outcome/short-term goals (include time frame)	Date/signature
	WEEK TO BUILD HIS SELF-ESTEEM AND SELF-CONCEPT AND TO PROVIDE HIM WITH A MORE ADAPTIVE STRUCTURED PLACE TO HELP HIM COPE WITH THE EXPERIENCE OF HIS ABUSE, GIVE HIM THE PERCEPTION OF CONTROL OVER HIS SELF AND BODY, AND IMBUE HIM WITH A HEALTHY SENSE OF CAUTION AND PERSONAL POWER	CEPT LEARNED IN THE CLUB; e.g., TAKE A BUDDY INTO THE PUBLIC RESTROOM ACCOMPANIED WITH A STAFF MEMBER ON UNIT. HE ALSO WILL SHOW A DECREASE IN SEX-PLAY, UNSAFE PLAY, AND AGGRESSION, AND WILL BEGIN TO DISCLOSE MORE IN HIS INDIVIDUAL THERAPY WITH REGARD TO WITNESSED TRAUMA AND SEXUAL ABUSE, BECAUSE OF LEARNING THAT IT IS "O.K. TO TELL"	
	-IN MILIEU, REINFORCE ALL SAFE, ASSERTIVE, EMPATHIC "BUDDY-TYPE" BEHAVIORS LEARNED IN "SAFETY KIDS CLUB" (e.g., "WHAT A GREAT SAFETY KID YOU ARE, A.J.! YOU SURE ARE LOOKING OUT FOR YOURSELF TODAY.") ENCOURAGE HIM TO IDENTIFY UNSAFE THINGS IN THE MILIEU (e.g., UNTIED SHOELACES). REASSURE HIM THAT HE IS SAFE AND VALUED HERE.		
	-TO ENSURE THAT A.J. DOES NOT DEVELOP AN EXAGGERATED VIEW OF A HOSTILE, DANGEROUS WORLD AND BECOME OVERLY FEARFUL, REVIEW AND CORRECT ANY MISCONCEPTIONS ABOUT DANGEROUS SITUATIONS THAT HE SPONTANEOUSLY MENTIONS AND DO NOT REINFORCE ERRONEOUS STEREOTYPES; e.g., ALL STRANGERS ARE BAD, UGLY, AND DRIVE BLACK CARS		
	-GIVE A.J. THE OPPORTUNITY TO CONSIDER POSITIVE FORMS OF TOUCHING, NURTURING, AND AFFECTION. USE PUPPETS TO ROLE PLAY		

Continued

Nursing Care Plan *continued*

Nursing diagnosis	Nursing intervention	Predicted outcome/short-term goals (include time frame)	Date/signature
	SCENES OF CONFUSING TOUCH TO HELP A.J. LEARN WHEN IT'S AP- PROPRIATE TO "TELL", "SAY NO", "GET HELP", "GET AWAY". MAKE A SAFETY PLAN WITH PARENT, OR "YELL" —ACKNOWLEDGE THAT BAD THINGS CAN HAPPEN, AND THAT THEY MAY GET WORSE IF HE KEEPS SECRETS. REINFORCE A.J.'S HEALTHY EXIST- ING SUPPORT SYSTEM WHEN HELPING HIM THINK OF "WHO COULD I TELL?" —APPROACH ALL TOPICS WITH THE INTENT TO INFORM WITHOUT UNDUE ALARM; USE A MATTER- OF-FACT, NONSENSA- TIONAL TONE OF VOICE AND MANNER —THROUGHOUT THE SES- SIONS, USE FAMILIAR WORDS RELATED TO HIS EVERYDAY LIFE EXPERIENCE		

was not able to express any direct feelings about his own victimization, which led to intrusive thoughts, nightmares, emotional regression, and acting-out behaviors. His loss of bodily control (enuresis), settling difficulties, overeating, and compulsive water activities all represented acute manifestations of his anxiety. Nevertheless, he remained responsive to praise and positive reinforcement and desired to be "a good boy" and be loved. He was able to reach out to others for assistance and accept limits when provided. Given a structured, predictable, nurturing environment, he exhibited good potential for making a successful emotional adjustment.

A.J. came from a chaotic, traumatized family environment that provided few nurturant resources and that had a hostile impact upon his emotional and physical development. Home discipline was weak and inconsistent; but although his mother did not act quickly on A.J.'s behalf to protect him, she recently evidenced a desire to correct the situation and had managed to seek assistance through the women's shelter. She showed some ability to use social services and resources, as evidenced by the job training in electronics, and kept a steady job. She cared deeply for A.J.'s welfare and, in an attempt to help him, began to share openly her own victimization.

SUMMARY

During A.J.'s first 3 days on the unit, he exhibited much compulsive, aggressive, sexual acting-out behavior. He attempted to disrobe, exhibited his buttocks and penis, and masturbated publicly. He made repeated reference to his "bone that moves" with accompanying grunts, snorts, flatulence, and sexual posturing, including groin thrusts. The second night, he urinated in a peer's bed and was found lying on a bed with another male peer with their pants down and giggling. On the third day, he compulsively attempted to lick the hind end of a bear statue encountered during a walk with staff on hospital grounds.

The multidisciplinary treatment plan was developed and implemented during a 30-day comprehensive acute treatment program. The primary therapist saw A.J. in individual psychotherapy to address intrapsychic issues. The primary therapist and social worker met with A.J.'s family to examine social network resources issues, address family dynamics contributing to A.J.'s problems, and facilitate DPSS legal casework completion.

The primary nurse implemented behavioral training techniques to help extinguish A.J.'s maladaptive compulsive sexual acting-out behaviors and reinforced self-care skills and socialization to build his self-esteem. The nurse also reviewed parent education on realistic home supervision expectations and discipline techniques.

A.J. was included in the "Safety Kids Club," a group therapy experience conducted by the clinical nurse specialist utilizing audio-visual materials on child sexual abuse prevention designed by Janeen Brady (1983). This therapeutic group, using concepts of abuse prevention to help shape improved self-concept, self-esteem, and bodily safety, provided a milieu management tool for dealing with the sexual and aggressive impulses A.J. expressed on the unit. As Adams (1984) points out, younger children "still believe adults are right, and continue to believe if something bad happens to them, it must have been their fault. They may also focus on wrong-doing they understand (such as telling lies or breaking rules) rather than sexual abuse.... Children in third through sixth grades are moving toward making independent judgments about people's behavior and the consequences of breaking rules." From a developmental perspective, A.J. was just becoming ready to consider the traumatic events of his life as being beyond his control and not his fault; he needed further nurturant guidance, in an outpatient residential therapy setting, to cognitively reconstruct his world view.

By discharge, A.J. showed improved adjustment in both his behavior and mood. He was no longer enuretic, he kept his hands to himself, and he masturbated privately in his room. He demonstrated a spontaneous awareness of rules for personal safety and asked to take his "Safety Kids" coloring book home with him. His posture was straighter, and he smiled when praised and complied with all unit rules within one verbal prompt. He had made no threats to himself or others nor any fire-setting attempts since admission. He was able to express anger at his stepfather but also talked about needing a daddy; his puppets were no longer mistreated victims, but instead "had problems and found people to help them." On his last day, A.J. expressed the wish to be a policeman when he grew up, "because they help keep people safe."

In summary, sexuality is a normal part of human development that needs expression throughout the life cycle. A.J. needed to learn the proper expression of various sexual behaviors within the social context, as a part of his developmental process. Even though he was a child, A.J. had a biological need for tension/sexuality outlets and needed direction to use these outlets in a socially acceptable manner. The multidisciplinary care plan developed for him helped provide this direction.

REFERENCES

Adams, C. "Considering Children's Developmental Stages in Prevention Education," *Child Sexual Abuse*. Edited by Finkelhor, D. New York: The Free Press, 1984.

Brady, J. *Safety Kids Club*. Salt Lake City: Brite Music Enterprises, 1983.

Edleson, J.L. "Working with Men Who Batter," *Social Work* 237-42, May/June 1984.

Sideleau, B.F. "Patterns of Abuse," in *Comprehensive Psychiatric Nursing*, 3rd ed. Edited by Haber, J., et al. New York: McGraw-Hill Book Co., 1987.

SELECTED BIBLIOGRAPHY

Anderson, C. "A History of the Touch Continuum," in *Child Sexual Abuse*. Edited by Finkelhor, D. New York: The Free Press, 1984.

Blos, P., Jr. "Children Think About Illness: Their Concepts and Beliefs," in *Psychosocial Aspects of Pediatric Care*. Edited by Gellert, E. New York: Grune & Stratton, 1978.

Gellert, E. "What Do I Have Inside Me? How Children View Their Bodies," in *Psychosocial Aspects of Pediatric Care*. Edited by Gellert, E. New York: Grune & Stratton, 1978.

Hutchinson, B., and Fridley, E. *My Personal Safety Coloring Book*. Fridley, Minnesota: Fridley Police Department, 1982.

Krause, E. *Speak Up, Say No!* Oregon City: Krause House, 1983.

Pynoos, R., and Eth, S. "Witness to Violence: The Child Interview," *Journal of the American Academy of Child Psychiatry* 25:306-19, 1986.

Nursing of Clients in the Home and Clinic

The following cases illustrate the work of the psychiatric–mental health nurse specialist in home and clinic settings. After graduate study and supervised clinical experience, these nurses practice at advanced competency levels, especially in the area of physical assessment skills. Nursing care plans conform to home health agency and clinical standards.

Jane:
Reversible Dementia

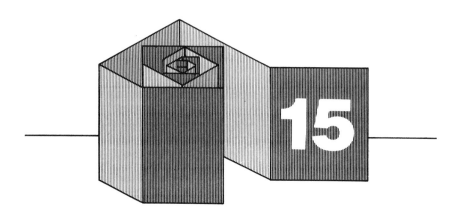

Marcia Pearson Miller, MS, RN

An estimated three million Americans over age 65 experience a clinically significant dementia; nearly 10% of these individuals reside at home (LaPorte, 1982). Just how many of these "at home" dementia cases are potentially reversible has yet to be studied. Nurses frequently are in a unique position to assess a client's functioning in the home. Public health nurses are particularly sensitive to the needs of the client who is treatable in the home. Often, the data received from the referring agent (for example, a physician or social worker) conflicts with the situation the nurse actually finds during the home visit. The misdiagnosis of a potentially reversible dementia as an irreversible Alzheimer's type dementia is a serious, yet common, error. This case exemplifies such a situation, in that the data presented to the nurse painted a grim picture for the client. In reality, however, expert assessment and nursing care were able to turn a seemingly irreversible problem into a return of the client to a more healthy state. Future health care trends indicate a need for improved health care efforts directed at the elderly population. While providing such care, psychiatric nurses must consider the reversible causes of dementia when performing home care assessments. A quick assumption about diagnostic labels may not only hinder the provision of proper care, but also result in what Dodson (1984) calls the "slow death" of an elderly client.

CASE STUDY

Jane, an 83-year-old white widow, was referred to a psychiatric clinical nurse specialist (PCNS) for home care evaluation. According to the referring physician, Jane's daughter, Mary, had contacted him with concerns about Jane's health. Mary described a 6-month history of Jane's progressive decline in self-care functioning and withdrawal from social activities, and questioned her mother's continued ability to live at home unsupervised. She also reported that her mother was displaying progressive confusion and memory loss. On the basis of this behavioral description, the physician tentatively diagnosed Jane as having Alzheimer's disease; he believed that home care interventions would be brief and crisis-oriented, and likely culminate in Jane's placement in a skilled nursing facility.

At the time of contact, Jane lived alone in a spacious two-bedroom apartment in a large suburban city. Her only child, Mary, lived 15 miles away; no other relatives lived nearby. Jane had no documented psychiatric history. Data for this case study was gathered from a wide variety of sources, including Jane's neighbors, friends, and immediate family.

Jane had retired from her job as a school teacher 20 years previously; her husband died 5 years later. From the time of her husband's death until 6 months prior to contact, Jane functioned well. She adjusted to widowhood by establishing a number of social contacts throughout her apartment complex, and she used her time productively, traveling often, joining in weekly bridge games, and participating in activities at the local Senior Citizen's Center. Gradually, however, Jane's neighbors began to notice a decline in her self-care abilities. Jane forgot scheduled appointments, later offering apologies for having slept through the appointments or having neglected to write them on her calendar. She frequently complained of her arthritis "acting up" and seemed unable to control her pain adequately with frequent doses of acetaminophen. As her pain worsened, she became progressively weaker and subsequently suffered loss of appetite and sleep, eventually losing weight and refusing to leave the apartment. Friends noticed she looked depressed, but although they offered help and support, Jane refused their visits. Her few social contacts noted a progressive worsening of her forgetfulness and confusion. At one point, a neighbor spotted smoke seeping from underneath Jane's apartment door; Jane had put a frozen dinner in the oven and gone to bed, forgetting all about it. This incident prompted Jane's friends to take swift action; they notified Mary of Jane's inability to maintain a safe environment.

Sue, Jane's closest neighbor and friend, was aware that Jane and Mary were rarely in contact; Jane had often complained of many personal differences with her daughter. Predictably, Mary was in no hurry to come to her mother's aid; rather, she promised to send her husband Mike over right away. Once Mike arrived, he recognized the need for a thorough evaluation of Jane and her home situation. He persuaded Mary to contact Jane's physician, who then referred the case to a PCNS at the local home health care agency.

For the initial interview, Jane insisted on Sue's presence "just in case I forget anything." Jane's chief complaint summarized her major concerns: "I think my daughter wants to put me in a home... I'll die if I have to go... They won't take pets and I can't get rid of my cat... I'll be all right with help... I just want to stay in my apartment."

Jane was clearly homebound due to extreme weakness, pronounced pain on ambulation, and the inability to accomplish basic activities of daily living. She described a 10-year history of osteoarthritis and was noticeably kyphotic with related joint deformities. She denied the presence of other chronic illnesses and claimed she took no medication except acetaminophen for joint pain and mineral oil for constipation. She had no allergies and abstained from alcohol and tobacco, although she enjoyed two cups of coffee a day. Her hearing, vision, touch, and overall sensory awareness all appeared intact. She denied any past hospitalizations, and her last physical examination, 7 months previous, was essentially unremarkable.

The physical examination performed by the PCNS revealed a blood pressure of 160/60 sitting and lying, and 130/60 standing. Jane was tachycardic at rest, 100 to 120 beats per minute with a regular apical rate. Her oral temperature was 38° C., with respirations of 24 at rest and 32 on exertion. Her mouth was in noticeably poor condition, with ill-fitting dentures, parched mucous membranes, furrowed tongue, and a pronounced odor of ketones. Her skin was warm and dry with poor turgor; the PCNS noted several old second-degree burns on both hands. Pulmonary auscultation revealed clear lungs; abdominal palpation and auscultation revealed a slightly hard and distended abdomen with hypoactive bowel sounds in all four quadrants; and digital rectal exam located a high fecal impaction. Jane's weight was 94 pounds; her height was 5 feet, 3 inches. The remainder of the physical examination, including gross neurological functioning, revealed no remarkable findings.

During the mental status examination, Jane presented as a thin, cachectic-looking woman dressed in a stained bathrobe. She attempted to greet the examiner appropriately although her facial expression appeared tense and strained. Jane's speech was coherent but somewhat halting, as if she were carefully searching for the correct responses to the examiner's questions. She made no attempts at confabulation; in fact, she volunteered very little information spontaneously. Her overall affect was blunted, with an occasional forced smile. She readily admitted to feeling "down" and discouraged about her memory loss and diminished functioning. She claimed she had not slept well in weeks, was not able to concentrate, and had no appetite. Her thought content was intact and pervaded with themes of hopelessness and helplessness. She was convinced that she might die if placed in a nursing home; such a placement was her greatest fear. She demonstrated no evidence of delusions or hallucinations. Her judgment appeared intact. She demonstrated good insight into the extent of her memory loss and readily agreed her safety would be in jeopardy if she did not get help.

To assess the extent of Jane's cognitive dysfunction, the PCNS performed the Cognitive Capacity Screening Exam (Jacobs, 1977), a 30-item test used to evaluate general cognitive orientation. Questions assess recent and remote memory, recall and recognition, abstraction, calculation, and conceptualization. A score of less than 20 indicates possible organic brain syndrome; Jane had a total score of 12.

While Jane was unable to identify the exact day, month, and date, with reminders she named the season and approximate month. She correctly identified her address. Her immediate recall was good, as evidenced by her ability to repeat four numbers in correct order. However, her recent memory was poor; she could not recall even one out of four items after 1 minute's time. Her remote memory was excellent; during the interview, she talked with less hesitation about her past than about any other subject. She also demonstrated the ability to grasp general information questions geared at knowledge of current events. She identified the location of personal possessions in the apartment and, although unable to perform serial sevens or threes, completed simple additions and subtractions accurately. Her ability to abstract and conceptualize was good; she correctly identified red and blue as colors, and correctly performed opposite identification (e.g., "the opposite of hard is soft"). Overall, her general ability to follow instructions was good.

Reader may now complete Recording the Data, Assigning Nursing Diagnoses, and Nursing Care Plan.

FORMULATION

On the basis of clinical findings, the PCNS questioned the physician's preliminary diagnosis of Alzheimer's disease. Certain findings, such as Jane's insight into the extent of her disability, her lack of confabulation, her verbalized themes of hopelessness, and vegetative signs, indicated the possibility that Jane's dementia was reversible.

The Alzheimer's disease–senile dementia complex, as described by
Continued on page 360

RECORDING THE DATA

After you have read the case, cluster significant data into functional health patterns.

Health management/health perception _____

_____

_____

_____

_____

Nutritional/metabolic _____

_____

_____

_____

Elimination _____

_____

_____

_____

Activity/exercise _____

_____

_____

_____

Cognitive/perceptual _____

_____

_____

_____

Sleep/rest _____

_____

_____

_____

Self-perception/self-concept _____

_____

_____

_____

Role relationship _____

_____

_____

_____

Sexuality/reproductive _____

_____

_____

_____

Coping/stress tolerance _____

_____

_____

_____

Value/belief _____

_____

_____

_____

ASSIGNING NURSING DIAGNOSES

Use your clustered data to select appropriate nursing diagnoses.

Health perception/health management

- ☐ Growth and Development, Altered (see Developmental Delay)
- ☐ Health Maintenance, Altered
- ☐ Infection, Potential for
- ☐ Injury (Trauma): Potential for
- ☐ Noncompliance (Specify)
- ☐ Poisoning: Potential for
- ☐ Suffocation: Potential for

Nutritional/metabolic

- ☐ Body Temperature, Potential Alteration in
- ☐ Developmental Delay: Physical Growth and Development
- ☐ Fluid Volume, Altered: Excess or Excess Fluid Volume
- ☐ Fluid Volume Deficit, Actual
- ☐ Fluid Volume Deficit, Potential
- ☐ Nutrition, Altered: Less Than Body Requirements or Nutritional Deficit (Specify)
- ☐ Nutrition, Altered: More Than Body Requirements or Exogenous Obesity
- ☐ Nutrition, Altered: Potential for More Than Body Requirements or Potential for Obesity
- ☐ Oral Mucous Membrane, Altered
- ☐ Skin Integrity, Impaired or Skin Breakdown
- ☐ Skin Integrity, Impaired or Potential Skin Breakdown
- ☐ Swallowing, Impaired or Uncompensated Swallowing Impairment
- ☐ Tissue Integrity, Impaired

Elimination

- ☐ Bowel Elimination, Altered: Constipation
- ☐ Bowel Elimination, Altered: Diarrhea
- ☐ Bowel Elimination, Altered: Incontinence

- ☐ Developmental Delay: Bowel/Bladder Control
- ☐ Incontinence: Functional
- ☐ Incontinence: Reflex
- ☐ Incontinence: Stress
- ☐ Incontinence: Total
- ☐ Incontinence: Urge
- ☐ Urinary Elimination, Altered Patterns of
- ☐ Urinary Retention

Activity/exercise

- ☐ Activity Intolerance
- ☐ Activity Intolerance, Potential
- ☐ Airway Clearance, Ineffective
- ☐ Breathing Pattern, Ineffective
- ☐ Cardiac Output, Altered: Decreased
- ☐ Developmental Delay: Mobility
- ☐ Developmental Delay: Self-Care Skills
- ☐ Diversional Activity Deficit
- ☐ Gas Exchange, Impaired
- ☐ Home Maintenance Management, Impaired (Mild, Moderate, Severe, Potential, Chronic)
- ☐ Mobility, Impaired Physical
- ☐ Self-Care Deficit: Feeding
- ☐ Self-Care Deficit: Bathing/Hygiene
- ☐ Self-Care Deficit: Dressing/Grooming
- ☐ Self-Care Deficit: Toileting
- ☐ Self-Care Deficit: Total
- ☐ Tissue Perfusion, Altered: (Specify)

Sleep/rest

- ☐ Sleep Pattern Disturbance

Cognitive/perceptual

- ☐ Comfort, Altered: Pain
- ☐ Comfort, Altered: Chronic Pain

☐ Developmental Delay: (Specify Cognitive Area; attention, decision making, etc.)
☐ Hypothermia
☐ Hyperthermia
☐ Knowledge Deficit (Specify)
☐ Sensory-Perceptual Alteration: Input Excess or Sensory Overload
☐ Sensory-Perceptual Alteration: Input Deficit or Sensory Deprivation
☐ Thermoregulation, Ineffective
☐ Thought Processes, Altered
☐ Unilateral Neglect

Self-perception/self-concept

☐ Anxiety
☐ Body Image Disturbance
☐ Fear
☐ Hopelessness
☐ Personal Identity Confusion
☐ Powerlessness (Severe, Low, Moderate)
☐ Self-Esteem Disturbance

Role relationship

☐ Communication, Impaired Verbal
☐ Developmental Delay: Communication Skills
☐ Developmental Delay: Social Skills
☐ Family Processes, Altered
☐ Grieving, Anticipatory
☐ Grieving, Dysfunctional
☐ Parenting, Altered: Actual or Potential

☐ Role Performance, Disturbance in
☐ Social Interactions, Impaired
☐ Social Isolation (Rejection)

Sexuality/reproductive

☐ Rape-Trauma Syndrome: Compounded
☐ Rape-Trauma Syndrome: Silent Reaction
☐ Sexual Dysfunction
☐ Sexuality Patterns, Altered

Coping/stress tolerance

☐ Adjustment, Impaired
☐ Coping, Ineffective Individual
☐ Coping, Ineffective Family: Compromised
☐ Coping, Ineffective Family: Disabling
☐ Coping, Family: Potential for Growth
☐ Developmental Delay (Specify area)
☐ Post-Trauma Response
☐ Violence, Potential for (Self-Directed or Directed at Others)

Value/belief

☐ Spiritual Distress (Distress of Human Spirit)

You are now ready to develop a nursing care plan for this client. Use the following blank pages to do so. Then refer to the author's formulation, diagnostic summary, care plan, and summary.

NURSING CARE PLAN

Complete the chart below to develop a nursing care plan for this client.

Discharge outcomes/long-term goals	

Nursing diagnosis	Nursing intervention	

	Predicted outcomes/short-term goals (include time frame)	Date/signature

Return to Formulation, page 353

nurse gerontologists Wolanin and Phillips (1981), is an irreversible condition of slow onset characterized by four cardinal symptoms: progressive aphasia (difficulty recalling simple words), progressive apraxia (inability to perform purposeful activity), progressive agnosia (difficulty recognizing objects), and progressive mnemonic disturbance (inability to remember recent events). While Jane showed elements of aphasia, apraxia, and mnemonic disturbance, her symptoms occurred within a relatively short time and were concurrent with evidence of significant depression and deterioration in her self-care abilities that resulted in a physical imbalance. In addition, her awareness of her memory loss represented an atypical finding in Alzheimer's disease. Many clients with Alzheimer's, particularly those in the later stages of the disease, use denial in varying degrees, yielding paranoid and defensive behavior—behavior that was absent in Jane's case.

Finally, until her recent social withdrawal, Jane had been able to maintain stable relationships with friends and neighbors and had routinely sought their support in times of need. Jane's wish to have her friend Sue present during her interview demonstrated her ability to draw on coping strategies to offset the stress of the interview. While Jane certainly needed medical follow-up to assess for potential underlying causes of her abrupt behavioral changes (such as an occult malignancy), the PCNS believed that nursing interventions delivered at home would probably reverse some of Jane's symptoms.

But which of the clinical findings were potentially reversible? Jane's overall appearance, verbalizations of hopelessness, insight into her memory loss, and vegetative signs indicate the existence of a primary or concurrent depressive disorder in addition to symptoms of Alzheimer's type dementia. Reisberg and Ferris (1982) discuss depression as providing the major differential diagnostic challenge in the assessment of older individuals experiencing cognitive deficits. Their review of studies shows that depressed individuals are more aware of their cognitive impairment than are those with Alzheimer's type dementia, and they more readily complain of anorexia, sleep disturbance, and emotional discomfort as a result of the condition. Furthermore, while no temporal predictors exist in the course of Alzheimer's type dementia, a very gradual onset and relatively stable downhill course is predictable in depression.

Pain is a second potentially reversible cause of acute confusional states in the elderly (Wolanin and Phillips, 1981). Pain can affect an individual's functional abilities, resulting in inactivity, weakness, fatigue, sleep deprivation, and depression; these symptoms often develop into a complex cycle of mental and physical disequilibrium. Jane's osteoarthritis caused her much pain, which could have contributed to her cognitive deficits.

Continued on page 375

DIAGNOSTIC SUMMARY FOR JANE

Data	Functional health pattern	Nursing diagnosis
—Refuses to leave her apartment —Experiences extreme weakness, pronounced pain on ambulation, and inability to accomplish basic activities of daily living —Has a 10-year history of osteoarthritis; is noticeably kyphotic with related joint deformities	Activity/Exercise	Activity intolerance related to homebound status secondary to malnutrition, depression and pain
—Has pronounced pain on ambulation —Seems unable to adequately control her pain with frequent doses of acetaminophen	Cognitive/Perceptual	Altered comfort: chronic pain related to severe osteoarthritis
—Exhibits a lack of awareness of environmental hazards (once left a frozen dinner cooking in the oven and had gone to bed)	Health Perception/ Health Management	Potential for injury related to sensory and motor deficits secondary to reversible brain syndrome
—Has a 6-month history of progressive decline in self-care functioning —Displays signs of confusion and memory loss —Forgets scheduled appointments —Wears stained clothing —Exhibits poor oral hygiene and ill-fitting dentures	Activity/Exercise	Self-care deficit: total related to cognitive impairments, depression, and physical status
—Parched mucous membranes, furrowed tongue, pronounced ketone breath odor —Warm, dry skin with poor turgor	Nutritional/ Metabolic	Fluid volume deficit related to decreased fluid intake secondary to cognitive impairment and depression
—Demonstrates a knowledge deficit on principles of basic nutrition —Lacks the ability to procure food for herself —Exhibits marked cachexia (weight, 94 lbs; height, 5′3″) —Has no appetite	Nutritional/ Metabolic	Alteration in nutrition: less than body requirements related to anorexia secondary to depression
—Expresses her greatest fear is placement in an extended care facility: "I think my daughter wants to put me in a home… I'll die if I have to go… They won't take pets and I can't get rid of my cat"	Coping/Stress Tolerance	Fear related to loss of functioning and potential loss of home and support system Ineffective individual coping related to depression secondary to stress of *Continued*

Diagnostic Summary for Jane *continued*

Data	Functional health pattern	Nursing diagnosis
—Demonstrates intact thought content with themes of hopelessness and helplessness —Refuses her friends' offers of help and support —Refuses to leave her apartment		physical illness and loss of control
—Relates poor contact with daughter Mary due to many personal differences (Mary was in no hurry to come to her mother's aid, but sent her husband Mike over right away.)	Coping/Stress Tolerance	Ineffective family coping: compromised, related to unmet psychosocial needs of parent by child
—Uses mineral oil to relieve constipation —High fecal impaction located on physical exam	Elimination	Altered bowel elimination: constipation related to poor nutrition and hydration status secondary to immobility and depression

NURSING CARE PLAN

Complete the chart below to develop a nursing care plan for this client.

Discharge outcome/long-term goals	
1. BY THE END OF 60 DAYS, OR AT THE TIME OF CASE CLOSURE JANE WILL NO LONGER BE HOMEBOUND AND WILL WALK TO THE STORE WITH ASSISTANCE.	

Nursing diagnosis	Nursing intervention	Predicted outcome/short-term goals (include time frame)	Date/signature
ACTIVITY INTOL- ERANCE RELATED TO HOMEBOUND STATUS SECOND- ARY TO MALNU- TRITION, DEPRES- SION, AND PAIN	—ENSURE A PHYSICAL THER- APY HOME EVALUATION FOR MUSCULOSKELETAL INTEG- RITY ASSESSMENT, STRENGTH- ENING EXERCISES, ACTIVITY STRUCTURING, AND ASSISTIVE DEVICES	—PHYSICAL THERAPY ASSESSMENT WILL BE COMPLETED IN 1 WEEK —JANE'S SIGNIFICANT OTHERS WILL BE MADE AWARE OF HER ACTIVITY SCHEDULE IN 2 WEEKS —JANE WILL TAKE 30 MINUTE WALKS DAILY WITH ASSISTANCE	1/15 MM
	—ENSURE THAT THE HOME CARE TEAM AND JANE'S SIGNIFICANT OTHERS EN- COURAGE ACTIVITY SCHEDULE	—BY CASE CLOSURE, JANE'S SIG- NIFICANT OTHERS WILL MAKE SURE THAT JANE WALKS AT LEAST EVERY OTHER DAY	
	—MAINTAIN A BALANCE OF ACTIVITY AND REST; e.g., AVOID ACTIVITY AFTER MEALS		
	—ALONG WITH THE PHYSICAL THERAPIST, EVALUATE JANE'S LIMITS AND TOLERANCES FOR SCHEDULING OF PRO- GRESSIVE ACTIVITIES		
	—SUMMARIZE ACTIVITY PROGRESS WITH JANE ON A WEEKLY BASIS AND PLAN FOR THE FOLLOWING WEEK'S ACTIVITY WITH A WRITTEN PLAN. MODIFY THE ACTIVITY PLAN ACCORD- ING TO SUBJECTIVE INDICA- TIONS OF JANE'S PAIN, FEAR, OR WEAKNESS		

Continued

Nursing Care Plan *continued*

Discharge outcome/long-term goals	
1. BY THE END OF 60 DAYS OR AT THE TIME OF CASE CLOSURE JANE WILL STATE THAT HER PAIN IS UNDER CONTROL.	

Nursing diagnosis	Nursing intervention	Predicted outcome/short-term goals (include time frame)	Date/signature
ALTERED COM- FORT: CHRONIC PAIN RELATED TO SEVERE OSTEOARTHRITIS	— CONFER WITH JANE'S PHYSICIAN REGARDING NEED FOR PAIN-RELIEF MEASURES, INCLUDING NONINVASIVE MODALITIES AND NONNARCOTIC, NON- STEROIDAL, AND ANTI-IN- FLAMMATORY MEDICATIONS	— IF MEDICATIONS ARE USED, JANE WILL EXPERIENCE NO SIDE EFFECTS — JANE'S PAIN WILL DECREASE, AS DESCRIBED ON A SCALE OF 1 TO 10 WITHIN 2 WEEKS — BY CASE CLOSURE, JANE WILL BE ABLE TO LEARN RELAXATION	1/15 MM
	— CONDUCT A PAIN ASSESS- MENT EACH VISIT, RATING PAIN ON SCALE FROM 1-10, OBSERVING VERBAL AND NONVERBAL CUES, DIURNAL VARIATIONS AND RELIEF OBTAINED FROM MEDS AND RELAXATION — INSTRUCT JANE ON RE- LAXATION EXERCISES (GUIDED IMAGERY MAY BE BEST, AS PROGRESSIVE RELAXATION TECHNIQUES MAY EXACERBATE PAIN)	TECHNIQUES AND USE THEM WITH ASSISTANCE	

Discharge outcome/long-term goals			
1 BY THE END OF 60 DAYS OR, AT THE TIME OF CASE CLOSURE: - JANE WILL IDENTIFY AT LEAST THREE POTENTIAL HAZARDS TO HOME SAFETY. - JANE WILL BE ABLE TO ACCOMPLISH		ACTIVITIES OF DAILY LIVING WITHOUT THREATS TO HOME SAFETY, AND HER FAMILY WILL AGREE SHE CAN BE MAINTAINED AT HOME SAFELY.	

Nursing diagnosis	Nursing intervention	Predicted outcome/short-term goals (include time frame)	Date/signature
POTENTIAL FOR INJURY RELATED TO SENSORY AND MOTOR DEFICITS SECONDARY TO REVERSIBLE BRAIN SYNDROME	- ENSURE AN OCCUPATIONAL THERAPY HOME EVALUATION FOR FINE MOTOR SKILLS AND INSTALLATION OF HOME SAFETY DEVICES, INCLUDING BATHROOM GRAB BARS, REMOVABLE SHOWER HEAD, TUB BENCH, AND TUB THERMOMETER - INSTRUCT JANE'S SIGNIFICANT OTHERS IN GENERAL PRINCIPLES FOR HOME SAFETY - TAKE SAFETY PRECAUTIONS: REMOVE JANE'S PORTABLE SPACE HEATER AND ELECTRIC BLANKET (WITH HER PERMISSION); CORRECT ANY OTHER FIRE HAZARDS; ENSURE THAT THE SMOKE ALARM IS FUNCTIONING - SET THE WATER HEATER AND THERMOSTAT AT SAFE TEMPERATURES; REMOVE ANY THROW RUGS OR PROTRUDING OBJECTS FROM ENVIRONMENT; ENSURE THAT A NIGHT LIGHT IS KEPT ON AT NIGHT; REMOVE MEDICATIONS FROM CHILDPROOF CONTAINERS AND STORE THEM SAFELY - CONSIDER KITCHEN MODIFICATIONS FOR COOKING IF JANE CANNOT DEMONSTRATE SAFE KITCHEN HABITS	- WITHIN 1 WEEK, THE PCNS AND OCCUPATIONAL THERAPIST WILL COMPLETE A HOME SAFETY ASSESSMENT - HOME HAZARDS WILL BE COMPLETELY CORRECTED BY CASE CLOSURE - SIGNIFICANT OTHERS WILL DEMONSTRATE AWARENESS OF HOME SAFETY PRECAUTIONS BY CASE CLOSURE	1/15 MM

Continued

Nursing Care Plan *continued*

Discharge outcome/long-term goals	
1. BY THE END OF 60 DAYS, OR AT THE TIME OF CASE CLOSURE: — JANE WILL BE ABLE TO REMAIN AT HOME WITH ASSISTANCE AND SUPERVISION.	— COGNITIVE CAPACITY SCREENING EXAM WILL NOT SHOW A DECLINE IN SCORES. — JANE WILL STATE SHE NO LONGER FEELS CONFUSED.

Nursing diagnosis	Nursing intervention	Predicted outcome/short-term goals (include time frame)	Date/signature
SELF-CARE DEFICIT: TOTAL RELATED TO COGNITIVE IMPAIRMENTS, DEPRESSION AND PHYSICAL STATUS	— ARRANGE FOR URGENT MEDICAL SOCIAL WORKER (MSW) REFERRAL FOR HOME HELP, PREFERABLY FOR 6 HOURS PER DAY FOR MEAL PREPARATION AND SUPERVISION (MSW WILL ALSO ASSIST WITH LONG-TERM PLANNING AND COUNSELING AND POSSIBLE PLACEMENT IN EXTENDED-CARE FACILITY IF LONG-TERM GOALS CANNOT BE REACHED)	— AN IN-HOME CARETAKER WILL BE HIRED WITHIN 2 WEEKS — JANE WILL BE DRESSED APPROPRIATELY DURING DAYLIGHT HOURS — JANE WILL ACCOMPLISH ALL ACTIVITIES OF DAILY LIVING, WITH THE CARETAKER'S HELP WITHIN 4 WEEKS	1/15 *MM*
	— ARRANGE FOR A HOME HEALTH AID TO VISIT JANE THREE TIMES PER WEEK UNTIL PERMANENT HELP IS OBTAINED		
	— ENCOURAGE JANE'S SIGNIFICANT OTHERS TO PROVIDE HER WITH STIMULATING VARIATIONS OF DAILY ACTIVITIES		
	— FOR JANE'S COGNITIVE IMPAIRMENTS: · ADMINISTER THE COGNITIVE CAPACITY SCREENING EXAM EACH WEEK, DOCUMENTING SCORES		
	· PROVIDE SIGNS AND VISUAL CUES TO HELP IMPROVE HER ABILITY TO RETAIN INFORMATION		
	· INSTRUCT SIGNIFICANT OTHERS ON REORIENTATION PROGRAM		
	· KEEP CLOCKS, CALENDARS, NEWSPAPERS, AND OTHER ORIENTATION DEVICES WITHIN HER VIEW		
	· INSTRUCT HER TO KEEP IMPORTANT PAPERS IN A CENTRAL LOCATION		
	· PROVIDE HER WITH ONGOING FEEDBACK ON HER PROGRESS		
	· WRITE ALL SCHEDULED		

Nursing diagnosis	Nursing intervention	Predicted outcome/short-term goals (include time frame)	Date/signature
	HOME CARE TEAM AND SIGNIFICANT OTHER VISITS ON THE CALENDAR		
	·POSITIVELY REINFORCE HER CORRECT RESPONSES TO YOUR QUESTIONS TESTING ORIENTATION		
	·REMEMBER THAT INSTRUCTION WILL REQUIRE REPETITION TO ENHANCE RETENTION		
	·GRADUALLY REINSTITUTE HER USEFUL COPING STRATEGIES, e.g., SOCIAL CONTACTS		
	·CONFER WITH JANE'S PHYSICIAN REGARDING IMPROVEMENTS OR REGRESSION IN COGNITIVE FUNCTIONING		

Continued

Nursing Care Plan *continued*

Discharge outcome/long-term goals			
		TIOHAL HABITS.	
1. BY THE END OF 60 DAYS, OR AT THE TIME OF CASE CLOSURE:		— JANE'S FLUID INTAKE WILL AVERAGE FROM 1500 TO 2000 cc PER DAY.	
— JANE AND/OR CARETAKER WILL DEMONSTRATE A KNOWLEDGE OF HEALTHY NUTRITIONAL AND HYDRA-			

Nursing diagnosis	Nursing intervention	Predicted outcome/short-term goals (include time frame)	Date/signature
FLUID VOLUME DEFICIT RELATED TO DECREASED FLUID INTAKE SECONDARY TO COGNITIVE IMPAIRMENT AND DEPRESSION	— CONFER WITH JANE'S PHYSICIAN REGARDING THE NEED FOR PERIODIC BLOOD CHEMISTRY DETERMINATIONS OF HER NUTRITIONAL AND HYDRATIONAL STATUS	— JANE'S REFRIGERATOR WILL CONTAIN A VARIETY OF FLUIDS FOR JANE'S REHYDRATION PROGRAM WITHIN 1 WEEK	1/15 MM
	— INSTRUCT JANE'S SIGNIFICANT OTHERS TO PUSH FLUIDS AND TO KEEP JUICES AND OTHER FLUIDS ON HAND	— AFTER 2 WEEKS, JANE WILL EXHIBIT NO SIGNS OF DEHYDRATION	
	— FOR VARIETY, CONSIDER USING NONLIQUID FORMS OF FLUIDS SUCH AS POPSICLES AND JELLO	— JANE AND HER SIGNIFICANT OTHERS WILL IDENTIFY AT LEAST THREE SIGNS AND SYMPTOMS OF DEHYDRATION BY CASE CLOSURE	
	— INSTRUCT JANE AND OTHERS TO LIMIT FLUIDS AFTER DINNER TO PREVENT NOCTURIA		
	— LIMIT, PREFERABLY ELIMINATE, JANE'S CAFFEINE INTAKE. ENCOURAGE ALTERNATIVE HOT BEVERAGES, i.e., DECAFFEINATED TEAS		
	— EACH VISIT, CAREFULLY PROVIDE SKILLED OBSERVATION FOR JANE'S SIGNS AND SYMPTOMS OF DEHYDRATION		
	— INSTRUCT JANE AND HER SIGNIFICANT OTHERS IN RECOGNIZING SIGNS AND SYMPTOMS OF DEHYDRATION (MUCOUS MEMBRANE INTEGRITY, URINE COLOR, ETC.)		
	— TAKE AND RECORD JANE'S VITAL SIGNS EACH VISIT		

Discharge outcome/long-term goals		DIET:	
1. BY THE END OF 60 DAYS, OR AT THE TIME OF CASE CLOSURE: —JANE WILL GAIN AT LEAST 5 POUNDS. —JANE WILL EAT A WELL-BALANCED			

Nursing diagnosis	Nursing intervention	Predicted outcome/short-term goals (include time frame)	Date/signature
ALTERATION IN NUTRITION: LESS THAN BODY REQUIRE-MENTS RELAT-ED TO ANOREXIA SECONDARY TO DEPRESSION	—ARRANGE FOR A HOME HEALTH AID TO ASSIST JANE WITH MEAL PREPARATION UNTIL A CARETAKER IS HIRED —INSTRUCT JANE AND HER SIGNIFICANT OTHERS TO PROVIDE NUTRITIOUS, PREPARED MEALS THAT JANE CAN QUICKLY HEAT AND EAT —ENSURE THAT THE CARETAKER OR HOME HEALTH AID SUPER-VISES TWO MEALS PER DAY; ENCOURAGE JANE'S FAMILY AND FRIENDS TO PHONE JANE WITH DINNER REMINDERS	—A CARETAKER WILL BE HIRED WITHIN 2 WEEKS —A NUTRITIONAL ASSESSMENT WILL BE COMPLETED BY JANE AND/OR HER SIGNIFI-CANT OTHERS WITHIN 2 WEEKS —WITHIN 1 MONTH, JANE WILL BE ABLE TO PREPARE FOOD SAFELY OR THE CARETAKER WILL PREPARE HER MEALS —JANE'S BLOOD CHEMISTRY RESULTS WILL DEMONSTRATE IMPROVED NUTRITIONAL STATUS BY CASE CLOSURE	1/15 MM
	—PROVIDE NUTRITIONAL ASSESSMENT DATA SHEET FOR 3-DAY LOG OF FOODS JANE EATS —CONFER WITH JANE'S PHYSICIAN REGARDING: ·PLACING JANE ON A HIGH-CALORIE, HIGH-PROTEIN, LOW-SALT DIET WITH ADDED FOODS RICH IN POTASSIUM AND IRON ·BEGINNING MULTIVIT-AMIN WITH IRON SUPPLEMENT ·ORDERING A COMPLETE BLOOD WORK PROFILE AND FOLLOW-UP APPOINT-MENTS WITH A DENTIST —INSTRUCT JANE AND HER SIGNIFICANT OTHERS ON THE ESSEN-TIALS OF BASIC NU-TRITION —WEIGH JANE ONCE PER WEEK IN THE SAME CLOTHES AND DOCUMENT —FOR MEALTIMES:		

Continued

Nursing Care Plan *continued*

Nursing diagnosis	Nursing intervention	Predicted outcome/short-term goals (include time frame)	Date/signature
	·BEGIN WITH SMALL FEED-INGS PROGRESSING TO LARGER; SCHEDULE MEALS AT JANE'S PRE-FERENCE		
	·USE APPEARANCE EN-HANCERS AND SPICES IN FOOD PREPARATION		
	·AVOID T.V. DINNERS AND HIGHLY PROCESSED FOODS		
	·PROVIDE CANNED NU-TRITIONAL SUPPLEMENTS (1/2 TO ONE CAN PER DAY) WITH INSTRUCTION ON PREPARATION, METHODS OF ENHANC-ING FLAVOR, AND POS-SIBLE SIDE EFFECTS		

Discharge outcome/long-term goals			
1. BY THE END OF 60 DAYS, OR AT THE TIME OF CASE CLOSURE JANE WILL ADMIT TO AN IMPROVED SENSE OF SELF-CONTROL.			

Nursing diagnosis	Nursing intervention	Predicted outcome/short-term goals (include time frame)	Date/signature
FEAR RELATED TO LOSS OF FUNCTIONING AND POTENTIAL LOSS OF HOME AND SUPPORT SYSTEM	—PROVIDE JANE WITH FREQUENT REASSURANCE THAT THE GOAL OF THE HOME CARE TEAM IS TO KEEP HER AT HOME —ASSIST JANE WITH PROBLEM-SOLVING EFFORTS TO ENHANCE HER FEELINGS OF SELF-CONTROL —HELP JANE TO DISCRIMINATE BETWEEN REALISTIC AND UNREALISTIC FEARS —ENLIST JANE'S SUPPORT IN THE CARE PLANNING PROCESS —SUMMARIZE WEEKLY PROGRESS WITH JANE, FOCUSING ON REALISTIC GOAL ATTAINMENT —PROVIDE JANE WITH ANTICIPATORY GUIDANCE —DEVELOP A COLLABORATIVE RELATIONSHIP WITH JANE BY PROMOTING HER INVOLVEMENT IN DECISIONS REGARDING HER CARE	—JANE WILL BE MADE AWARE OF FUTURE PLANS AND PROGRESS ON AN ONGOING BASIS —JANE WILL SHOW EVIDENCE OF INCREASED PROBLEM-SOLVING ABILITY WITHIN 1 MONTH —JANE WILL RECOGNIZE THREE BEHAVIORAL INDICATORS OF DECREASED FEAR WITHIN 1 MONTH	1/15 MM

Continued

Nursing Care Plan *continued*

Discharge outcome/long-term goals		
	DIMINISH AND SHE WILL RENEW SOCIAL CONTACTS.	
1. BY THE END OF 60 DAYS, OR AT THE TIME OF CASE CLOSURE:		
—JANE WILL VOICE FEELINGS OF HOPE ABOUT HER FUTURE.		
—JANE'S VEGETATIVE SIGNS WILL		

Nursing diagnosis	Nursing intervention	Predicted outcome/short-term goals (include time frame)	Date/signature
INEFFECTIVE INDIVIDUAL COPING RELATED TO DEPRESSION SECONDARY TO STRESS OF PHYSICAL ILLNESS AND LOSS OF CONTROL	—PROVIDE AT LEAST ONE 20-MINUTE PRIVATE ONE-TO-ONE SESSION EACH VISIT FOR ASSESSMENT AND INTERVENTION OF JANE'S COPING ABILITIES —ENCOURAGE HER TO USE HELPFUL COPING MECHANISMS TO OFFSET FURTHER DECLINE; e.g., ENCOURAGE SOCIAL CONTACTS AND ACTIVITY, KEEPING BUSY, AND TEACH RELAXATION TECHNIQUES TO ENHANCE SLEEP —INSTRUCT JANE AND HER SIGNIFICANT OTHERS IN RECOGNIZING THE SIGNS AND SYMPTOMS OF DEPRESSION AND UNDERSTANDING THE NEED FOR REALISTIC APPRAISAL —SEEK FEEDBACK FROM OTHERS REGARDING JANE'S FUNCTIONING —CONSIDER REFERRING JANE TO A PSYCHIATRIST FOR EVALUATION FOR POSSIBLE MEDICATION TRIAL	—JANE'S SLEEP PATTERN AND APPETITE WILL IMPROVE WITHIN 2 WEEKS —JANE WILL STATE SHE FEELS LESS DEPRESSED WITHIN 1 MONTH —PSYCHIATRIC REFERRAL WILL BE SOUGHT IMMEDIATELY SHOULD JANE'S EMOTIONAL STATUS DETERIORATE OR NOT IMPROVE, AS JUDGED BY THE RNS, CARETAKERS, OR JANE HERSELF	1/15 MM

Discharge outcome/long-term goals			
1. BY THE END OF 60 DAYS, OR AT THE TIME OF CASE CLOSURE JANE'S FAMILY WILL HAVE DEVELOPED A COLLABORATIVE RELATIONSHIP WITH THE PCNS			

Nursing diagnosis	Nursing intervention	Predicted outcome/short-term goals (include time frame)	Date/signature
INEFFECTIVE FAMILY COPING: COMPROMISED RELATED TO UNMET PSYCHO-SOCIAL NEEDS OF PARENT BY CHILD	—ACTIVELY INVOLVE DAUGHTER MARY IN JANE'S CARE (IF MARY WISHES)	—MARY WILL NOT REFUSE TO DISCUSS HER CONCERNS WITH THE PCNS	1/15 MM
	—WITH JANE'S PERMISSION TELEPHONE MARY AND MIKE WITH WEEK-LY PROGRESS REPORTS ON JANE'S CONDITION	—MIKE WILL CONTINUE TO BE INVOLVED IN HIS MOTHER-IN-LAW'S CARE EVEN IF MARY CHOOSES NOT TO BE INVOLVED	
	—CONDUCT AN ONGOING INVESTIGATION OF JANE AND MARY'S IN-TERPERSONAL DIFFI-CULTIES; CORRECT MIS-CONCEPTIONS OR AS-SUMPTIONS IF EX-PRESSED		
	—DEVELOP A COLLABOR-ATIVE RELATIONSHIP WITH JANE'S FAMILY		
	—CONSIDER CALLING A FAMILY MEETING IF RESISTANCE CONTINUES TO BE A PROBLEM, OR CONSIDER REFERRAL TO PSYCHIATRIST OR FAMILY THERAPIST IF APPROPRIATE		
	—STRESS THE CONTINUED NEED FOR JANE TO HAVE SOCIAL SUPPORT IF SHE IS TO REMAIN AT HOME		

Continued

Nursing Care Plan *continued*

Discharge outcome/long-term goals			
1. BY THE END OF 60 DAYS, OR AT THE TIME OF CASE CLOSURE JANE WILL DEMONSTRATE KNOWLEDGE OF MEASURES TO COUNTERACT CONSTIPATION			

Nursing diagnosis	Nursing intervention	Predicted outcome/short-term goals (include time frame)	Date/signature
ALTERED BOWEL ELIMINATION: CONSTIPATION, RELATED TO POOR NUTRITIONAL AND HYDRATION STATUS SECONDARY TO IMMOBILITY AND DEPRESSION	—ESTABLISH AND MAINTAIN JANE'S PERSONAL BOWEL HABITS —CONFER WITH JANE'S PHYSICIAN REGARDING MANUAL DISIMPACTION AND THE ONGOING NEED FOR STOOL SOFTENERS OR LAXATIVES —INSTRUCT JANE AND HER SIGNIFICANT OTHERS ON SAFE LAXATIVE USE —ENCOURAGE NATURAL LAXATIVE FOODS AND METHODS —INSTRUCT JANE AND HER SIGNIFICANT OTHERS TO RECORD HER BOWEL MOVEMENTS ON A CALENDAR FOR PCNS's REVIEW	—JANE WILL BE PLACED ON A BOWEL-TRAINING PROGRAM AS SOON AS POSSIBLE —JANE AND HER SIGNIFICANT OTHERS WILL VERBALIZE AT LEAST TWO NATURAL LAXATIVE METHODS WITHIN 2 WEEKS —JANE WILL HAVE REGULAR BOWEL MOVEMENTS AND WILL NOT STRAIN TO DEFECATE WITHIN 2 WEEKS	1/15 ヤヤヤ

Poor nutritional and hydrational self-care practices follow as dangerous sequelae of depression and pain. Jane's weight loss, poor skin turgor, ketotic halitosis, and dry mucous membranes all pointed to acute starvation and dehydration. These factors, along with associated fecal impaction, also contributed to the deterioration of her cognitive abilities and decline in functioning.

Based on this assessment, the PCNS predicted that skilled nursing interventions would effectively reverse the etiological factors in Jane's dementia and allow her to remain safely at home. With this goal in mind, the following nursing care plan was developed.

SUMMARY

The PCNS scheduled skilled nursing visits for three times per week for the first 2 weeks, followed by twice-per-week visits thereafter. A physical therapist, Sally, provided a walker and a schedule of written gait training and strengthening exercises. Jane's first exercise attempts took place within her apartment, but within 2 weeks of beginning therapy she progressed to short walks outdoors. Sally helped to initiate Jane's walks at least every other day and offered verbal direction for Jane's daily exercises.

One week after Jane started therapy, her family hired a caretaker, Mrs. Mullins, to come to her apartment from 10 AM to 4 PM each day to prepare her meals and assist her with activities of daily living. An occupational therapist installed grab bars, a removable shower head, and a tub bench in Jane's bathtub to enable her to bathe independently with Mrs. Mullins's verbal directions and supervision only.

After the PCNS's clinical findings, Jane's physician ordered ibuprofen 400 mg three times daily for pain control, a multivitamin supplement with iron, a stool softener, and baseline blood chemistries (complete blood count and "chem-12" panel). Predictably, baseline blood chemistries revealed that Jane was anemic, dehydrated, hypokalemic, and hyperalbuminemic—findings indicating malnutrition and dehydration.

To facilitate proper medication administration, the PCNS provided Jane with a medication reminder box. Concurrently, the PCNS instructed Jane and Mrs. Mullins on the name, dosage schedule, side effects, and precautions of the new medications. Within the first 2 weeks of therapy, Jane experienced a significant relief from pain.

Mrs. Mullins prided herself in preparing nutritious meals that Jane could later heat and eat. Jane enjoyed the meals Mrs. Mullins prepared and even began to experiment with some of the newer foods on the market; she especially loved frozen fruit juice bars and tropical fruit nectars. She was not able to tolerate canned nutritional supplements, claiming that they were too sweet even when adequately chilled. She also eliminated coffee from her diet. Gradually, her appetite improved, and she began to gain weight on the average of 1 pound per week; by case closure, Jane had gained 7 pounds and was beginning to assist Mrs. Mullins in food preparation and shopping trips.

The PCNS corrected all home safety hazards within the first 3 weeks of opening the case. Unfortunately, Jane was unable to learn to use her stovetop and oven safely; consequently, the PCNS, home aid, and Jane agreed that Jane's cooking attempts should center around the microwave and toaster oven. (With other apartment residents to consider, all potential fire hazards needed to be eliminated.)

As Jane's nutritional and hydrational status improved, so did her appearance and overall health status. Her skin tone became firmer and more elastic, and her mucous membranes regained a normal, well-hydrated appearance. Her initial tachycardia eventually stabilized to a resting pulse of 96, and her blood pressure averaged 140/90 over the final three visits and no longer fluctuated with posture. Final blood chemistry determinations taken before case closure revealed all levels within normal limits. After initial fecal disimpaction efforts by the PCNS, Jane was able to regulate her bowel movements solely through dietary modifications and stool softeners. Appointments were scheduled for continued medical and dental follow-up at the time of case closure.

Within the first 2 weeks of the PCNS's contact, Jane's affect began to improve. This improvement concurred with Jane's pain reduction and a return to her former activities of daily living. As she improved, she expressed a renewed interest in her surroundings and in reestablishing her network of social contacts. She looked forward to her one-to-one sessions with the PCNS and used her time productively, demonstrating an increasing ability to make more complex independent decisions for future planning purposes. As Jane began to identify her progress and newly found strength, her prior hopelessness changed to a renewed sense of hope. By the time of case closure, Jane no longer demonstrated evidence of the behavioral vegetative signs she had presented with at the beginning of therapy.

Most important, Jane's gross memory deficits and forgetfulness gradually improved as her depression abated. Although at case closure Jane continued to evidence some mild forgetfulness, her Cognitive Capacity Screening Exam scores had increased from 12 on contact to 22 at closure. As demonstrated by these scores, Jane's cognitive deficits had been almost entirely reversed.

The PCNS closed Jane's case 6 weeks after opening it. All of her long-term goals had been met, except one. While Mary was so pleased with her mother's progress that she eventually abandoned the plan to place Jane in a skilled nursing facility, she never established a trusting relationship with the PCNS to share her feelings about her mother's experience, despite the PCNS's attempts to engage her. The quality of Jane and Mary's relationship never changed. Mike believed his wife's and mother-in-law's troubles were so ingrained as to offer little hope of a reconciliation. The PCNS never determined the basis of Jane and Mary's continued resistance to each other.

REFERENCES

Dodson, J. "The Slow Death: Alzheimer's Disease," *Journal of Neurosurgical Nursing* 16:270-73, 1984.

Jacobs, J.W., et al. "Screening for Organic Mental Syndromes in the Medically Ill," *Annals of Internal Medicine* 86:40-46, 1977.

LaPorte, H.J. "Reversible Causes of Dementia: A Nursing Challenge," *Journal of Gerontological Nursing* 8(2):74-80, 1982.

Reisberg, B.S., and Ferris, S. "Diagnosis and Assessment of the Older Patient," *Hospital and Community Psychiatry* 33:104-10, 1982.

SELECTED BIBLIOGRAPHY

Boss, B.J. "The Dementias," *Journal of Neurosurgical Nursing* 15(2):87-97, 1983.

Charles, R., et al. "Alzheimer's Disease: Pathology, Progression, and Nursing Process," *Journal of Gerontological Nursing* 8(2):69-73, 1982.

Dietsche, L.M., and Pollman, J.N. "Alzheimer's Disease: Advances in Clinical Nursing," *Journal of Gerontological Nursing* 8(2):97-100, 1982.

Langston, N.F. "Reality Orientation and Effective Reinforcement," *Journal of Gerontological Nursing* 7(4):224-27, 1981.

Mackey, A.M. "OBS and Nursing Care," *Journal of Gerontological Nursing* 9(2):74-84, 1983.

Rabins, P.V. "Reversible Dementia and the Misdiagnosis of Dementia: A Review," *Hospital and Community Psychiatry* 34:830-35, 1983.

Rathmann, K.L., and Conner, C.S. "Alzheimer's Disease: Clinical Features, Pathogenesis, and Treatment," *Drug Intelligence and Clinical Pharmacy* 18:684-89, 1984.

Wolanin, M.O., and Phillips, L.R. *Confusion Prevention and Care*. St. Louis: C.V. Mosby Co., 1981.

Clara:
Medically Ill Client with Associated Depression

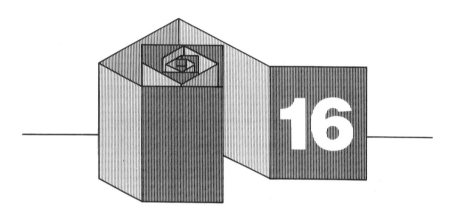

Susan Abbott Gierszewski, MS, RN, PHN

Nurses in the public health arena frequently assist medically ill clients who also have underlying psychological problems. Since many of these clients deny psychological symptoms (such as anxiety or depression), the nurse's work must focus on the integration of psychiatric–mental health nursing skills into the physiological care of the client and family. Through a well-established nurse-client-family relationship, defensiveness and resistance toward the thought of possible psychopathology may lift as the client and family come to acknowledge and respect the therapeutic efforts of the professional nurse.

This case study illustrates the interrelated nature of a client's physical and emotional status and the well-being of her family system. To reestablish equilibrium within the client's personal and family systems, nursing interventions needed to be directed toward her multiple physical and psychosocial problems.

The case also illustrates the effectiveness of some nursing interventions with a client who refused constructive feedback in almost all areas, and demonstrates the fact that, even with consistent, firm direction and guidance, some clients just will not respond or adhere to recommended therapeutic interventions.

CASE STUDY

Clara, a 55-year-old white female, lived in a small northeastern city. Clara never married but lived with a male friend, Harry, for 10 years in the ground-floor apartment of a small house. Both Clara and Harry were on welfare and could not remember when they last worked. However, they stated that many years ago they ran a small restaurant. Neither completed high school, and, although they both professed religious faith, neither was affiliated with any church. Clara denied having any family or friends other than Harry.

Clara was referred to home health care by her physician due to severe stasis dermatitis and ulcers. These skin conditions had progressed to the point that Harry, in "poor health" himself, could no longer manage Clara's required twice-daily dressing care. The physician had wanted to hospitalize Clara for treatment of her infected ulcers, but she had refused.

According to Clara's physician, Clara was grossly obese, weighing approximately 450 pounds; had been noncompliant with a 1400-calorie-per-day reducing diet; and had not walked for 2 years. She was also depressed but had refused any medication or other treatment. Her prescribed medications were an antibiotic and an analgesic; she had no known allergies.

At the nurse's first home visit, both Clara and Harry were very receptive to services. Both stated that Harry could no longer perform the dressing changes because of the strong, foul odor. Clara reported that she had been healthy until 2 years previously (and in fact could not remember ever receiving any previous medical care). At that time, she had noticed some discoloration, tingling, and small ulcers on her lower legs and feet, which she attributed to "bites." She did not seek medical treatment until she could barely walk with the pain in her legs and feet, at which time her physician agreed to make home visits.

On examination of Clara's legs and feet, the nurse found reddened, shiny, edematous skin from the knees down, including the bottoms of the feet, oozing serous fluid punctuated by multiple ulcers (up to 5 cm × 10 cm in size) draining copious, purulent, foul-smelling material. While the nurse soaked and dressed the affected areas, Clara continued relaying her history, weeping openly as she did so. She turned her head away and would not look at her feet or legs. She complained of the constant aching in her legs and feet and of having been confined to the wheelchair and her home for the past 2 years. She was fearful that Harry had become exasperated with her care and might leave her, which would surely result in her placement in a nursing home. She had lost all interest in the hobbies and pastimes she formerly enjoyed and spent her days looking out the window. Tearfully, she wondered aloud why she had been afflicted with this deforming condition and questioned whether her struggle was worth it.

The nurse's assessment uncovered two areas worthy of further investigation. While discussing her nutritional status, Clara became very defensive and angry at the nurse's suggestion that obesity was aggravating her condition. According to Clara, although she had always been overweight, her skin condition had developed only over the last 2 years. Clara and Harry (who was slightly underweight) became very hostile towards the nurse. Harry jumped to Clara's defense, asking the nurse, "Wouldn't you eat a lot if you were stuck in a chair all day?" Clara added, "Just do your job and don't talk to me about diets." Over the course of visits, the nurse frequently found Clara eating calorie-rich foods. Both she and Harry emphatically denied any use of alcohol.

The nurse elicited yet another angry, hostile response when she questioned Clara about her personal hygiene. Clara's face and upper extremities (she refused examination of her torso) were coated with baby powder, and her skin was dry and flaking. Clara stated that she kept herself clean with a daily application of powder and explained that bathing would be harmful because her skin would absorb water, which would then increase the drainage from her legs and feet. She refused the nurse's offer to arrange for home health aid services to assist with her personal care. Over subsequent visits the nurse continued to find Clara dressed in the same soiled housecoat and still coated with baby powder.

During the initial visit, Harry was very restless, getting up from his chair frequently and pacing about the house. As the nurse examined Clara's legs and feet, Harry made derogatory remarks, to which Clara responded with angry retorts. They argued about the cost of dressing supplies and the date of the doctor's last visit. At one point, Harry remarked that now that Clara had a nurse, he was obviously not needed anymore; he then left the house, slamming the door behind him. Clara passed this event off as his customary behavior.

In fact, Clara was dependent on Harry for most activities of daily living, including transferring, toileting, and dressing. She frequently summoned him to bring her something to eat or an article that she could not reach from her chair. Harry did all the housekeeping without any outside assistance. During the initial visit, he repeatedly stated that he did not feel well and needed to "slow down."

During later visits, the nurse learned that Clara and Harry had known each other since their teens. However, Clara had continued to live with her family until 10 years before, when her mother had died. At that point, she had "no one," and so moved in with Harry. According to Clara, she and Harry "needed each other." She declined to discuss any former or current sexual contacts.

Approximately 1 week after care was initiated, the nurse noted a change in Clara's affect. Upon arriving for a home care visit, the nurse found Clara in her customary position, sitting in her wheelchair looking out the window. But this time, Clara greeted her with a bright smile and a jovial hello. She had applied some lipstick and had arranged her hair more carefully than previously. She reported that the physician had visited her and found her ulcers much improved, and expressed confidence that she would be walking within a few weeks. On examination, however, the nurse found Clara's ulcers unchanged. Clara maintained her bright outlook throughout the visit, but the following day her mood was again depressed and she wept quietly throughout her dressing change.

Reader may now complete Recording the Data, Assigning Nursing Diagnoses, and Nursing Care Plan.

FORMULATION

Clara had a severely disabling and disfiguring medical condition that for 2 years had confined her to a wheelchair at home and caused her chronic pain. Her predominant affect, appearance, and mood were indicative of moderate depression. Developmentally, she was at a stage where she should have been able to perform activities of daily living (ADL) independently and take an active role in the home and community. Instead, she was dependent on a male friend for twice-daily treatments and most ADL. The friend, himself in ill health, began to feel overwhelmed by the burden of providing all of Clara's care and performing all home maintenance. He started making angry and derogatory remarks and leaving the home unannounced.

Clara's depression appeared to relate to several factors: a long-term lack of ability and function, which cut her off from all social contact except Harry; the breakdown in her relationship with Harry; the unsightly appearance and odor of her body; and chronic physical pain.

Her primary method of coping with her condition and resulting functional disabilities appeared to be overeating. She denied any relationship between her weight and her physical condition, becoming angry and defensive at the suggestion. She also appeared to deny periodically the seriousness and long-term nature of her condition and, in fact, had refused hospitalization for it.

The initial priority for Clara's care was to promote ulcer healing and resolution of infection and thus relieve pain, while also establishing

Continued on page 388

RECORDING THE DATA

After you have read the case, cluster significant data into functional health patterns.

Health management/health perception _____

_____

_____

_____

_____

Nutritional/metabolic _____

_____

_____

_____

Elimination _____

_____

_____

_____

Activity/exercise _____

_____

_____

_____

Cognitive/perceptual _____

_____

_____

_____

Sleep/rest _____

_____

_____

_____

Self-perception/self-concept _____

_____

_____

_____

Role relationship _____

_____

_____

_____

Sexuality/reproductive _____

_____

_____

_____

Coping/stress tolerance _____

_____

_____

_____

Value/belief _____

_____

_____

_____

ASSIGNING NURSING DIAGNOSES

Use your clustered data to select appropriate nursing diagnoses.

Health perception/health management

- [ ] Growth and Development, Altered (see Developmental Delay)
- [ ] Health Maintenance, Altered
- [ ] Infection, Potential for
- [ ] Injury (Trauma): Potential for
- [ ] Noncompliance (Specify)
- [ ] Poisoning: Potential for
- [ ] Suffocation: Potential for

Nutritional/metabolic

- [ ] Body Temperature, Potential Alteration in
- [ ] Developmental Delay: Physical Growth and Development
- [ ] Fluid Volume, Altered: Excess or Excess Fluid Volume
- [ ] Fluid Volume Deficit, Actual
- [ ] Fluid Volume Deficit, Potential
- [ ] Nutrition, Altered: Less Than Body Requirements or Nutritional Deficit (Specify)
- [ ] Nutrition, Altered: More Than Body Requirements or Exogenous Obesity
- [ ] Nutrition, Altered: Potential for More Than Body Requirements or Potential for Obesity
- [ ] Oral Mucous Membrane, Altered
- [ ] Skin Integrity, Impaired or Skin Breakdown
- [ ] Skin Integrity, Impaired or Potential Skin Breakdown
- [ ] Swallowing, Impaired or Uncompensated Swallowing Impairment
- [ ] Tissue Integrity, Impaired

Elimination

- [ ] Bowel Elimination, Altered: Constipation
- [ ] Bowel Elimination, Altered: Diarrhea
- [ ] Bowel Elimination, Altered: Incontinence

- [ ] Developmental Delay: Bowel/Bladder Control
- [ ] Incontinence: Functional
- [ ] Incontinence: Reflex
- [ ] Incontinence: Stress
- [ ] Incontinence: Total
- [ ] Incontinence: Urge
- [ ] Urinary Elimination, Altered Patterns of
- [ ] Urinary Retention

Activity/exercise

- [ ] Activity Intolerance
- [ ] Activity Intolerance, Potential
- [ ] Airway Clearance, Ineffective
- [ ] Breathing Pattern, Ineffective
- [ ] Cardiac Output, Altered: Decreased
- [ ] Developmental Delay: Mobility
- [ ] Developmental Delay: Self-Care Skills
- [ ] Diversional Activity Deficit
- [ ] Gas Exchange, Impaired
- [ ] Home Maintenance Management, Impaired (Mild, Moderate, Severe, Potential, Chronic)
- [ ] Mobility, Impaired Physical
- [ ] Self-Care Deficit: Feeding
- [ ] Self-Care Deficit: Bathing/Hygiene
- [ ] Self-Care Deficit: Dressing/Grooming
- [ ] Self-Care Deficit: Toileting
- [ ] Self-Care Deficit: Total
- [ ] Tissue Perfusion, Altered: (Specify)

Sleep/rest

- [ ] Sleep Pattern Disturbance

Cognitive/perceptual

- [ ] Comfort, Altered: Pain
- [ ] Comfort, Altered: Chronic Pain

- [ ] Developmental Delay: (Specify Cognitive Area; attention, decision making, etc.)
- [ ] Hypothermia
- [ ] Hyperthermia
- [ ] Knowledge Deficit (Specify)
- [ ] Sensory-Perceptual Alteration: Input Excess or Sensory Overload
- [ ] Sensory-Perceptual Alteration: Input Deficit or Sensory Deprivation
- [ ] Thermoregulation, Ineffective
- [ ] Thought Processes, Altered
- [ ] Unilateral Neglect

Self-perception/self-concept

- [ ] Anxiety
- [ ] Body Image Disturbance
- [ ] Fear
- [ ] Hopelessness
- [ ] Personal Identity Confusion
- [ ] Powerlessness (Severe, Low, Moderate)
- [ ] Self-Esteem Disturbance

Role relationship

- [ ] Communication, Impaired Verbal
- [ ] Developmental Delay: Communication Skills
- [ ] Developmental Delay: Social Skills
- [ ] Family Processes, Altered
- [ ] Grieving, Anticipatory
- [ ] Grieving, Dysfunctional
- [ ] Parenting, Altered: Actual or Potential

- [ ] Role Performance, Disturbance in
- [ ] Social Interactions, Impaired
- [ ] Social Isolation (Rejection)

Sexuality/reproductive

- [ ] Rape-Trauma Syndrome: Compounded
- [ ] Rape-Trauma Syndrome: Silent Reaction
- [ ] Sexual Dysfunction
- [ ] Sexuality Patterns, Altered

Coping/stress tolerance

- [ ] Adjustment, Impaired
- [ ] Coping, Ineffective Individual
- [ ] Coping, Ineffective Family: Compromised
- [ ] Coping, Ineffective Family: Disabling
- [ ] Coping, Family: Potential for Growth
- [ ] Developmental Delay (Specify area)
- [ ] Post-Trauma Response
- [ ] Violence, Potential for (Self-Directed or Directed at Others)

Value/belief

- [ ] Spiritual Distress (Distress of Human Spirit)

You are now ready to develop a nursing care plan for this client. Use the following blank pages to do so. Then refer to the author's formulation, diagnostic summary, care plan, and summary.

NURSING CARE PLAN

Complete the chart below to develop a nursing care plan for this client.

Discharge outcomes/long-term goals	

Nursing diagnosis	Nursing intervention	

	Predicted outcomes/short-term goals (include time frame)	Date/signature

Return to Formulation, page 381

an effective pain management regimen. At the same time, ineffective individual and family coping also presented significant problems; the nurse needed to encourage Clara and Harry to express their feelings and assist them, along with the social worker, in developing further means of support. Additional measures needed to improve Clara's physical and emotional comfort included promoting improved body image and role performance, encouraging appropriate personal hygiene, and working with physical therapy to prevent hazards of immobility and to increase her ability to move about her home and outside. Since Clara's obesity represented a significant long-term problem that she refused to acknowledge, the nurse first needed to establish a trusting relationship and focus on other nursing problems before initiating any related interventions.

SUMMARY

Clara was visited by the home health nurse over an 8-month period, with frequency gradually decreasing from twice a day to daily to five times per week, and so on, until eventually she was seen one time per week for assessment of healing. The decreased nursing frequency became possible due to the success of the nursing interventions directed towards wound healing and pain management, along with a gradual lifting of Clara's depression and a more harmonious, effective family situation.

Clara was readily able to express her feelings of anger, depression, and frustration to the nurse, but only after many weeks of encouragement was she able to begin initiating any purposeful activities or social contact. This was somewhat expected due to her long-term sick role. Somewhat unexpected, however, were the ambivalent feelings roused in Harry by her eventual ability to take on more appropriate role performance. Consequently, the nurse and social worker helped Harry to recognize his feelings related to the loss of Clara's dependence on him, and encouraged him to facilitate her efforts toward further independence and broadening of her social network. As both Clara and Harry developed sources of support and socialization outside their family system, they were better able to support and communicate with each other. During later visits, the nurse observed gestures of affection between the two, gestures that had been entirely absent at the beginning of care.

Significant to the improvement in individual and family coping were the resources that were brought into the home. After about 1 month, after Harry had resumed the evening dressing changes and again was feeling overwhelmed and fatigued, Clara and Harry finally agreed to accept homemaker assistance through their social worker. The home-

Continued on page 399

DIAGNOSTIC SUMMARY FOR CLARA

Data	Functional health pattern	Nursing diagnosis
—Exhibits reddened, shiny, edematous skin from the knees down to and covering the bottoms of the feet, oozing serous fluid punctuated by multiple ulcers draining copious, purulent, foul-smelling material	Nutritional/ Metabolic	Impaired skin integrity related to ulceration of both lower extremities and feet secondary to stasis dermatitis
—Complains of constant aching pain in her legs and feet, and confinement to a wheelchair for the past 2 years	Cognitive/Perceptual	Altered comfort: pain, related to stasis dermatitis, ulcers, and immobility
—Weeps openly while relaying her history —Has lost interest in all hobbies and pastimes she formerly enjoyed; spends her days looking out the window —Displays a defensive and angry interpersonal style	Coping/Stress Tolerance	Ineffective individual coping related to depression secondary to loss of mobility and function, altered relationship with significant other, chronic pain, and poor self-concept
—Her friend Harry obviously restless during initial assessment; gets up from his chair frequently and paces about the house —Counters Harry's derogatory remarks with angry retorts —Argues with Harry about the cost of dressing supplies —Describes Harry's leaving the house angrily as customary behavior	Coping/Stress Tolerance	Ineffective family coping: compromised related to demands of client's care and changed role performance
—Tearfully wonders aloud why she has been afflicated with this deforming condition, and questions whether her struggle is worth it —Is dependent on Harry for most activities of daily living, including transferring, toileting, and changing clothes	Self-Perception/Self-Concept	Body image disturbance and disturbance in role performance related to lower extremity ulcers and odor, lack of mobility and function, and obesity
—Coats her face and upper extremities with baby powder; skin is dry and flaking —States she keeps herself clean with daily applications of baby powder —Believes bathing would be	Activity/Exercise	Self-care deficit: bathing/ hygiene related to lack of mobility, beliefs re: harm of bathing, and obesity

Continued

Diagnostic Summary for Clara *continued*

Data	Functional health pattern	Nursing diagnosis
harmful because water absorbed by her skin would increase the drainage from her legs and feet —Wears same soiled housecoat day after day		
—Has not walked for 2 years —Is wheelchair-bound	Activity/Exercise	Impaired physical mobility related to painful foot ulcers, obesity, and long-term inactivity
—Is grossly obese—weighs 450 pounds —Is noncompliant with a 1400-calorie-per-day reducing diet —Is frequently "caught" eating calorie-rich foods —Rationalizes overeating: "Wouldn't you eat a lot if you were stuck in a chair all day?"	Nutritional/Metabolic	Altered nutrition: more than body requirements related to long-term eating habits, inactivity, and boredom

NURSING CARE PLAN

Complete the chart below to develop a nursing care plan for this client.

Discharge outcome/long-term goals	
1. WITHIN 6 MONTHS, CLARA'S ULCERS WILL HEAL. 2. WITHIN 6 MONTHS, CLARA AND HARRY WILL PROVIDE CARE TO AFFECTED AREAS TO PREVENT FURTHER ULCERS.	

Nursing diagnosis	Nursing intervention	Predicted outcome/short-term goals (include time frame)	Date/signature
ALTERED SKIN INTEGRITY RELATED TO ULCERATION OF BOTH LOWER EXTREMITIES AND FEET SECONDARY TO STASIS DERMATITIS	— SOAK AFFECTED AREAS AND APPLY OINTMENTS AND DRESSINGS AS PRESCRIBED BY PHYSICIAN — EVALUATE HEALING (NOTE SIZE AND DEPTH OF ULCERS; AMOUNT, NATURE, AND ODOR OF DRAINAGE; GRANULATION; EDEMA; ERYTHEMA; SIGNS/SYMPTOMS OF INFECTION) — INSTRUCT CLARA REGARDING ANTIBIOTIC MEDICATION REGIMEN (SCHEDULE, PURPOSE, SIDE EFFECTS) AND ASSESS HER COMPLIANCE — INSTRUCT CLARA AND HARRY REGARDING THE HEALING PROCESS AND SIGNS/SYMPTOMS OF INFECTION — INSTRUCT CLARA TO ELEVATE HER FEET WHENEVER POSSIBLE, 4 TIMES A DAY FOR PERIODS OF 1 HOUR EACH — ASSESS HARRY'S WILLINGNESS TO RESUME RESPONSIBILITY FOR SOME OF CLARA'S DRESSING CHANGES; INSTRUCT AND SUPERVISE HIM AS NECESSARY	— INFECTION WILL RESOLVE WITHIN 2 WEEKS — WITHIN 3 DAYS, CLARA AND HARRY WILL DESCRIBE HEALING PROCESS AND SIGNS/SYMPTOMS OF INFECTION APPROPRIATELY — WITHIN 2 TO 3 WEEKS, HARRY WILL RESUME AT LEAST ALL THE EVENING DRESSING CHANGES — CLARA WILL ELEVATE HER FEET FREQUENTLY, BEGINNING IN 2 DAYS	6/4

Continued

Nursing Care Plan *continued*

Discharge outcome/long-term goals	
1. CLARA WILL BE COMFORTABLE WITHOUT USE OF ANALGESICS. 2. CLARA WILL IDENTIFY AT LEAST TWO SOURCES OF EMOTIONAL SUPPORT IN ADDITION TO HARRY AND NURSE.	3. CLARA WILL RESUME AT LEAST TWO PASTTIMES OR HOBBIES. 4. CLARA WILL DESCRIBE FEELINGS OF HOPE CONSISTENT WITH DEGREE OF HEALING, RESTORATION OF FUNCTION, AND PAIN RELIEF.

Nursing diagnosis	Nursing intervention	Predicted outcome/short-term goals (include time frame)	Date/signature
ALTERED COMFORT: PAIN RELATED TO STASIS DERMATITIS AND ULCERS	—TEACH CLARA ABOUT PAIN MANAGEMENT: TIMELY, REGULAR ADMINISTRATION OF ANALGESICS, SIGNS/SYMPTOMS OF SIDE EFFECTS —ASSESS HER COMPLIANCE WITH AND THE EFFECTIVENESS OF PAIN MANAGEMENT REGIMEN —TEACH RELAXATION TECHNIQUES TO AUGMENT PHARMACOTHERAPY	—CLARA WILL REPORT SATISFACTORY (DECREASED LEVEL OF PAIN TO A TOLERABLE LEVEL) MANAGEMENT OF PAIN WITHIN 3 DAYS —CLARA WILL UTILIZE RELAXATION TECHNIQUES WITHOUT PROMPTS IN 1 MONTH	6/4 JL
INEFFECTIVE INDIVIDUAL COPING RELATED TO DEPRESSION SECONDARY TO LOSS OF MOBILITY AND FUNCTION, ALTERED RELATIONSHIP WITH SIGNIFICANT OTHER, CHRONIC PAIN, AND POOR SELF-CONCEPT	—INITIATE A THERAPEUTIC RELATIONSHIP: ·EXPLAIN ROLE OF HOME HEALTH NURSE TO CLARA AND HARRY ·REVIEW CLARA'S AND HARRY'S EXPECTATIONS OF SERVICES ·ARRANGE A MUTUALLY SATISFACTORY SCHEDULE OF VISITS AND FOLLOW-THROUGH ·IDENTIFY GOALS FOR CARE WITH CLARA AND HARRY —ASSESS CLARA'S MOOD AND CAUSATIVE FACTORS: ·EXPLORE HER FEELINGS RELATED TO LOSS OF MOBILITY AND FUNCTION, BODY IMAGE, RELATIONSHIP WITH HARRY, AND PAIN ·ACKNOWLEDGE NORMALCY OF DEPRESSED FEELINGS IN RESPONSE TO SITUATION ·ENCOURAGE CLARA TO IDENTIFY AND EXPRESS HER FEELINGS AT EACH VISIT ·NOTIFY PHYSICIAN OF ANY SIGNIFICANT CHANGES IN HER CONDITION AND	—FROM THE START OF THERAPY, CLARA WILL VERBALIZE FEELINGS TO NURSE —WITHIN 1 WEEK, CLARA WILL IDENTIFY DEPRESSION AS A NORMAL RESPONSE TO HER CONDITION —WITHIN 1 WEEK, SHE WILL IDENTIFY HARRY AND NURSE AS SOURCES OF SUPPORT —SHE WILL VERBALIZE HER FEELINGS TO HARRY WITHIN 2 WEEKS —WITHIN 3 WEEKS, SHE WILL BE ABLE TO DESCRIBE ACTUAL HEALING PROCESS ACCURATELY AND IDENTIFY REALISTIC GOALS WITH NURSE'S ASSISTANCE	6/4 JL

Nursing diagnosis	Nursing intervention	Predicted outcome/short-term goals (include time frame)	Date/signature
	CONSIDER THE NEED FOR FURTHER TREATMENT		
	—DETERMINE CLARA'S PREVIOUS COPING METHODS AND EFFECTIVENESS; ASSIST HER IN DEVELOPING NEW COPING METHODS AS NECESSARY		
	—REINFORCE YOUR SUPPORT AND WILLINGNESS TO LISTEN AT EACH VISIT		
	—EDUCATE HARRY ABOUT CLARA'S NEED TO VERBALIZE HER FEELINGS AND ENCOURAGE HIS EFFORTS TO FACILITATE THIS		
	—ASSESS CLARA'S PREVIOUS PASTTIMES AND HOBBIES AND ENCOURAGE HER TO RESUME THOSE APPROPRIATE TO HER LEVEL OF MOBILITY		
	—ENCOURAGE CLARA TO BROADEN HER SOCIAL NETWORK VIA RENEWAL OF OLD FRIENDSHIPS (THROUGH THE USE OF THE TELEPHONE IF OTHERS ARE UNABLE TO VISIT) AND/OR ACCEPTANCE OF A FRIENDLY VISITOR PROGRAM		
	—PROVIDE CLARA WITH ACCURATE INFORMATION REGARDING THE PROGRESS OF HEALING		
	—REFER CLARA TO A SOCIAL WORKER FOR COUNSELING AND REFERRAL TO COMMUNITY RESOURCES		

Continued

Nursing Care Plan *continued*

Discharge outcome/long-term goals	
1. HARRY WILL SOCIALIZE OUTSIDE OF HOME AT LEAST TWICE PER WEEK.	3. CLARA AND HARRY WILL EXPRESS SATISFACTION WITH THEIR RELATIONSHIP.
2. HARRY WILL VERBALIZE FEELINGS OF CONTROL AND ABILITY TO MANAGE HOME AND CLARA'S CARE DEMANDS.	4. CLARA AND HARRY WILL SHARE THEIR FEELINGS WITHOUT PROMPTING.

Nursing diagnosis	Nursing intervention	Predicted outcome/short-term goals (include time frame)	Date/signature
INEFFECTIVE FAMILY COPING: COMPROMISED RELATED TO DEMANDS OF CLIENT'S CARE AND CHANGED ROLE PERFORMANCE	—ASSESS HARRY'S FEELINGS RELATED TO CLARA'S LOSS OF FUNCTION, ILLNESS, AND DEMANDS FOR CARE	—WITHIN 1 TO 2 WEEKS HARRY WILL EXPRESS HIS FEELINGS RELATED TO CLARA'S LOSS OF FUNCTION, ILLNESS, AND CAREGIVING DEMANDS	6/4 🔏
	—ASSESS HARRY'S PHYSICAL, MENTAL, AND EMOTIONAL ABILITY TO COPE WITH HOME MAINTENANCE AND CLARA'S CARE	—WITHIN 1 WEEK, HE WILL IDENTIFY NURSE AS A SOURCE OF SUPPORT	
	—REFER HARRY TO A SOCIAL WORKER FOR ASSESSMENT AND REFERRAL TO APPROPRIATE AGENCIES FOR IN-HOME SUPPORTIVE SERVICES AND SOCIAL OUTLETS FOR CLARA	—WITHIN 2 TO 3 WEEKS, HE WILL RESUME AT LEAST EVENING DRESSING CHANGES	
	—ENCOURAGE HARRY TO EXPRESS HIS FEELINGS AT EACH VISIT	—HE WILL ACCEPT NEEDED ASSISTANCE IN HOME (ALONG WITH CLARA) IN 3 WEEKS	
	—ENCOURAGE HARRY TO SOCIALIZE OUTSIDE OF THE HOME AT LEAST TWICE PER WEEK (IN CONJUNCTION WITH COMPANIONSHIP PROGRAM FOR CLARA)		
	—FACILITATE COMMUNICATION OF FEELINGS BETWEEN CLARA AND HARRY		
	—TEACH HARRY ABOUT THE WOUND-HEALING PROGRESS AND ENCOURAGE GRADUAL RESUMPTION OF WOUND CARE AS HE FEELS ABLE		

Discharge outcome/long-term goals			
1. CLARA WILL OBSERVE ULCERS AND DESCRIBE THE HEALING PROCESS REALISTICALLY.			

Nursing diagnosis	Nursing intervention	Predicted outcome/short-term goals (include time frame)	Date/signature
BODY IMAGE DISTURBANCE AND DISTURBANCE IN ROLE PERFORMANCE RELATED TO LOWER EXTREMITY ULCERS AND ODOR, LACK OF MOBILITY AND FUNCTION, AND OBESITY	—ASSESS CLARA'S PERCEIVED VS. IDEALIZED BODY IMAGE AND ROLE FUNCTION —ACKNOWLEDGE NORMALCY OF CLARA'S DISTRESS IN RESPONSE TO APPEARANCE AND ODOR OF WOUNDS AND LOSS OF FUNCTION —OBSERVE AND DRESS WOUNDS WITHOUT INDICATING DISTASTE —DISCUSS HOUSEHOLD ACTIVITIES THAT CLARA COULD PERFORM WHILE IN WHEELCHAIR (eg, CUTTING VEGETABLES, MENDING) AND ENCOURAGE/REINFORCE HER PARTICIPATION IN THESE ACTIVITIES —ENCOURAGE HARRY IN HIS EFFORTS TO DEMONSTRATE HIS ACCEPTANCE OF CLARA'S STATUS AND HIS AFFECTION FOR HER	—WITHIN 3 WEEKS, CLARA WILL EXPRESS FEELINGS REGARDING APPEARANCE AND ODOR OF LOWER EXTREMITIES AND LOSS OF FUNCTION —WITHIN 1 MONTH, SHE WILL ASSIST WITH TWO PURPOSEFUL HOUSEHOLD ACTIVITIES PER DAY	6/4 JM

Continued

Nursing Care Plan *continued*

Discharge outcome/long-term goals		2. CLARA WILL DRESS IN CLEAN CLOTHING
1. CLARA WILL BATHE AND MOISTURIZE ALL PARTS OF HER BODY UNAFFECTED BY STASIS DERMATITIS WITH ASSISTANCE FROM HARRY AND/OR HOME HEALTH AID, AS NEEDED.		DAILY.

Nursing diagnosis	Nursing intervention	Predicted outcome/short-term goals (include time frame)	Date/signature
SELF-CARE DEFICIT: BATHING/HYGIENE RELATED TO LACK OF MOBILITY, BELIEFS REGARDING HARM OF BATHING, AND OBESITY	—EDUCATE CLARA ON THE IMPORTANCE OF BATHING AND MOISTURIZING THE SKIN —TEACH CLARA ABOUT THE NORMAL SKIN BARRIER THAT PREVENTS WATER ABSORPTION —INSTRUCT CLARA ABOUT POTENTIAL FOR DRYING AND INFECTION FROM CONTINUED APPLICATION AND BUILD-UP OF POWDER ON SKIN —IDENTIFY AND DISCUSS DEPRESSION AS ONE FACTOR CAUSING LACK OF INTEREST IN BATHING AND CHANGING CLOTHES —ENCOURAGE CLARA TO TRY BATHING AND MOISTURIZING A SMALL AREA OF SKIN AND OBSERVING RESULTS —ENCOURAGE HER TO CHANGE INTO CLEAN CLOTHING DAILY —OFFER CLARA THE PERIODIC SERVICES OF HOME HEALTH AID TO ASSIST WITH PERSONAL HYGIENE AND SOME LIGHT HOUSEKEEPING	—WITHIN 2 TO 3 WEEKS, CLARA WILL DESCRIBE THE BENEFITS OF BATHING AND MOISTURIZING SKIN AND DANGER IN CONTINUED APPLICATION OF POWDER —CLARA WILL IDENTIFY DEPRESSION AS A FACTOR IN HER LACK OF INTEREST IN PERSONAL HYGIENE AND GROOMING WITHIN 2 TO 3 WEEKS —WITHIN 1 MONTH, SHE WILL BATHE AT LEAST BOTH HANDS AND LOWER ARMS AND APPLY MOISTURIZING LOTION AS NEEDED	6/4 *JC*

Discharge outcome/long-term goals			
1. CLARA WILL DEMONSTRATE AN ABILITY TO PREVENT BREAKDOWN ON PRESSURE AREAS. 2. CLARA WILL MOVE OUTSIDE OF HER HOME VIA HER WHEELCHAIR.			

Nursing diagnosis	Nursing intervention	Predicted outcome/short-term goals (include time frame)	Date/signature
IMPAIRED PHYSICAL MOBILITY RELATED TO PAINFUL FOOT ULCERS, OBESITY AND LONG-TERM INACTIVITY	—TEACH CLARA THE IMPORTANCE OF MAXIMAL MOBILITY WITHIN THE LIMITS OF HER CONDITION —ENCOURAGE HER TO SHIFT POSITION IN WHEELCHAIR AT LEAST HOURLY, AND TEACH HER TO DO ACTIVE UPPER EXTREMITY ROM EXERCISES AT LEAST THREE TIMES PER DAY —ARRANGE A REFERRAL TO A PHYSICAL THERAPIST TO TEACH CLARA SAFE TRANSFER TECHNIQUES, ORDER ADAPTIVE EQUIPMENT, AND PROGRESS AMBULATION AS ULCERS HEAL —DISCUSS WITH CLARA AND HARRY THE POSSIBILITY OF OBTAINING A RAMP TO ENABLE CLARA TO LEAVE THE HOME IN HER WHEELCHAIR —ASSESS PRESSURE AREAS FOR SKIN BREAKDOWN AT EACH VISIT, TEACH HARRY HOW TO DO THIS ASSESSMENT	—IN 3 DAYS TIME, CLARA WILL DESCRIBE IMPORTANCE OF INCREASING MOBILITY —WITHIN 3 TO 5 DAYS, SHE WILL CHANGE POSITION IN WHEELCHAIR HOURLY, DO UPPER EXTREMITY ROM EXERCISES, AND TRANSFER SAFELY	6/4 DK

Continued

Nursing Care Plan *continued*

Discharge outcome/long-term goals	
1. CLARA WILL COMPLY WITH HER PRE-SCRIBED DIET.	
2. CLARA WILL LOSE WEIGHT WITHIN THE GUIDELINES ESTABLISHED BY HER PHYSICIAN.	

Nursing diagnosis	Nursing intervention	Predicted outcome/short-term goals (include time frame)	Date/signature
ALTERED NUTRI-TION: MORE THAN BODY RE-QUIREMENTS RELATED TO LONG-TERM EATING HABITS, INACTIVITY, AND BOREDOM	—EXPLAIN THE RELATION-SHIP BETWEEN IMMOBIL-ITY, FEELINGS OF BORE-DOM AND DEPRESSION, AND WEIGHT GAIN —REQUEST CLARA TO KEEP A 3-DAY DIARY OF ALL FOOD CONSUMED —INSTRUCT CLARA AND HARRY ABOUT THE FOUR FOOD GROUPS AS THEY RELATE TO THE PRE-SCRIBED 1400-CALORIE DIET —INSTRUCT CLARA AND HARRY ABOUT THE RELA-TIVE IMPORTANCE OF VITAMINS, MINERALS, AND PROTEIN FOR HEALING, AS OPPOSED TO CALORIES —ASSESS CLARA'S FOOD PREFERENCES AND FOODS CURRENTLY IN HOME; EXPLAIN WAYS IN WHICH THESE MAY BE INCORPORATED INTO PRESCRIBED DIET —INSTRUCT CLARA AND HARRY AND PERIODICALLY REMIND THEM OF BEN-EFITS OF WEIGHT LOSS FOR IMPROVING MOBIL-ITY AND SKIN STATUS —ENCOURAGE AND REIN-FORCE FEWER CALORIES AND IMPROVED BALANCE AMONG FOOD GROUPS —ASSIST CLARA IN IDENTIFYING OTHER ACTIVITIES WHICH COULD SUBSTITUTE FOR EATING WHEN SHE'S FEELING BORED OR UPSET —PACE INFORMATION AS PER CLARA'S INTEREST; DO NOT BOMBARD HER WITH INFORMATION ALL AT ONCE	—WITHIN 1 MONTH, CLARA WILL KEEP A 3-DAY FOOD DIARY —WITHIN 5 WEEKS, SHE WILL BE ABLE TO DESCRIBE FOUR FOOD GROUPS AND EXPLAIN THE IMPORTANCE OF EATING FOODS FROM EACH GROUP DAILY —IN 6 WEEKS TIME, SHE WILL BE ABLE TO IDENTIFY FACTORS OTHER THAN HUNGER AS CAUSATIVE OF HER EATING AND WILL IDENTIFY AT LEAST THREE ACTIVITIES WHICH COULD SUBSTITUTE FOR EAT-ING —WITHIN 6 WEEKS, SHE WILL IDENTIFY BENEFITS OF WEIGHT LOSS AND WILL IDENTIFY PRINCIPLES OF REDUCING DIET	6/4 SL

maker provided companionship and socialization for Clara, and Harry eventually followed through with the social worker's suggestion to investigate activities at the local community center.

Clara demonstrated improved acceptance of her condition and body image about 3 weeks into her care when the nurse informed her of a noticeable decrease in the amount of drainage and size of two of her ulcers. By this time, the odor was less foul, and Harry had begun to do some evening dressing changes. From that point on, Clara actually took an interest in observing the ulcers and verifying with the nurse her perceptions of progress.

Clara's mobility improved when, at about 6 months into her care, her left foot healed sufficiently to allow limited weight-bearing on that side. The physical therapist instructed her in the use of crutches, and by the end of care, she was able to move from her living area to the kitchen for meals. She had been able to leave her home via her wheelchair several times, after volunteers from a community group for the handicapped had made the necessary adjustments to her doorway. The physical therapist planned to resume treatment when healing progressed such that Clara could bear weight on both sides.

Despite her improvements in the areas of healing, socialization, acceptance, and mobility, throughout care Clara remained almost totally resistant to change in the areas of personal hygiene and eating habits. She would correctly repeat the nurse's instructions, but repeatedly became angry and hostile when asked to make any changes in her behavior. The nurse focused on these problems at intervals, hoping that, with intermittent "rests," Clara would eventually become more receptive. However, after about 3 months, the nurse discontinued all of her efforts in these areas for fear of angering Clara to the point that she would refuse services entirely. The nurse then hoped that Clara might change her hygiene and eating habits as she became more active and socially involved, and so targeted nursing interventions in these areas. Indeed, these interventions helped improve Clara's grooming and her mood, but her powdering and eating habits remained unchanged. The nurse finally had to accept the fact that Clara was making an informed decision and that no intervention could ensure a change in behavior.

Clara's resistance to change and lack of insight into her problems frustrated the nurse greatly. From the beginning of care, the nurse had set goals and timeframes in accordance with Clara's feelings and wishes. In spite of this, Clara did not meet all the goals of her care. During the course of care, the nurse shared her frustrations and perceptions with the other team members caring for Clara. In addition, she periodically discussed Clara's case with nursing colleagues to obtain their suggestions and support. One of these conferences prompted her to arrange for occasional visits to Clara by other nurses, which provided her with brief respite periods and with direct feedback regarding Clara's status and the appropriateness of her nursing care plan.

In summary, the nursing interventions designed for Clara met with moderate to good success in conjunction with the efforts of the physician, social worker, physical therapist, and several community agencies. Clara's case clearly illustrates the interrelatedness of the physical and psychosocial realms and the benefits to be gained when the multidisciplinary home health–community team addresses and integrates interventions in these areas.

SELECTED BIBLIOGRAPHY

Carmack, B. "Guidelines for Assessing Mental/Psychosocial Status," *Occupational Health Nurse* 30(5):24-34, 1982.

Clements, I.W., and Roberts, F.B., eds. *Family Health: A Theoretical Approach to Nursing Care*. New York: John Wiley & Sons, 1983.

Connelly, C.E. "Patient Compliance: A Review of the Research with Implications for Psychiatric–Mental Health Nursing," *Journal of Psychiatric Nursing and Mental Health Services* 16(10):15-18, 1983.

Flaskerud, J., and Van Servellin, G.M. *Community Mental Health Nursing: Theories and Methods*. East Norwalk, Conn.: Appleton-Century-Crofts, 1985.

Pelletier, L.R. and Cousins, A. "Depression Update," *Journal of Emergency Nursing* 10(1):315-18, 1984.

Tinkham, C.W., and Voorhies, E.F. *Community Health Nursing: Evolution and Process*. East Norwalk, Conn.: Appleton-Century-Crofts, 1977.

Bob:
Dementia

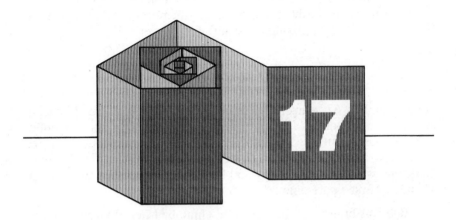

Kathleen J. Faude, MN, RN, CS
Jill Shapira, MN, RN,C, ANP

Dementia is defined as a clinical syndrome characterized by acquired persistent impairment in at least three spheres of mental activity: language, memory, visuospatial skills, emotion, or personality and cognition (abstraction, calculation, judgment, etc.) (Cummings et al., 1980). This definition stresses several key concepts. The persistence of dementia distinguishes it from acute confusional states caused by toxic or metabolic conditions (e.g., alcohol intoxication). The intellectual limitations are acquired rather than congenital in origin, as in the mental retardation syndromes. By requiring an involvement of several types of intellectual abilities, the definition excludes disorders that affect only one type of mental activity (i.e., cerebral infarct causing only the inability to speak). Finally, dementia is a syndrome, not a diagnosis, and applies to reversible as well as irreversible conditions. Some dementias can be cured completely, and others can be stopped from progressing further.

For accurate diagnosis, the cause of intellectual decline suffered by an elderly client must be determined. Too often, a diagnosis of progressive, irreversible dementia is given before other possibilities are excluded. Principal disorders to be considered in the differential diagnosis of dementia include Alzheimer's disease, multiple stroke syndromes, extrapyramidal disorders, depression, and chronic confusional states.

The victims of dementia extend beyond the client to include family members and friends. Spouse, adult and adolescent children, and young grandchildren are exposed to burden and grief as the family strives to cope with this devastating disease. The goal of nursing care is to identify emerging problems in the client or family members and to support the client and family by utilizing community resources.

CASE STUDY

Robert Lamb, a 62-year-old white male, lived with his wife, Michelle, in a large metropolitan area. Both "Bob" and Michelle were Catholic, although neither attended church regularly. Bob had a Master's degree in business administration and was a senior vice-president in charge of marketing when he retired at age 60 from a large insurance corporation. Michelle worked part-time as a real estate sales agent.

Bob was brought to an outpatient clinic by Michelle for evaluation of a "memory problem." She wondered if he might have Alzheimer's disease, which she had learned about from television. Bob doesn't understand what "all the fuss" is about, but will do whatever Michelle says he should.

According to Michelle, Bob was well until 4 years previously, when he began to notice increasing difficulty carrying out his duties at work. He forgot appointments and had trouble balancing the annual budget. About 3 years prior to admission, he became lost while driving to a business appointment and called Michelle from a city 100 miles away. He was able to drive himself home that evening. Bob and Michelle both thought he must have been under stress from his job at the time. A year after this incident, Bob's employers recommended that he leave the company with an early retirement. The couple had eagerly anticipated this retirement; Bob enjoyed woodworking and gardening, and both had been eager to travel to foreign cities the next year when Michelle decreased her work schedule. But Michelle was surprised at how little Bob seemed to accomplish during his 2 years of retirement. He showed no interest in his hobbies, preferring to watch television unless encouraged by Michelle to pursue an activity.

About 6 months prior to admission, Bob and Michelle had toured Europe for 4 weeks. According to Michelle, during their trip Bob seemed "confused" and could not remember the names of their hotels or even what city they were currently visiting. Since their return, he remained somewhat "out-of-touch" with his environment; he had trouble remembering what he did during the day, occasionally had difficulty finding the words he wanted to say, and twice got lost while driving. He was able to dress himself without difficulty, but had trouble deciding what shirt to wear with a particular pair of pants. Michelle explained that she worked 2 days each week; Bob telephoned her 10 to 12 times each day asking when she was coming home. When she was not at home for a meal, he was able to prepare sandwiches or warm up a leftover dish in the oven. Bob slept 8 to 9 hours each night and had a good appetite.

Bob denied previous psychiatric hospitalization or psychiatric contact of any kind. He had no family history of psychiatric illness. He denied sleep disturbance, depression, appetite change, or weight loss.

Bob's medical history was positive for the usual childhood diseases without sequelae. He had a tonsillectomy and adenoidectomy at age 5 and an appendectomy at age 14. He had no history of hypertension, diabetes, cancer, cardiovascular, pulmonary, or liver disease, or head injury. Never a heavy drinker, he limited his alcohol consumption to one to two glasses of wine each night with dinner. He smoked one pack of cigarettes per day for 30 years, but stopped smoking completely at age 52. On initial evaluation, he was taking no medications.

Bob was born and raised on a farm in the midwest. After graduating with honors from high school, he enlisted in the Army and served in Italy during World War II as a clerical assistant to a general. He saw little actual combat, and left the army with the rank of sergeant after 4 years. After his discharge, he attended college and graduate school in business administration. He worked for several small business firms for several years after graduation until his last position, which he held for 26 years until retirement.

Both of Bob's parents were long since deceased. His father died of colon cancer at age 72; his mother, of "senility" at age 80 in a nursing home. According to Bob, his mother didn't know him for the last 5 years of her life. Bob has one younger sister, age 58, who is alive and well except for mild arthritis and lives on the family farm with her husband. Bob married his first wife at age 22 and had two sons; the marriage ended in divorce after 18 years. The older son, age 44, is a dentist and lives in a city 350 miles away. He is married with three children. Bob sees this son three to four times a year and maintains monthly telephone contact. Bob's younger son, age 42, is a foreign news correspondent and is unmarried; Bob sees him yearly.

Bob married his second wife, Michelle, 12 years ago. Michelle had a daughter, age 39, from a previous marriage, who lives in a nearby city. Michelle described Bob as a "brilliant" man who was well-liked by everybody. They had a warm and loving relationship until 4 years ago, when he lost interest in sex. The frequency of their sexual activity gradually decreased over the years; they had had no sexual relations during the 18 months prior to admission, but still enjoyed "cuddling together" at night. Michelle related a gradual change in her attitude towards Bob, to the point where she felt "more like a mother than a wife." She stated that she's "scared to death" to learn that Bob might have Alzheimer's disease, but realized she must learn what she's "up against."

Bob's mental status examination revealed a neatly dressed Caucasian male who appeared somewhat younger than his stated age of 62 years. He was cooperative and attempted to answer all questions, although he allowed Michelle to do most of the talking. Eye contact was good, and rapport was easily established. He was alert and attentive and able to repeat six digits forward and four digits backward and spell the word "world" backwards without error. Although he was oriented to year and month, he incorrectly stated the day of the week and the date. He knew he was in an outpatient clinic, but could not recall the floor. When asked to remember three words for 5 minutes, he could recall none of the words spontaneously and only one word with multiple-choice clues. His memory of past events was good, but knowledge of current events was mildly impaired. His spontaneous speech was fluent, with no dysarthria or paraphasic errors. He was able to name common objects without difficulty, but had some difficulty naming low-frequency words, e.g., cuff, watch stem, door hinge. Compared to a normal finding of 18 to 22 names, he could generate a list of only 9 animals in 1 minute. He was able to follow one- and two-step commands only. He could copy a sentence from dictation and also spontaneously write a sentence describing the weather. Although he was able to do simple calculations, he could not perform a more complex word problem. He was able to copy simple drawings, but could not maintain the three-dimensional aspect of more complex constructions. He could explain simple idioms, but provided concrete responses to more complex abstractions.

Bob's neurological exam findings were within normal limits: cranial nerves I–XII were intact; muscle strength was $5+/5+$ bilaterally; sensation was intact bilaterally; coordination and gait were normal; reflexes were symmetric; both toes were down-gains; and frontal systems tests were normal.

Laboratory test results revealed normal white blood count hemoglobin, hematocrit, sedimentation rate, calcium phosphorus, VDRL, electrolytes, glucose, blood urea nitrogen, liver function tests, thyroid function tests, and B12 and folate levels. An electrocardiogram and chest X-ray were normal, as was an electroencephalogram. A computed tomography (CT) scan and magnetic resonance imaging (MRI) revealed no lesions, masses, or structural abnormalities.

Reader may now complete Recording the Data, Assigning Nursing Diagnoses, and Nursing Care Plan.

FORMULATION

This case evaluation is consistent with a dementia as defined by Cummings and Benson (1983): "an acquired persistent compromise of intellectual function with impairments in at least three of the following spheres of mental activity: language, memory, visuospatial skills, personality, cognition (abstraction, mathematics)." In terms of differential diagnosis, no evidence existed of a focal lesion affecting only one side of the brain. Bob's movements were normal; he had neither the shuffling gait and hand tremor of the client with Parkinson's disease nor the choreic movements and family history associated with Huntington's disease. He exhibited no indication of depression. His normal physical examination and laboratory findings tended to rule out a chronic confusional state due to metabolic or toxic disorders, and the CT scan and MRI revealed no ventricular enlargement (hydrocephalus) or other structural abnormalities.

Bob demonstrated the classical clinical characteristics of impaired memory, mild language disturbance, impaired cognitive abilities (calculations and abstractions), visuospatial difficulties (becoming lost; inability to copy three-dimensional drawings), and personality change (apathy/indifference). These impairments would gradually worsen.

Bob's intellectual impairment and poor memory and abstracting abilities required that he be placed in a consistent structured environment, such as a day care center that specializes in caring for clients with dementing disorders. He could not safely remain alone while his wife worked, and could not safely drive any longer because of his visuospatial impairments.

At this stage of his illness, Bob required supervision with activities of daily living. He also needed encouragement to do as much for himself as possible without becoming frustrated. Pursuing his previous hobbies of woodworking and gardening with direct supervision would allow him to maintain a level of self-esteem.

Staff realized the importance of evaluating the coping skills of Bob's family members. Home care of a client with Alzheimer's disease places great psychological and physical stress on the care-givers. Michelle could anticipate experiencing many feelings, such as loneliness, discouragement, sadness, guilt, anger, and fatigue. For this reason, staff referred her to a support group for families of clients with dementia. In such a support group, Michelle would learn about Alzheimer's disease and its progression and could gain some insight into her feelings and the reasons behind them.

Continued on page 420

RECORDING THE DATA

After you have read the case, cluster significant data into functional health patterns.

Health management/health perception _____

_____

_____

_____

_____

Nutritional/metabolic _____

_____

_____

_____

Elimination _____

_____

_____

_____

Activity/exercise _____

_____

_____

_____

Cognitive/perceptual _____

_____

_____

_____

Sleep/rest _____

_____

_____

_____

Self-perception/self-concept _____

_____

_____

_____

Role relationship _____

_____

_____

_____

Sexuality/reproductive _____

_____

_____

_____

Coping/stress tolerance _____

_____

_____

_____

Value/belief _____

_____

_____

_____

ASSIGNING NURSING DIAGNOSES

Use your clustered data to select appropriate nursing diagnoses.

Health perception/health management

☐ Growth and Development, Altered (see Developmental Delay)
☐ Health Maintenance, Altered
☐ Infection, Potential for
☐ Injury (Trauma): Potential for
☐ Noncompliance (Specify)
☐ Poisoning: Potential for
☐ Suffocation: Potential for

Nutritional/metabolic

☐ Body Temperature, Potential Alteration in
☐ Developmental Delay: Physical Growth and Development
☐ Fluid Volume, Altered: Excess or Excess Fluid Volume
☐ Fluid Volume Deficit, Actual
☐ Fluid Volume Deficit, Potential
☐ Nutrition, Altered: Less Than Body Requirements or Nutritional Deficit (Specify)
☐ Nutrition, Altered: More Than Body Requirements or Exogenous Obesity
☐ Nutrition, Altered: Potential for More Than Body Requirements or Potential for Obesity
☐ Oral Mucous Membrane, Altered
☐ Skin Integrity, Impaired or Skin Breakdown
☐ Skin Integrity, Impaired or Potential Skin Breakdown
☐ Swallowing, Impaired or Uncompensated Swallowing Impairment
☐ Tissue Integrity, Impaired

Elimination

☐ Bowel Elimination, Altered: Constipation
☐ Bowel Elimination, Altered: Diarrhea
☐ Bowel Elimination, Altered: Incontinence

☐ Developmental Delay: Bowel/Bladder Control
☐ Incontinence: Functional
☐ Incontinence: Reflex
☐ Incontinence: Stress
☐ Incontinence: Total
☐ Incontinence: Urge
☐ Urinary Elimination, Altered Patterns of
☐ Urinary Retention

Activity/exercise

☐ Activity Intolerance
☐ Activity Intolerance, Potential
☐ Airway Clearance, Ineffective
☐ Breathing Pattern, Ineffective
☐ Cardiac Output, Altered: Decreased
☐ Developmental Delay: Mobility
☐ Developmental Delay: Self-Care Skills
☐ Diversional Activity Deficit
☐ Gas Exchange, Impaired
☐ Home Maintenance Management, Impaired (Mild, Moderate, Severe, Potential, Chronic)
☐ Mobility, Impaired Physical
☐ Self-Care Deficit: Feeding
☐ Self-Care Deficit: Bathing/Hygiene
☐ Self-Care Deficit: Dressing/Grooming
☐ Self-Care Deficit: Toileting
☐ Self-Care Deficit: Total
☐ Tissue Perfusion, Altered: (Specify)

Sleep/rest

☐ Sleep Pattern Disturbance

Cognitive/perceptual

☐ Comfort, Altered: Pain
☐ Comfort, Altered: Chronic Pain

☐ Developmental Delay: (Specify Cognitive Area; attention, decision making, etc.)

☐ Hypothermia

☐ Hyperthermia

☐ Knowledge Deficit (Specify)

☐ Sensory-Perceptual Alteration: Input Excess or Sensory Overload

☐ Sensory-Perceptual Alteration: Input Deficit or Sensory Deprivation

☐ Thermoregulation, Ineffective

☐ Thought Processes, Altered

☐ Unilateral Neglect

Self-perception/self-concept

☐ Anxiety

☐ Body Image Disturbance

☐ Fear

☐ Hopelessness

☐ Personal Identity Confusion

☐ Powerlessness (Severe, Low, Moderate)

☐ Self-Esteem Disturbance

Role relationship

☐ Communication, Impaired Verbal

☐ Developmental Delay: Communication Skills

☐ Developmental Delay: Social Skills

☐ Family Processes, Altered

☐ Grieving, Anticipatory

☐ Grieving, Dysfunctional

☐ Parenting, Altered: Actual or Potential

☐ Role Performance, Disturbance in

☐ Social Interactions, Impaired

☐ Social Isolation (Rejection)

Sexuality/reproductive

☐ Rape-Trauma Syndrome: Compounded

☐ Rape-Trauma Syndrome: Silent Reaction

☐ Sexual Dysfunction

☐ Sexuality Patterns, Altered

Coping/stress tolerance

☐ Adjustment, Impaired

☐ Coping, Ineffective Individual

☐ Coping, Ineffective Family: Compromised

☐ Coping, Ineffective Family: Disabling

☐ Coping, Family: Potential for Growth

☐ Developmental Delay (Specify area)

☐ Post-Trauma Response

☐ Violence, Potential for (Self-Directed or Directed at Others)

Value/belief

☐ Spiritual Distress (Distress of Human Spirit)

You are now ready to develop a nursing care plan for this client. Use the following blank pages to do so. Then refer to the author's formulation, diagnostic summary, care plan, and summary.

NURSING CARE PLAN

Complete the chart below to develop a nursing care plan for this client.

Discharge outcomes/long-term goals	

Nursing diagnosis	Nursing intervention	

	Predicted outcomes/short-term goals (include time frame)	Date/signature

Return to Formulation, page 405

DIAGNOSTIC SUMMARY FOR BOB

Data	Functional health pattern	Nursing diagnosis
—Often becomes lost when driving —Is oriented to year and month, but not to day or date —Is unable to recall three words in 5 minutes —Demonstrates mildly impaired knowledge of current events —Has difficulty naming "low-frequency" words —Demonstrates poor word list generation —Can only follow two-step commands —Is unable to perform complex mathematical word problems —Can not maintain the three-dimensional aspect of more complex constructions —Exhibits evidence of concreteness on complex abstractions	Cognitive/Perceptual	Altered thought processes related to progressive deterioration in brain functioning secondary to Alzheimer's disease
—Took an early retirement from employment —Has little interest in pursuing hobbies —Has trouble remembering what he does during the day —Often gets lost when driving —Had difficulty making decisions about what clothes to wear —Is unable to cook a balanced meal by himself	Activity/Exercise	Self-care deficit: Feeding, Bathing/Hygiene, Dressing/Grooming, related to progressive dysfunction in memory secondary to disease process
—Early retirement caused loss or decrease of finances and status —Wife has become more of a "mother" to him as his dependency increases —Couple has experienced loss of sexual relationship —Wife "scared to death" of Alzheimer's disease	Coping/Stress Tolerance	Ineffective family coping: compromised related to client's progressive dysfunction in memory secondary to Alzheimer's disease

NURSING CARE PLAN

Complete the chart below to develop a nursing care plan for this client.

Discharge outcome/long-term goals			
1. BOB WILL CONTINUE TO FUNCTION INDE-PENDENTLY IN AREAS THAT HE CAN SAFELY DEMONSTRATE COMPETENCE. 2. MICHELLE WILL VERBALIZE PHYSICAL/EMOTIONAL SIGNS AND SYMPTOMS THAT		WOULD REQUIRE IMMEDIATE PROFES-SIONAL ATTENTION. 3. MICHELLE WILL VERBALIZE AN UNDER-STANDING OF THE COURSE OF ALZ-HEIMER'S DISEASE AND BE ABLE TO IDENTIFY AVAILABLE RESOURCES AND	

Nursing diagnosis	Nursing intervention	Predicted outcome/short-term goals (include time frame)	Date/signature
ALTERED THOUGHT PRO-CESSES RELATED TO PROGRESSIVE DETERIORATION IN BRAIN FUNC-TIONING SEC-ONDARY TO ALZHEIMER'S DISEASE	—REORIENT BOB TO DAY AND DATE OF MONTH EVERY MORNING —PROVIDE REORIENTATION MATERIALS SUCH AS CLOCKS AND CALENDARS IN BOB'S ROOM AND IN COMMON AREAS —ALLOW BOB ACCESS TO RADIO, TELEVISION, NEWS-PAPERS, AND MAGAZINES AS ANOTHER MEANS OF REORIENTATION TO CURRENT EVENTS —ONLY USE ONE- OR TWO-STEP COMMANDS AS BOB BECOMES CON-FUSED WITH MORE COM-PLEX COMMANDS —PROVIDE CONSISTENCY IN ROUTINE ACTIVITIES FROM DAY TO DAY TO PREVENT AS MUCH CONFUSION, ANXIETY, AND FRUSTRA-TION AS POSSIBLE. AVOID THOSE ACTIVITIES OR SET-TINGS THAT APPEAR TO OVERSTIMULATE BOB. PROVIDE BOB AND HIS WIFE WITH A SCHEDULE OF THERAPEUTIC ACTIVITIES —CONTINUE TO ASSESS FOR EVIDENCE OF DEPRESSION (WHICH IS NOT UNCOMMON IN STAGE I). ASSESS VEGETATIVE SYMPTOMS OF DEPRESSION SUCH AS LOSS OF APPETITE/ WEIGHT, SLEEP DISTUR-BANCE, AHERGIA, DE-CREASED CONCENTRATION, EVIDENCE OF ANHEDONIA, AND DECREASED SEX DRIVE. NOTIFY THE PRI-MARY PHYSICIAN IF THESE SYMPTOMS ARE EVIDENT —ASSESS BOB'S KNOW-LEDGE AND UNDER-	—BOB WILL VERBALIZE WITH PROMPTS DAILY —BOB WILL CONTINUE TO FUNC-TION WITH TWO-STEP COM-MANDS AND MINIMAL SUPER-VISION DURING STAGE I OF ILLNESS —BOB WILL NOT VERBALIZE THE SIGNS OR SYMPTOMS OF DE-PRESSION DURING STAGE I OF ILLNESS. IF HE DOES BECOME DEPRESSED, HE WILL VERBAL-IZE THIS TO HIS WIFE, MICHELLE AND SEEK TREATMENT FOR DEPRESSION —BOB WILL VERBALIZE THE KNOWLEDGE THAT HE HAS ALZHEIMER'S DISEASE AND WILL SHARE FEELINGS AND CONCERNS ABOUT THIS WITH MICHELLE AND TREATMENT TEAM DURING STAGE I OF ILLNESS —BOB AND MICHELLE WILL VER-BALIZE UNDERSTANDING OF TEACHING AND THE NEED TO CONTINUE TO ASSESS FOR PO-TENTIAL FUTURE NEEDS. THIS WILL BE AN ONGOING PROCESS	4/19 JS KF

Continued

Nursing Care Plan *continued*

Discharge outcome/long-term goals	
SUPPORT SYSTEMS.	

Nursing diagnosis	Nursing intervention	Predicted outcome/short-term goals (include time frame)	Date/signature
	STANDING OF THE ILL-NESS. ALLOW HIM TO ASK QUESTIONS AND BE OPEN AND HONEST WITH HIM. ALLOW HIM TIME DURING ONE-TO-ONE INTERACTIONS TO SHARE FEELINGS SUCH AS ANGER AND FRUSTRATION, FEAR OF DYING AND DEATH, SENSE OF BEING A BURDEN, AND LOSS OF ROLE		
	– HEALTH TEACHING WITH BOB, MICHELLE, AND ANY OTHER INVOLVED FAMILY TO INCLUDE ALL OF THE ABOVE. ALSO DO ANTIC-IPATORY TEACHING RE-GARDING HIS GRADUAL PROGRESSIVE DECLINE IN FUNCTIONING AND POTENTIAL FUTURE NEEDS, SUCH AS CON-SERVATORSHIP, NURSING HOME PLACEMENT, AND SUPPORT SYSTEMS FOR THE FAMILY SUCH AS ALZHEIMERS DISEASE AND RELATED DISORDERS ASSOCIATION (ADRDA)		

Discharge outcome/long-term goals			
	AS DISEASE PROGRESSES.		
1. BOB'S FAMILY WILL VERBALIZE THAT ADDITIONAL SUPERVISION WITH ADLs MAY BE REQUIRED AND ADDITIONAL HELP IN THE HOME MAY BE NECESSARY AS BOB BECOMES MORE DYSFUNCTIONAL			
Nursing diagnosis	Nursing intervention	Predicted outcome/short-term goals (include time frame)	Date/signature
SELF-CARE DEFI-CIT: FEEDING, BATHING/HY-GIENE, AND DRESSING/ GROOMING RE-LATED TO PRO-GRESSIVE DYS-FUNCTION IN MEMORY SEC-ONDARY TO DIS-EASE PROCESS	—ASSESS BOB'S ABILITY TO PERFORM ACTIVITIES OF DAILY LIVING (ADLs). ALLOW HIM TO FUNCTION INDEPENDENTLY IN THOSE AREAS WHERE HE CAN SAFELY DO SO, BUT SUPERVISE WHEN UN-SAFE, BOB SHOULD BE SUPERVISED WITH ADLs. HE SHOULD ALSO BE SUPERVISED IF HE BE-COMES MORE INATTENTIVE TO ADLs	—DURING STAGE I OF ILLNESS, BOB WILL BE ABLE TO PER-FORM ADLs WITH MINIMAL PROMPTS AND/OR SUPERVISION —BOB WILL ACTIVELY PARTICI-PATE IN A HOBBY OF HIS CHOICE AT LEAST THREE TIMES A WEEK —BOB WILL NO LONGER DRIVE A CAR AND WILL VERBALIZE HIS FEELINGS OF ANGER AND LOSS SURROUNDING THIS ISSUE	4/19 JS KF
	—ENCOURAGE BOB TO PUR-SUE A HOBBY THAT HE ENJOYED IN THE PAST (THIS AVOIDS HAVING TO LEARN A NEW HOBBY AND ASSISTS HIM IN STRUC-TURING TIME) —BEGIN TO WORK WITH BOB TO HELP HIM COME TO TERMS WITH THE LOSS OF ABILITY TO DRIVE DUE TO VISUO-SPATIAL IMPAIRMENT AND BECOMING LOST		

Continued

Nursing Care Plan *continued*

Discharge outcome/long-term goals	
1. AS BOB'S DISEASE PROGRESSES, MICHELLE WILL CONTINUE INVOLVEMENT IN ADRDA. 2. MICHELLE WILL CONTINUE WITH ANTICIPATORY PLANNING AS THE DISEASE PROGRESSES.	

Nursing diagnosis	Nursing intervention	Predicted outcome/short-term goals (include time frame)	Date/signature
INEFFECTIVE FAMILY COPING, COMPROMISED, RELATED TO CLIENT'S PROGRESSIVE DYSFUNCTION IN MEMORY SECONDARY TO ALZHEIMER'S DISEASE	—ENCOURAGE MICHELLE TO ATTEND A DEMENTIA FAMILY EDUCATION GROUP TO OBTAIN INFORMATION ABOUT ALZHEIMER'S DISEASE, WHICH WILL IN TURN AID HER IN PROBLEM-SOLVING. AREAS TO BE COVERED SHOULD INCLUDE CAUSES OF THE ILLNESS, MEDICAL TREATMENT, AND WHAT THE ILLNESS DOES TO BOB'S BEHAVIOR	—MICHELLE WILL ATTEND DEMENTIA FAMILY EDUCATION GROUP AND COMPLETE WITHIN 6 WEEKS —MICHELLE WILL BEGIN TO VERBALIZE AT COMPLETION OF FAMILY EDUCATION GROUP THAT BOB'S TROUBLING BEHAVIOR IS RELATED TO HIS DISEASE AND IS NOT INTENTIONAL	4/19 JS
	—DO NOT DISSUADE MICHELLE FROM PURSUING CURES BUT ENCOURAGE HER TO VIEW THE DRUGS AS AN EXPERIMENT AND NOT TO PLACE MUCH HOPE IN THEM		
	—ASSIST MICHELLE IN EXPLAINING AND RELABELING BOB'S TROUBLING BEHAVIOR CAUSED BY HIS ILLNESS; e.g., THAT BOB IS NOT ASKING REPETITIVE QUESTIONS ON PURPOSE. TEACH HER THAT BOB'S MEMORY LOSS IS NOT THE RESULT OF HIS LACK OF EFFORT		
	—ENCOURAGE MICHELLE TO ALLOW BOB TO DO AS MUCH FOR HIMSELF AS POSSIBLE AND TO INTERVENE ONLY WHEN THERE IS OBVIOUS DANGER	—BOB WILL NO LONGER DRIVE CAR, BUT MICHELLE WILL CONTINUE TO ALLOW HIM TO DO AS MANY OTHER THINGS FOR HIMSELF AS POSSIBLE	
	—ALLOW MICHELLE TO DISCUSS HER FEARS OF FINANCIAL BURDEN, ISOLATION, AND ROLE REVERSAL AS BOB BECOMES INCREASINGLY DEPENDENT	—MICHELLE WILL BEGIN DISCUSSING FEARS OF HER OWN FUTURE WITHIN 1 WEEK	
	—PROVIDE FACTS ABOUT WHAT IS AND IS NOT		

Nursing diagnosis	Nursing intervention	Predicted outcome/short-term goals (include time frame)	Date/signature
	KNOWN ABOUT ALZHEI-MER'S DISEASE, AS THE FAMILY MAY BE FRIGHTENED BY THE PROSPECT OF GENETIC LINKAGES		
	—ENCOURAGE MICHELLE TO MAKE BOB'S ENVI-RONMENT ROUTINE, SAFE, PREDICTABLE, AND FAILURE-FREE FOR BOB. (THIS AVOIDS DRAINING ENERGY OF BOTH CLIENT AND WIFE AND MAY HELP TO AVOID CATASTROPHIC REACTIONS.) ALSO, RE-ASSIGNING TASKS AND CHANGING HER EXPEC-TATIONS OF BOB ARE CRUCIAL ENVIRONMENTAL STRATEGIES FOR PRE-VENTING CATASTROPHIC REACTIONS	—BOB WILL HAVE ONLY ONE CATAS-TROPHIC REACTION PER WEEK AS VERBALIZED BY MICHELLE	
	—DETERMINE MICHELLE'S THEORIES OF CAUSATION OF BOB'S ILLNESS. EX-PLAIN THAT SHE IS NOT TO BLAME FOR HIS ILL-NESS, THEREBY ALLE-VIATING SOME OF HER GUILT	—WITHIN 1 WEEK, MICHELLE WILL VERBALIZE THAT SHE DOES NOT FEEL GUILTY AS SHE KNOWS SHE DID NOT CAUSE BOB'S DISEASE	
	—TEACH MICHELLE THAT THE ACCUMULATION OF STRESS CAN BE UPSETTING. HELP HER DEVELOP A PLAN TO RELIEVE TENSION e.g., GOING INTO A ROOM BY HERSELF, GOING FOR A WALK, OR BRINGING SOME-ONE INTO THE HOUSE TO STAY WITH BOB WHILE SHE GOES OUT	—WITHIN 1 WEEK, MICHELLE WILL BE ABLE TO VERBALIZE STRATEGIES TO PROVIDE SOME RESPITE FOR HERSELF	
	—ASCERTAIN MICHELLE'S FEELINGS ABOUT ASKING FOR HELP IN CARING FOR BOB. ENCOURAGE HER TO SEEK INFORMAL SUPPORT FROM FAMILY AND FRIENDS AND FORMAL SUPPORT FROM SOCIAL SERVICE AGENCIES	—WITHIN 1 WEEK, A FAMILY MEETING WILL BE HELD TO DISCUSS FORMAL AND INFOR-MAL SUPPORT FOR MICHELLE	
	—ENCOURAGE BOB'S FAMILY'S INVOLVEMENT IN FAMILY MEETINGS AS A WAY TO PROVIDE		

Continued

Nursing Care Plan *continued*

Nursing diagnosis	Nursing intervention	Predicted outcome/short-term goals (include time frame)	Date/signature
	SUPPORT TO MICHELLE. ENCOURAGE PARTICIPA- TION AS FAMILY MEET- INGS WILL BE A PLACE TO ANSWER QUESTIONS, TO IDENTIFY MICHELLE'S MOST PRESSING NEEDS, AND TO PROBLEM-SOLVE WITH THE FAMILY SUPPORT SYSTEM		
	—ENCOURAGE MICHELLE TO BECOME INVOLVED IN AN ADRDA (ALZ- HEIMER'S DISEASE AND RELATED DISORDERS ASSOCIATION) SUPPORT GROUP. THIS WILL ENABLE	—WITHIN 6 WEEKS, MICHELLE WILL VERBALIZE THAT SHE HAS BECOME ACTIVE IN ADRDA	
	HER TO SHARE INFOR- MATION AND TO UNDER- STAND THAT OTHER CAREGIVERS EXPERIENCE SIMILAR FRUSTRATIONS, AND ALSO TO SEEK RE- COGNITION THAT SHE MAY NOT GET FROM BOB. THE SUPPORT GROUP CAN ALSO HELP HER DEAL WITH		
	ANTICIPATORY GRIEF, FEELINGS OF ISOLATION, THE PRESSURE OF COP- ING WITH BOB'S PROB- LEM BEHAVIORS, AND DISAPPOINTMENT AT THE CRUSHED EX- PECTATIONS OF BOB'S RETIREMENT YEARS		
	—BEGIN ANTICIPATORY PLANNING WITH MICHELLE EXPLAIN THAT THE DISEASE IS PROGRESSIVE AND IRREVERSIBLE AND THAT BOB WILL NOT IM- PROVE. OFFER INFORMA- TION ABOUT HOME HEALTH CARE AND DAY CARE SERVICES. ENCOURAGE HER TO EXPLORE RE- SPITE CARE, AND EX- PLAIN THAT EVENTUALLY BOB MAY NEED TO BE INSTITUTIONALIZED. OFFER SUPPORT TO MICHELLE AS SHE EXPLORES FEELINGS OF GRIEF AND LOSS SUR- ROUNDING BOB'S EVENTUAL		

Nursing diagnosis	Nursing intervention	Predicted outcome/short-term goals (include time frame)	Date/signature
	DEATH —ASSIST BOB IN EXPLOR- ING COMMUNITY RE- SOURCES, SUCH AS ADRDA AND LEGAL AND FINANCIAL PLAN- NING EXPERTS FOR ITEMS SUCH AS ESTATE PLANNING AND DESIG- NATING POWER OF ATTORNEY	—WITHIN 6 WEEKS, MICHELLE WILL VERBALIZE THE NEED FOR ANTICIPATORY PLANNING AND WILL EXPLORE LEGAL AND FINANCIAL OPTIONS	

Referral to legal counseling would enable Michelle to make informed decisions about issues such as guardianship, conservatorship, and durable power of attorney.

A family meeting was arranged with Bob's children to inform them of the diagnosis and to answer any questions they might have. The children were also referred to an Alzheimer's disease support group.

SUMMARY

Bob and Michelle returned to the outpatient department 3 months after the initial assessment. At this time, Michelle reported a further decline in Bob's memory and language abilities. He now had trouble remembering his children's names and recently began repetitive questioning. Michelle had purchased an I.D. bracelet, which Bob wore in the event he became lost while walking the dog around the block.

Bob stated that he enjoyed attending the day care program 4 days a week. He was able to assist those more impaired than he, which made him feel useful. The program also allowed Michelle to continue her part-time work.

Although Bob was no longer able to pursue woodworking, he did enjoy drawing with charcoal. Michelle eventually hired a gardener but Bob still helped care for the roses.

Shortly after Bob's initial assessment, Michelle began to attend a weekly support group, at which she learned that Bob's repetitive questioning was caused by his illness and was not done purposefully to irritate her. In this group, she was able to discuss *her* fears of her future as it related to Bob's future as he became increasingly dependent on her, such as fears of financial hardship, isolation, loneliness, and role reversal.

She learned that Alzheimer's disease is a chronic progressive illness for which no treatment exists and decided to keep Bob at home as long as she could physically and emotionally care for him and he was ben-efitting from day care activities. Michelle came to realize that she needed more time for herself and was willing to ask her daughter to stay with Bob one day a week so she could shop, go to dinner with friends, and engage in other activities that gave her pleasure.

Although Bob's children lived some distance away, they showed support by increasing their telephone calls and providing financial as-sistance for Bob's care.

Bob and Michelle were followed by the physician/nurse team at 6-month intervals. Bob's condition steadily worsened over the following 2 years. He became agitated, with constant pacing during the day and an average of only 3 hours of sleep a night. Eventually, he could no longer attend the day care center, as he wandered away and got lost on several occasions. He also began to have episodes of urinary incontinence.

Although Bob still recognized Michelle, she was emotionally and physically exhausted and she felt he needed more care than she was able to provide. Finally, with support from Bob's children, she decided to place Bob in a long-term care facility. In her support group, Michelle had discussed her guilt feelings associated with this placement. With the help of her group and with weekly sessions with the nurse from the outpatient departments, Michelle came to realize that she needed to make an individual decision, that there is no "right" or "wrong" answer when placement is at issue. Bob's sons were understanding and agreed to provide financial assistance for the nursing home care.

Eighteen months after the nursing home admission, Bob was admitted to the acute care medical center with aspiration pneumonia. Although supportive care was initiated, Bob died 3 days later. After his death, Michelle decided to co-lead a newly formed support group for families of Alzheimer's victims and became active in seeking supportive legislation for Alzheimer's disease victims and their families.

REFERENCES

Cummings, J.L., and Benson, D.F. *Dementia: A Clinical Approach*. Boston: Butterworths, 1983.

Cummings, J.L., et al. "Reversible Dementia," *Journal of the American Medical Association* 243:2434–39, 1980.

SELECTED BIBLIOGRAPHY

Abrahams, J.P., and Crooks, V.J., eds. *Geriatric Mental Health*. New York: Grune & Stratton, 1984.

Barnes, R., and Raskind, M. "Long-Term Clinical Management of the Dementia Patient," in *Geriatric Mental Health*. Edited by Abrahams, J.P., and Crooks, V.J. New York: Grune & Stratton, 1984.

Carpenito, L.J. *Nursing Diagnosis: Application to Clinical Practice*. Philadelphia: J.B. Lippincott Co., 1983.

Edinberg, M.A. *Mental Health Practice with the Elderly*. Englewood Cliffs, N.J.: Prentice–Hall, 1985.

Feldman, R.G., and Cummings, J.L. "Treatable Dementias," in *Geriatric Neurology*. Edited by Slade, W.R. New York: Futura, 1981.

Fishbach, F.T. "Easing Adjustment to Parkinson's Disease," *American Journal of Nursing* 1:66–69, 1978.

Folstein, M.F., et al. "Mini-Mental State: A Practical Method for Grading the Mental State of Patients for the Clinician," *Journal of Psychiatric Research*, 12:189–98, 1975.

Goldman, L.S., and Luchins, D.J. "Depression in the Spouses of Demented Patients," *American Journal of Psychiatry* 141(11):1467–68, 1984.

Gwyther, L.P., and Matteson, M.A. "Care for the Caregivers," *Journal of Gerontological Nursing* 9(2):17–21, 1983.

Hachinski, V.C., et al. "Cerebral Blood Flow in Dementia," *Archives of Neurology* 32:632–37, 1975.

Kim, M.J., and Moritz, D.A. *Classification of Nursing Diagnosis: Proceedings of the Third and Fourth National Conferences.* New York: McGraw-Hill Book Co., 1982.

Kim, M.J., et al. *Classification of Nursing Diagnosis: Proceedings of the Fifth National Conference.* St. Louis: C.V. Mosby Co., 1984.

McHugh, P.R., and Folstein, M.F. "Psychiatric Syndromes of Huntington's Chorea: A Clinical and Phenomenologic Study," in *Psychiatric Aspects of Neurological Disease.* Edited by Benson, D.F., and Blumer, D. New York: Grune & Stratton, 1975.

Mortimer, J.A., et al. "Epidemiology of Dementing Illness," in *The Epidemiology of Dementia.* Edited by Mortimer, J.A., and Schuman, L.M. New York: Oxford University Press, 1981.

Perlmutter, I., and Gobles, C. "Subdural Hematoma in Older Patients," *Journal of the American Medical Association* 176:212–14, 1961.

Plum, F. "Dementia: An Approaching Epidemic," *Nature* 279:372-73, 1979.

Rabins, P.V., et al. "The Impact of Dementia on the Family," *Journal of the American Medical Association* 248(3):333–35, 1982.

Shapira, J., et al. "Distinguishing Dementias," *American Journal of Nursing* 86:698–702, 1986.

Steffle, B.M., ed. *Handbook of Gerontological Nursing.* New York: Van Norstrand Reinhold Co., 1984.

Strub, R.L., and Black, F.W. *The Mental Status Examination in Neurology,* 2nd ed. Philadelphia: F.A. Davis Co., 1985.

Stuteville, P., and Welch, K. "Subdural Hematoma in the Elderly Person," *Journal of the American Medical Association* 168:1445–49, 1958.

Wells, C.E. "A Deluge of Dementia," *Psychosomatics* 22:837–38, 1981.

Zarit, S.H. *Aging and Mental Disorders: Psychological Approaches to Assessment and Treatment.* New York: Free Press, 1980.

Zarit, S.H., and Zarit, J.M. "Families Under Stress: Interventions for Caregivers of Senile Dementia Patients," *Psychotherapy Theory, Research and Practice* 19(4):461–71, 1982.

Zarit, S.H., et al. *The Hidden Victims of Alzheimer's Disease: Families Under Stress.* New York: New York University Press, 1985.

Zarit, S.H., et al. "Relatives of the Impaired Elderly: Correlates of Feelings of Burden," *Gerontologist* 20:649–55, 1980.

Nursing of Clients in Outpatient Psychiatric Settings: The Work of Clinical Nurse Specialists

The following cases illustrate the work of the psychiatric–mental health nurse specialist. After graduate study and supervised clinical experience, these nurses practice at advanced competency levels. Those nurses working in private practice are self-employed and may gain compensation for psychotherapeutic services either through direct fees or through third party reimbursement.

Although clinical nurse specialists adopt the nursing process as the foundation of their practice, they also employ psychotherapeutic techniques based upon other behavioral sciences.

In this section, cases are presented differently from those for the generalist nurse. These cases do not contain nursing care plans, but rather include descriptions of assessment data, formulation and problem description, course of treatment, and summary. This format reflects the current practice of advanced psychiatric–mental health nurses.

Karen:
Adjustment Disorder
with Mixed Emotional Features

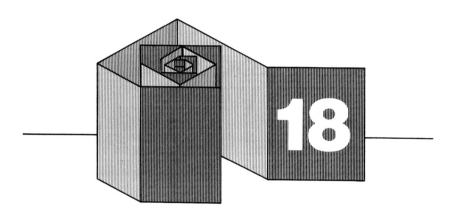

Carole J. Singer, MSN, RN, CS

This case study illustrates the work of a clinical nurse specialist in treating a client with an adjustment disorder over a period of 7 months. Negotiation of the therapeutic contract, explanation of specific therapeutic techniques used, and evaluation of progress throughout the three phases of treatment are outlined. The nursing diagnoses represented in this case include:
• Disturbance in self-esteem related to fear of failure and self-deprecation secondary to adjustment disorder.
• Sleep pattern disturbance related to difficulty falling asleep and early morning awakening secondary to depression.
• Anxiety related to chronic sense of failure secondary to poor parental role model introjects.
• Grieving related to compromised physical status secondary to thyroiditis.

CASE STUDY

Karen, a 33-year-old twice-divorced white woman, presented to a community mental health clinic for the first time. She lived alone in an apartment in a Boston suburb and had just quit her job with a computer firm 2 weeks before contact. She had held a managerial position with the firm in Miami and had moved, secondary to a transfer within the company, to an upgraded management position in Boston 2 months prior to her intake appointment.

On contact, Karen described a long-standing depression and poor self-esteem. These feelings culminated in her resignation from her new job, secondary to her own self-doubts and fears of failure, even though she stated that her supervisor had been quite pleased with her work.

The Christmas holidays appeared to be the direct precipitant that led Karen to contact the clinic. Her expression of feeling depressed and alone had caused a friend to refer her.

Karen was born in Atlanta, Georgia, the youngest child of four. At the time of contact, her 40-year-old brother, diagnosed with manic-depressive illness and stabilized on lithium carbonate therapy, was living in North Carolina with his family. Her sister, 37 years old and single, was living and working in New York City. According to Karen, both her brother and sister were "doing well." Another brother, 3 years older than Karen, died in a boating accident 10 years before at age 26.

Karen described her childhood as chaotic and unhappy. Her parents were both alcoholics, and her father often beat her mother. The children were not physically abused, but often witnessed their parents' fights and received verbal abuse.

Both parents were of Irish-Catholic descent. The family was not very religious, but attended church on holidays. Karen did not practice her religion, and felt only minimal ties to it.

Karen described her mother as a passive, long-suffering woman who lacked courage and skills to better her home situation. She often threatened divorce, but never followed through. In Karen's view, she was the more involved, caring parent, and often tried to protect the children from their father. Karen felt closer to her than she did to her father.

Karen's father was a maintenance man in a nearby apartment building, and worked relatively steadily. Karen's mother worked off-and-on as a part-time secretary once the children started school.

Karen got along well with her siblings, and in fact felt somewhat protected from the family strife because she was the youngest. When asked about the impact of her brother's death 10 years earlier, Karen replied it was extremely difficult, though she cannot remember much from that period. However, she began to drink excessively shortly after his death.

Karen had the usual childhood diseases without significant incident. She attended school regularly, where she received average-to-good grades and made friends easily. She displayed no history of behavioral problems associated with childhood. She began to date in groups at age 14, and described herself as being a shy, "good teen." But she felt ashamed about bringing friends home because of the messy state of the house and her parents' conflicts. Karen began menstruating at age 13 and has experienced a regular cycle since then.

When Karen was 14 years old, her father committed suicide by taking an overdose of barbiturates. He was 40 years old. Karen stated that she does not remember much about this period, except that her mother found her father in the bathroom and told Karen when she returned from playing at a friend's house. Karen remembered that her older brother took the news harder than anyone else in the family.

Shortly after her father's death, the family moved to Charlotte, North Carolina, to live in their former summer home. Her mother was originally from North Carolina and had family there. At this time, Karen's two brothers were working and living on their own and her sister was living at home, working as a secretary. During the interview, Karen described this period of her life as her happiest. Her home life was calmer, she became closer to her mother's relatives, and she developed new friendships.

After Karen completed high school, she attended two junior colleges in North Carolina, each for a period of 1 year. She studied computer science mainly because she knew job opportunities were readily available if she completed her studies. However, she quit each school because she felt she "never fit in, I couldn't compete." She then added, "All I seem to do is quit."

At age 20, Karen moved to Miama, Florida, with a friend and obtained work as a secretary. She lived and worked in Miami for the next 13 years, until her move to Boston. Karen lived with this roommate for 3 years following her move; she described this as a good experience. Karen began dating and had her first sexual experience at age 21—an experience she described as "OK." She used the contraceptive pill for birth control.

Through this roommate, Karen met her first husband, a police officer. According to Karen, he was a "nice man" but "I never really loved him." During their 2-year-long marriage, Karen developed a drinking problem that adversely affected the relationship. According to Karen, the marital breakup was amicable, and she kept in touch with her ex-husband (who subsequently remarried) periodically for a few years afterwards.

Following the breakup of her first marriage, Karen lived alone and continued working. At a party, she met her second husband, a salesman who was also alcoholic and lonely. According to Karen, "by being together, we were two halves making a whole." They married when Karen was age 27, but divorced 2 years later. Karen described alcoholism as the major problem with this marriage; eventually she realized that she did not have much else in common with her husband. Karen ended this marriage and had not been in contact with her ex-husband since the breakup. At the time of her second divorce, Karen began to realize that she had an alcohol problem. Consequently, she began attending Alcoholics Anonymous (AA) meetings on her own and has been sober since that time, a total of 4 years. Karen maintained a strong alliance with AA in Miami and formed several close friendships through the organization. Upon her arrival in Boston, she immediately sought out the support of a local AA chapter and met some new friends. At the time of admission, she was not dating, however.

According to Karen, her brother did not have an alcohol problem and her sister was a "teetotaler." She denied any family history of abuse of other drugs.

At age 30, Karen took a position as a secretary in a computer firm. She was taught data processing along with other computer skills, and performed so well that she was promoted several times over the next 3 years. She found this pleasing, although somewhat surprising. She described the promotion that caused her transfer to Boston as something she had to accept; to not have done so would have meant career stagnation.

Over the years, Karen kept in touch with her mother, brother, and sister, although not as closely as in earlier years. Her mother's health began to deteriorate secondary to alcoholism, and she died of cirrhosis 1½ years ago at age 57. Karen felt that she had not fully grieved-through this loss.

One year ago, Karen saw a clinical psychologist in Miami for bimonthly treatment over a 6-month period. This was related to depression following her mother's death. She found this treatment only moderately helpful and stated that her therapist terminated it, saying he felt she was doing better.

Karen had a number of physical problems in recent years. She was diagnosed as having thyroiditis 3 years ago. The following year, lupus was diagnosed, and 3 months later she had a kidney biopsy secondary to excessive edema. Finally, a year ago she had an ovarian cyst removed. At the time of contact, she was taking two medications: prednisone, 5 mg/day, and levothyroxine sodium (Synthroid), 5 mg/day. She was seeing a specialist at Metropolitan General Hospital under continuing care; her records were requested to complete this evaluation.

On mental status examination, Karen presented as a very thin, attractive female looking younger than her stated age. She was well-groomed and neat in appearance. She was very pleasant and cooperative, almost ingratiating, with the intake process and did not seem particularly anxious.

Her speech was clear and coherent and of normal rhythm and tone. Her content of thought was focused on her overall depression and the struggle to "stay on top of it." Throughout the interview, she displayed a full range of affect and was able to call upon her sense of humor. However, she also tended to be self-deprecating.

She was oriented to time, place, person, and situation. Her recent and remote memory was intact. She displayed no evidence or history of psychotic process. She did display moderate signs of vegetative depression: difficulty falling asleep, early morning awakening, and a recent weight loss of 4 pounds, although Karen reported this was all worse during the 2 months she had held her new job. Her appetite had remained stable. For 2 days following her resignation, Karen felt suicidal, but had no plans. She did not think of drinking and had not felt suicidal or homicidal since.

Karen was judged to be of above-average intelligence, with fair insight. Her cognitive functioning appeared to be intact and appropriate. Her coping strategies included using supports known to be helpful (AA), and asking for help when indicated.

FORMULATION

Karen grew up in a household that suffered from her parents' alcoholism and fighting. Both parents drank as long as Karen could remember. In her father, Karen found a hostile, distant man who was a poor role model. His death when Karen was age 14 came at a crucial time in her development, when she was first dealing with a budding interest in heterosexual activities. Karen characterized her mother as a depressed, weak person who was not able to assert herself; thus, Karen was also deprived of a strong female image. Karen spoke of feeling ashamed of her parents' home and behavior while growing up, and at times feeling sorry for herself. Her childhood years, characterized by a lack of nurturance and consistency, marked the beginning of Karen's chronic depression. As a young adult, Karen attempted to fill this narcissistic wound with hurried marriages and alcohol abuse. As Renner (1979) points out, one common way that an individual deals with such feelings is through drug abuse.

Growing up, Karen kept her anger about her family situation inward, as if expressing it might mean total loss of any parental affection and interest. As a child of alcoholics, Karen undoubtedly felt left out and abandoned, which led to feelings of low self-worth and guilt and possibly to feelings that she must have done something wrong to warrant such poor treatment. Psychodynamically, Karen's childhood experiences left her with a poorly developed ego. Her father's suicide served to increase her sense of guilt because, to her mind, she clearly failed him by not preventing his desperate act. Her father's death was never discussed in the family, which left Karen to internalize her anger and sadness.

From the biological and family systems points of view (Burkhalter, 1975), Karen's alcoholism came as no surprise. Within the context of her family, Karen learned a particular style of handling anxiety and emptiness—distancing into a substance for comfort. Karen made an attempt to separate from her unhappy home life by moving to another state. However, an individual cannot flee his or her family's problems; unless dealt with, they remain, as Karen was to see with her own alcoholism. With this self-destructive behavior, Karen perpetuated her feelings of low self-esteem into young adulthood. Bibring (1968) emphasized a loss of self-esteem as the crucial element in depression, stating that "the emotional expression of a state of helplessness and powerlessness of the ego, irrespective of what may have caused the breakdown of the mechanisms which establish the self-esteem, constitutes the essence of the condition."

Karen's first marriage represented an attempt to solidify her life; unfortunately, she chose a man she never loved, and the marriage ended in divorce. Undoubtedly, her lack of self-worth sabotaged her effort by not enabling her to choose a better-suited partner. By the time of her second marriage, Karen was deeper into her depression and chose a man she knew was an alcoholic, the only thing they had in common.

Because Karen had never been involved in a satisfactory intimate relationship, she was never able to master Erikson's (1963) sixth developmental stage, the establishment of a sense of intimacy versus isolation. This is the central issue of young adulthood.

Karen spoke of her difficulty completing things in life, and referred in particular to her aborted attempts at finishing college. From a cultural standpoint, Karen's background was lower-middle class Irish Catholic, a tradition that, to her parents' generation, stressed that a young woman marry and raise a family rather than obtain an education and career. In addition, secondary to her poor self-esteem, Karen harbored deep-rooted fears of failure, having introjected the role models her parents afforded her. This sense of failure was exacerbated by her two marriages and culminated in her recent job loss. Exploring the other side of this issue, Karen also unconsciously feared success, as this was not familiar to her. While Karen had a strong work history, her previous positions were mainly ones she "fell into." Her recent promotion required that she make a substantial move towards a more independent and assertive role. Karen's ego deficits in the area of self-esteem thus yielded compromised functioning in both the interpersonal and broader social systems of her life.

Karen's characteristic defense style was one of denial, as if not dealing with unpleasant feelings would make them go away. This is clearly demonstrated by her difficulty in remembering and focusing on the deaths of her father, brother, and mother. Denial is a mechanism Karen grew up with; her family made great use of it, specifically around their alcoholism and in their response to her father's death.

Karen also utilized the defense mechanism of self-deprecation, in which she ridiculed herself continually. In this manner, she sent messages to herself and others that not much can be expected of her, which served to diminish any future disappointments. This defense also elevated others to a higher status in comparison to Karen, which, when combined with her ingratiating manner, helped to secure other people around her. This style of relating appeared to be a life stance Karen adopted many years ago.

Karen had to deal with several medical problems in recent years, some severe. This had an impact on her emotionally as well as physically, and presented a source of ongoing concern. Although Karen's lupus and general health were stable at the time of contact, she undoubtedly experienced anxiety related to the future course of the illness and restrictions it may pose. Because of her long-standing poor self-esteem, some part of Karen may have secretly felt she deserved to be saddled with illness or an early death like her parents.

Despite her background, Karen had considerable strengths. She had sustained numerous losses during her life and still managed to push forward. Her work history and recent sobriety evidences much tenacity and the capacity to learn and integrate new skills. She was able to ask for help and had clearly decided that she would not go the route of her parents. Overall, the interviewer got the sense that she believed in her capacity for growth and change, which is a prerequisite for any successful therapy.

Interpersonally, Karen demonstrated warmth and charm. These skills enabled Karen to engage well with people, providing her with the tools necessary to both enjoy and improve her personal and professional life.

COURSE OF TREATMENT

Karen requested individual treatment from the clinic. My assessment data and staff input corroborated with this strategy, as Karen expressed her needs and problems clearly and demonstrated the motivation required for successful individual treatment. In addition, Karen was in somewhat of a crisis, having lost most anchors in her life. She needed immediate access to a supportive, caring relationship that would help guide her through the crisis period and hopefully settle her into the work of insight-oriented psychotherapy. Because Karen had access to a supportive group situation through AA, individual work was thought to offer a good balance. The fact that the clinical team and Karen shared the same thoughts regarding her treatment needs helped to validate Karen's feelings, thus increasing her trust.

In addressing the goals of Karen's treatment, a negotiated approach incorporating the nursing process was utilized, with her input and responses dictating the course of treatment.

Together, Karen and I outlined the short-term goals of treatment as centering on the overall relief of her presenting symptoms: decrease in anxiety and vegetative signs of depression and stabilization of her social/vocational functioning. As her therapist, I also included as a goal the establishment of a therapeutic relationship.

In relation to long-term goals, Karen felt it was time to examine her deep-seated fears and insecurities in the hope of resolving them. This resolution, along with the maintenance of Karen's health status, would enable her to function most optimally in the different areas of her life.

Karen settled into the Beginning Phase of treatment well and was able to relate comfortably. Early in the course of treatment, she made use of the mental health center's crisis services, calling when feeling very anxious and overwhelmed. During this time, I worked collaboratively with the crisis team staff in providing services to Karen. Karen's use of the crisis team subsided over a few weeks' period as her feelings of anxiety abated.

Karen's style of relating was based on self-denigration and ingratiation to others. In therapy, this represented a defensive block. Karen was quick to use her denigrations as her all-encompassing reason for failure, thus warning me not to expect more. By being ingratiating, she was working hard to please me and get me to like her, as she was too frightened to let me see her real self. This *modus operandi* was Karen's transference to me, operating under the assumption that by being extremely nice she would give me less reason to reject or leave her, as others had done from early on in her life. This behavior in turn evoked countertransference feelings in me of wanting to take care of Karen, as well as frustration at her continual and predictable manner of self-denigration. I realized that I should not act out these feelings, but instead should point out and clarify what I observed. Assuring Karen that I could handle her anger and aggression was a vital aspect of treatment at this time. To help accomplish this, I utilized the technique of self-disclosure—

the nurse's revealing of her own experiences, thoughts, ideas, values, attitudes, or feelings in the context of the relationship (Sundeen et al., 1981). Using this technique with discretion, I was able to provide Karen with a model of a real person who could understand her concerns. This promoted a sense of mutuality in our relationship, helping Karen see that her experiences were not foreign to the understanding of others.

Treatment progressed into the Working Phase. At one point early in the third month of this phase, Karen responded to her fears of abandonment by attempting to get me to reject her. In the Working Phase, periods of growth typically alternate with periods of resistance, during which the client continues with or reverts to earlier behaviors (Sundeen et al., 1981). Karen began arriving late for sessions, then missed some, evidently hoping that I would become annoyed and close her case. If I did so, she would be able to maintain her familiar, albeit painful, feelings of depression. For Karen, this prospect was less frightening than remaining in a relationship and facing fears of abandonment. Her strategy also helped to maintain the consistency of her negative world view.

When I confronted Karen with her behavior, along with my hypothesis of what was happening, she broke down in tears and acknowledged her feelings. This session proved to be a turning point for Karen, as she was able to break through her resistance and experience emotional insight, an experiential understanding of self (Lego, 1985).

Early in treatment, I utilized behavioral therapy in teaching Karen the techniques of relaxation and positive affirmation. This helped her by giving her something concrete to do when she felt anxious, as well as by slowly increasing her self-esteem. She quickly adopted these techniques. Because of her alcoholism, I wanted to refrain, if possible, from recommending the use of antianxiety medications. Utilization of behavioral techniques in lieu of medications also offered Karen alternative methods of dealing with stress and depression.

Over the next 4 months of treatment, Karen focused on the numerous losses and failures in her life. Discussions also explored past and present relationships with her family members. Karen evidenced significant insight into her thoughts and behaviors and was increasingly able to internalize a more realistic and positive view of herself. Her self-deprecation decreased and, as she grew more trusting of me, her ingratiating defense lessened.

Karen demonstrated increasing growth in the way in which she incorporated the insights and techniques learned in treatment into her life. She used the behavioral techniques often with success, and even passed them on to a friend who was in need. Karen noted feeling more secure with herself, which enabled her to be more open and honest with her feelings, first with herself and then with others. Dealing with the loneliness brought on by starting a new life in a strange city was a focus for Karen at this time.

During the Beginning Phase of treatment, Karen was able to obtain part-time employment in secretarial positions through a temporary employment agency. As her therapy continued and her self-esteem improved, she was offered and accepted a full-time administrative position at an advertising agency.

Karen maintained her sobriety and membership in AA, and although she missed her Miami network and a group she had helped start there, she clearly drew a great deal of strength from the organization. She also kept a close watch on her medical concerns, following through with appointments and her medication regimen. We did some grief work on the loss of physical health Karen faced, as well as the threat of a worsening condition. She appreciated the opportunity to discuss her physical problems with a nurse.

At the end of her 7th month of treatment, Karen related that a friend in Miami had offered her the use of her apartment for several months while she was on sabbatical. During her stay in Boston, Karen had kept in close touch with her Miami friends, whom she found to be very supportive. Immediately following her job resignation, these friends encouraged her to return to Miami, but Karen felt she should stick it out in Boston. But her friend's offer caused Karen to reconsider this decision; she felt that even though she was functioning better, she still missed her friends and home base. In addition, Karen was closer to her brother than her sister, and missed the accessibility she had to him and his family when she lived in Florida.

Karen felt she had reached the point where she was able to forgive herself for her recent career loss and no longer felt embarrassed about it. She was leaning towards returning to Miami, where she would search for a job in a new field and would have her social supports. Over the next 2 weeks she displayed ambivalence about this decision but finally decided to move.

Karen followed-through with Termination nicely, which in itself was a new experience for her. She was able to relate our termination to previous times that she failed to follow-through with others, feeling sad for the past but pleased for her present effort. Karen spoke of what she learned in treatment and how it helped to change her life through new understanding and behavior, and thanked me for my efforts on her behalf. At our last appointment, she gave me a scarf she had knit and asked if she could contact me at some later time.

SUMMARY

Karen's course of treatment proved successful in helping her obtain her short-term goals, and also made an impact on her long-term goals. Because of her decision to return to Miami, these goals vis-à-vis current treatment had to be reassessed. Karen stated she planned to seek out treatment in Miami to continue her work towards greater self-understanding and growth. In our work together, Karen worked hard in letting go of her denial and allowing herself to examine problems and feelings she had never addressed previously, such as her experiences with rejection, death, anger, and fear. This enabled her to take the initial steps toward increasing her self-esteem and asserting herself. In future treatment, Karen could solidify this, building a stronger ego that would afford her a continually rewarding life.

A major area not touched on in our treatment was that of romantic relationships. Hopefully, when Karen feels better about herself, she will choose more appropriate men. Another focus for Karen might be the continuation of her education.

Karen was a pleasure to work with, as she approached her treatment seriously, had an attractive personality, and readily showed improvement. As her therapist, I was provided with an opportunity to feel rewarded by her progress.

The input from staff peer review yielded agreement that Karen had made a significant start and numerous gains in treatment. Overall, she made an excellent adjustment to the stresses facing her and was able to engage in a trusting therapeutic relationship that by nature is often anxiety-producing. Most staff agreed it was best for her to return to the security of her home base, as feeling secure was a rare experience for her. Staff commended the use of behavioral techniques along with insight-oriented psychotherapy in this case, as well as the therapist's use of self through self-disclosure. One staff member raised the question of how Karen viewed the therapist's acceptance of her gift: did it show that she had to continue giving and being nice to people in order to be liked? Staff also wondered how she would have reacted had the gift been refused. The majority of staff, however, felt Karen's gift was appropriate and expressed heartfelt thanks for her successful therapy experience.

REFERENCES

Bibring, E. *The Meaning of Despair*. New York: Science House, 1968.

Burkhalter, P.K. *Nursing Care of the Alcoholic and Drug Abuser*. New York: McGraw-Hill Book Co., 1975.

Erikson, E.H. *Childhood and Society,* 3rd ed. New York: W.W. Norton & Co., 1963.

Lego, S. "Psychoanalytically Oriented Individual and Group Therapy with Adults," in *The Clinical Specialist in Psychiatric Mental Health Nursing: Theory, Research, and Practice.* Edited by Critchley, D.L., and Maurin, J.T. New York: John Wiley & Sons, 1985.

Renner, J.A., Jr. "Drug Abuse," in *Outpatient Psychiatry—Diagnosis and Treatment.* Edited by Lazare, A. Baltimore: Williams & Wilkins Co., 1979.

Sundeen, S.J., et al. *Nurse-Client Interaction: Implementing the Nursing Process.* St. Louis: C.V. Mosby Co., 1981.

SELECTED BIBLIOGRAPHY

Adams, C.G., and Macione, A., eds. *Handbook of Psychiatric–Mental Health Nursing.* New York: John Wiley & Sons, 1983.

Burgess, A.W. *Psychiatric Nursing in the Hospital and the Community,* 4th ed. Englewood Cliffs, N.J.: Prentice-Hall, 1985.

Lancaster, J. *Adult Psychiatric Nursing.* New Hyde Park, N.Y.: Medical Examination Publishing Co., 1980.

Mendels, J. *Concepts of Depression.* New York: John Wiley & Sons, 1970.

Miller, J.B. *Toward a New Psychology of Women.* Boston: Beacon Press, 1976.

Nemiah, J.C. *Foundations of Psychopathology.* New York: Oxford University Press, 1961.

Rogers, C.R. *Client-Centered Therapy.* Boston: Houghton Mifflin, 1951.

Mrs. Brown:
Major Depression

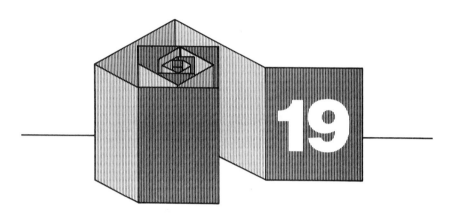

Ellen C. Drever, MS, RN, CS

The following case exemplifies the work of a clinical nurse specialist in treating a depressed client.

The following nursing diagnoses are represented in this case study:
- Ineffective family coping: compromised, related to strained marital relationship secondary to wife's illness.
- Altered parenting related to wife's feelings of inadequacy secondary to major depression.
- Impaired verbal communication related to husband's fear of upsetting wife secondary to wife's vulnerability.

CASE STUDY

Mrs. Brown, a 36-year-old, white, Catholic female, lived with her husband, an insurance broker, and their 2-year-old daughter in a suburban town outside a major western city. Although she held a bachelors degree in retailing and had worked previously selling women's garments, Mrs. Brown had not worked outside the home since the birth of her daughter.

Mrs. Brown was referred to a psychiatric clinical nurse specialist in the hospital's outpatient department after a 3-week hospitalization on the adult unit. Two weeks prior to this hospitalization, while out to dinner with her husband and another couple, she had felt a sudden, alarming sense of dread. The group had been discussing the difficulties of adjusting to a new baby in the house. Mrs. Brown became noticeably anxious and upset, and she and her husband left the dinner party abruptly. She was unable to sleep that night and reported recurring thoughts centering on her inability to properly care for her infant daughter and thoughts that her husband would leave her if he knew how poorly she performed. Mr. Brown became alarmed and took her to her former psychiatrist, who prescribed alprazolam (Xanax), 0.5 mg every 4 hours as needed for anxiety, and arranged biweekly appointments. But despite these interventions, Mrs. Brown became increasingly fearful and withdrawn and reported thoughts of wanting her "life to be over." Thus, hospitalization was arranged.

During hospitalization, desipramine hydrochloride (Norpramin) was instituted and therapeutic blood levels achieved on a dose of 200 mg daily. Her sleeping patterns and appetite improved, her fearfulness remitted, and she steadily increased her ability to participate in the unit's activities. However, an evaluation of her and her husband's interpersonal patterns revealed significant communication problems, especially relating to the discipline and care of their daughter. In spite of an improvement in her mood and daily functioning, Mrs. Brown continued to report a lack of self-confidence, a tendency to devalue herself, and a dissatisfaction with her role as wife and mother. Consequently, she was referred to outpatient therapy for medication management and for assistance in improving her interpersonal relationships, caring for her child, and developing a more realistic self-appraisal.

Mrs. Brown had been hospitalized twice before for symptoms of depression, once at age 22 and then again at age 28. Both hospitalizations followed significant psychosocial stressors. The first occurred after the suicide of her mother from a drug overdose at age 54. During this episode, Mrs. Brown was treated with low doses of thioridazine (Mellaril) for symptoms of increased fearfulness, generalized anxiety, poor sleep, and feelings of extreme guilt and self-incrimination. She was released after 4 days and followed in twice-weekly psychotherapy for a period of 2 years.

Mrs. Brown's second hospitalization occurred at age 28. At the time, she reported progressive sleeplessness, decreased appetite, and marital conflicts. She was treated with amitriptyline hydrochloride (Elavil), 100 mg q.d., and was followed in outpatient therapy for 6 months. She resumed her full work schedule and sought no psychiatric treatment until 9 months before her latest hospitalization. At that time, problems relating to the care of their daughter and their marriage led Mr. and Mrs. Brown to seek family counseling. A 3-week separation occurred during this period. Mr. Brown moved to an apartment but returned after he became distressed that the separation would lead to divorce.

During her outpatient evaluation interview, Mrs. Brown denied any previous medical hospitalizations, surgeries, or major illnesses. She reported episodes of asthma as a child that ceased during her teenage years. She denied excessive alcohol or drug use, but admitted smoking marijuana while in college. She had experienced a miscarriage 1 year prior to the pregnancy that produced her 2-year-old daughter. She displayed normal menstrual cycles, and used a diaphragm with spermicidal gel as her method of contraception.

Mrs. Brown described her childhood as "unhappy." Although she did well in school and had several friends, her home life was often disrupted by the absence of her mother and father. Her mother was a withdrawn and demanding woman who pushed Mrs. Brown to achieve in school and to be socially popular. Looking back, Mrs. Brown described her mother's mood as depressed. (Her mother actually had sought treatment for depression—a fact Mrs. Brown did not learn until she was an adult.) Her father, a patent attorney, often was absent from the home for business purposes and was generally emotionally remote from Mrs. Brown and her mother. Mrs. Brown's maternal grandmother encouraged her to go away to college to escape her problems at home, and actually paid for her education. Mrs. Brown earned a B.A. in retailing from an eastern university; she did not see her parents at all during her college years. She spent the summer between her junior and senior years in France and reported this as one of her happiest memories.

As mentioned before, Mrs. Brown's mother died at age 54 of a drug overdose. Her father died of a heart attack at age 56. She had one brother, 2 years younger, an attorney living in Boston with his wife and two sons. She described him as bright and successful and expressed a wish to see him and his family more frequently.

On mental status examination, Mrs. Brown presented as an attractive, small-framed woman looking younger than her stated age. She was dressed in a casual blouse and skirt and sat quietly in a relaxed posture with her hands clasped. Her speech was well modulated and of normal quantity and speed. Her intellectual functioning was intact, and her fund of knowledge congruent with her level of education. Her concentration was good, and she was cooperative throughout the interview. She displayed a wide range of emotion. Her main concern was her fear of coping with the increasing demands of her daughter; she expressed feeling "overwhelmed" by the task. She became tearful when relating the events that led to the trial separation from her husband and expressed concern about caring for her daughter if her husband ever left again. She denied suicidal ideation and agreed to report such thoughts should they recur.

FORMULATION

Mrs. Brown reported symptoms of dysphoria, decreased appetite and sleep, loss of energy, fatigue, diminished concentration, and thoughts of wishing she were dead for a period of 2 weeks prior to hospitalization. This symptom constellation meets the *DSM-III* criteria for major depression (APA, 1980; see *Diagnostic Criteria for Major Depressive Episode,* pages 446 and 447). The disorder was in remission after a 3-week hospitalization and daily oral administration of desipramine, 200 mg. The dependent features of Mrs. Brown's personality became more prominent when she was depressed. She passively allowed others to assume major responsibility for areas of her life and displayed a severe lack of self-confidence. She was fearful of jeopardizing close relationships by making demands, and thus withdrew from friends and family. The concept of "learned helplessness" defines these behaviors as an individual's perceived lack of control over environmental reinforcement. The behaviors include withdrawal, loss of motivation for any activity, and a lowered ability to learn or attempt new behaviors that could result in future environmental control (Gordon and Ledray, 1985). Feminine values, economic dependency, and stressful processes of marriage, separation, and child-bearing are thought to contribute to the woman's feelings of powerlessness and learned helplessness.

Weissman and Klerman (1982) examined learned helplessness as one explanation for the preponderance of depressive illness in women. They found a 2:1 sex ratio upheld across studies in the United States and in most foreign countries. Women in their reproductive years run the greatest risk. The authors also reviewed findings on genetic transmission, female endocrine physiology, and social status. They concluded that findings on genetic transmission needed further examination and that the data on the relationship of endocrine function to clinical depressed states was inconsistent. They did, however, find much evidence linking the postpartum period to increased depression.

Mrs. Brown had experienced several severe environmental stressors—most notably marital discord, and changes in her role resulting from motherhood, which created a lack of structure and social rewards as were previously provided by her employment outside the home. Weissman (1980) describes marital difficulty as "the most commonly reported event in the 6 months prior to the onset of depression and the most frequent problem presented by depressed women in outpatient treatment." Brown and Harris (1978) found "a confiding, intimate relationship with the spouse was the most important protection against depression in the face of life stress"; however, Gove and Tudor (1973) concluded marriage had a positive effect on males but a detrimental effect on females. Another pertinent study found that one important variable that separated depressive from nondepressive married women was employment outside the home (Gordon and Ledray, 1985).

Mrs. Brown's level of adaptive functioning for the previous year was judged only fair, based on prolonged social withdrawal, a lack of pleasurable leisure pursuits, and a decline in her ability to manage the increasing demands of her healthy and active daughter. Wotman and Nadelson (1980) define pregnancy and childbirth as normal conditions, yet also as developmental crises because they require adaptation. The individual is confronted with new conflicts that may "precipitate the reemergence of earlier unsettled conflicts." The physical and psychological changes are stressful, yet present the new mother with the opportunity for further growth and maturation. Anxieties typically arise about changes in roles and the impact on the marriage relationship and career aspirations. The new mother's early relationship with her own mother is crucial to role enactment.

Mrs. Brown's own experience was deprived. Her mother was often depressed, demanding, and emotionally distanced, and emphasized achievement rather than emotional closeness. This negative mothering experience inadequately prepared Mrs. Brown for child-raising. Wotman and Nadelson (1980) recommend that the therapeutic interventions "involve the parents with help in working through earlier unresolved conflicts and differentiate them from current concerns." Consequently, the nurses caring for Mrs. Brown stressed the importance of her recognition of ambivalence during this period, as expectations are often unrealistic.

COURSE OF TREATMENT

The treatment plan developed by the psychiatric clinical nurse specialist (PCNS) involved the client and her husband in weekly conjoint sessions, each preceded by a 10-minute period focusing on Mrs. Brown's medication management and symptom monitoring. Because Mrs. Brown had responded well to medication therapy and psychotherapy during her two previous episodes of depression, she was deemed readily able to seek, accept, and follow-through with treatment. This pointed to a good prognosis for recovery from this latest episode. Because of the specific interpersonal problems identified in this case—namely marital conflicts related to parental/child interpersonal and behavioral problems—the PCNS thought it appropriate to include Mr. Brown in developing and implementing problem-solving strategies.

The goals of treatment were to provide a forum for practical applications of clear, direct, and open communication; to support the verbalization of individual thoughts, feelings, and desires; and to develop a consistent approach to resolution of conflicts. Pertinent issues included the discipline and care of the couple's 2-year-old daughter, the nature of their interactions, the satisfying and unsatisfying aspects of their marriage relationship, and the role of early depressive symptoms as a consequence of interpersonal disputes as well as their effects on the relationship.

The PCNS met with Mrs. Brown individually to present the treatment plan and explore her perceptions of problem areas. Because of Mrs. Brown's concerns over the possibility of endangering the marital relationship, it was decided to have the client raise less-threatening issues first and then move on to more central issues. Mr. Brown agreed to participate. He had been responsible for the care of their daughter while his wife had been hospitalized and wanted to be a part of the problem-solving process.

In the Beginning Phase of treatment, a model of problem-solving and open communication was developed to meet the couple's needs. They were encouraged to discuss the changes brought about by the birth of their daughter. Mr. Brown revealed that he had kept his concerns to himself because he feared they would make his wife more depressed. Mrs. Brown reported that she interpreted his reluctance to talk with her as evidence of his opinion that she was incapable of working out the problems and that, subsequently, she became more depressed. At first, the couple was reluctant to problem-solve outside the therapy session, and on two occasions Mr. Brown left the home feeling angry and rejected, yet unable to talk with his wife. These behaviors ceased after consistent replaying of the scenes and implementing the problem-solving process in sessions. The couple negotiated plans for establishing a consistent bedtime for their daughter, arranging for child care three days a week so Mrs. Brown could return to classes and part-time work, and managing evening meals. Subsequently, after implementing these plans, Mrs. Brown demonstrated renewed energy in dealing with her daughter, and Mr. Brown began to ask for quality time with his wife away from home.

During Working Phase sessions, the couple revealed a willingness to confront issues but required assistance to seek resources outside of the marital dyad. They spent some sessions evaluating gains, and others seeking support for feelings of loss and sadness related to the changes they had experienced.

Termination proved difficult. Mr. Brown wanted therapy to end on the scheduled date, but Mrs. Brown wanted the support to continue. During the final session, the couple and the clinical nurse specialist discussed satisfactions and feelings of loss. A review of the treatment process revealed that a substantial number of issues had been identified and resolved and that Mr. and Mrs. Brown now had the tools to deal with their problems. They were aware that the problem-solving process involved energy and time and a commitment to working together. At termination, they were informed that they could call or return for subsequent sessions if they ever felt the need.

SUMMARY

The course of treatment extended 3 weeks beyond the target date of 3 months. After termination, Mrs. Brown's medication monitoring was to continue bimonthly up to 6 months and was then to be reevaluated. During therapy, Mr. and Mrs. Brown were able to achieve their goals of developing a consistent approach to resolving conflicts. They also became aware of the symptoms of early depression and felt better equipped to handle the challenge of caring for their daughter.

Throughout the course of the Browns' therapy, ongoing supervision for the clinical specialist had been provided by the medical resident for medication management. Supervision for the couple's therapy was provided weekly by the nursing director, an expert in family therapy. The clinical specialist received valuable assistance with appropriate discipline strategies to meet the developmental needs of a 2-year-old from the child psychiatric clinical nurse specialist on the children's service.

REFERENCES

Abramson, L.T., et al. "Learned Helplessness in Humans: Critique and Reformulation," *Journal of Abnormal Psychology* 87:49-74, 1978.

American Psychiatric Association. *Diagnostic and Statistical Manual of Mental Disorders,* 3rd ed. Washington, D.C.: American Psychiatric Association, 1980.

Brown, G.W., and Harris, T. *The Social Origins of Depressions: A Study of Psychiatric Disorder in Women.* London: Tavistock, 1978.

Gordon, V.C., and Ledray, L.E. "Depression in Women," *Journal of Psychosocial Nursing and Mental Health Services* 23(1):26-34, 1985.

Gove, N.R., and Tudor, J.F. "Adult Sex Roles and Mental Illness," *American Journal of Sociology* 78:812-35, 1973.

Weissman, M.M. "Depression," in *Women and Psychotherapy.* Edited by Brodsky, A.M., and Hare-Mustin, R.T. New York: The Guilford Press, 1980.

Weissman, M.M., and Klerman, G.L. "Depression in Women: Epidemiology, Explanations, and Impact on the Family," in *The Woman Patient.*

Edited by Wotman, M.T., and Nadelson, C. New York: Plenum Press, 1982.

Wotman, M.T., and Nadelson, C. "Reproductive Crises," in *Women and Psychotherapy*. Edited by Brodsky, M., and Hare-Mustin, R.T. New York: The Guilford Press, 1980.

SELECTED BIBLIOGRAPHY

Hauser, M.J. "Cognition Commands Change," *Journal of Psychosocial Nursing and Mental Health Services* 11:19-26, 1981.

Klerman, G.L., and Weissman, M.M. "Depressions among Women: Their Nature and Causes," in *Mental Health of Women*. Edited by Guttenberg, M., et al. New York: Academic Press, 1980.

Seligman, M. *Helplessness: On Depression, Development, and Death*. San Francisco: Freeman, 1975.

Weissman, M.M., and Klerman, G.L. "Sex Differences and the Epidemiology of Depression," *Archives of General Psychiatry* 34:98-111, 1977.

DIAGNOSTIC CRITERIA FOR MAJOR DEPRESSIVE EPISODE

A. Dysphoric mood or loss of interest or pleasure in all or almost all usual activities and pastimes. The dysphoric mood is characterized by symptoms such as the following: depressed, sad, blue, hopeless, low, down in the dumps, irritable. The mood disturbance must be prominent and relatively persistent, but not necessarily the most dominant symptom, and does not include momentary shifts from one dysphoric mood to another dysphoric mood, e.g., anxiety to depression to anger, such as are seen in states of acute psychotic turmoil. (For children under age 6, dysphoric mood may have to be inferred from a persistently sad facial expression.)

B. At least four of the following symptoms have each been present nearly every day for a period of at least 2 weeks (in children under age 6, at least three of the first four):
(1) poor appetite or significant weight loss (when not dieting) or increased appetite or significant weight gain (in children under age 6, consider failure to make expected weight gains)
(2) insomnia or hypersomnia
(3) psychomotor agitation or retardation (but not merely subjective feelings of restlessness or being slowed down) (in children under 6, hypoactivity)
(4) loss of interest or pleasure in usual activities, or decrease in sexual drive not limited to a period when delusional or hallucinating (in children under 6, signs of apathy)
(5) loss of energy; fatigue
(6) feelings of worthlessness, self-reproach, or excessive or inappropriate guilt (may be delusional)
(7) complaints or evidence of diminished ability to think or concentrate, such as slowed thinking, or indecisiveness not associated with marked loosening of associations or incoherence
(8) recurrent thoughts of death, suicidal ideation, wish to be dead, or suicide attempt.

C. Neither of the following dominate the clinical picture when an affective syndrome (i.e., criteria A and B above) is not present, that is, before it developed or after it has remitted:
(1) preoccupation with a mood-incongruent delusion or hallucination (see definition below)
(2) bizarre behavior.

D. Not superimposed on either schizophrenia, a schizophreniform disorder, or a paranoid disorder.

E. Not due to any organic mental disorder or uncomplicated bereavement.

Fifth-digit code numbers and criteria for subclassification of major depressive episode.
(When psychotic features and melancholia are present, the coding system requires that the clinician record the single most clinically significant characteristic.)
6. in remission
4. with psychotic features
3. with melancholia
2. without melancholia
0. unspecified

American Psychiatric Association Diagnostic and Statistical Manual of Mental Disorders, 3rd edition. Washington, D.C., © APA, 1980. Used with permission.

Jean and Ed:
Substance Abuse in Adult Children of Alcoholics

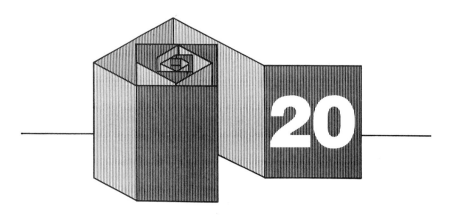

Jill Ione Lomax, MN, RN

Over the last several years, much has been written about the special problems faced by adult children of alcoholics. To truly understand the interpersonal dynamics learned by children in alcoholic families, the nurse must become familiar with the characteristic communication patterns and methods of relating found in such families.

The following case study, written by a clinical nurse specialist who is herself the child of an alcoholic family, illustrates an approach to couples therapy for two adult children of alcoholics. In this case, the treatment plan was based on the following nursing diagnosis:
• Ineffective family coping: compromised, related to ambivalent commitment in a relationship secondary to early maturational deficits in both partners.

CASE STUDY

Married for 7 years, divorced for 2, and now living together again, Jean and Ed entered couples therapy to explore whether they could resolve their relationship problems and successfully remarry.

Jean and Ed were 38 and 36 years old, respectively, and childless by choice. Both were intelligent and psychologically sophisticated middle-class Anglo-Americans from Protestant upbringings. Jean was a pediatric nurse with a stable work history; before meeting Ed, she had led a basically celibate life. Ed, unemployed at the beginning of therapy, had a highly erratic and unstable work history. None of his various jobs had lasted more than 6 months, and he sometimes went extended periods without working. Prior to meeting Jean, he had a few romantic relationships, but none had lasted more than a month.

Both Jean and Ed reported lonely, chaotic, and unstable childhoods as the emotionally abandoned only children of alcoholic fathers and co-alcoholic mothers. Asked to describe a scene that characterized her childhood, Jean recollected sitting alone on her front porch for hours at a time, feeling sad and isolated as she watched the neighborhood children play. She wanted to join them but was forbidden to leave her yard and was reluctant to invite them into her yard because of the shouting and turmoil reverberating from inside her home. Jean tearfully described feeling "old before my time. I felt so responsible for everything. But powerless.... I tried so hard to be a good girl—to please my parents and help them get along and not be any trouble to them. But I got yelled at anyway. No matter what I did, it wasn't good enough not to get yelled at. I would go to my room and cry...I didn't have anyone to talk to and didn't feel understood. I never felt really happy or secure. I still don't.

"I grew up in an autocratic family where children were to be seen and not heard. It wasn't OK to act like a regular child—to play or be silly. I was 'Mother's little helper'—very responsible. Sometimes I'd help her put dad to bed after he passed out. Sometimes I'd do it by myself if she was at work. I never really knew until recently that all this wasn't normal—that I was an abused child. Not physically or sexually—but emotionally abused. I thought I was bad—or crazy. Even though I know better now, sometimes I still feel that way."

If Jean questioned her parents, they either ignored or rebuked her or gave answers that frequently seemed to hide rather than reveal information. She learned early not to trust what they told her and to feel guilty, inadequate, and unsure of herself. Although her tears and apologies sometimes escalated the tension in the house, more often than not they provoked a temporary respite from criticism. She also learned to minimize her needs and to stifle any direct expression of anger over unfulfilled needs.

Ed described similar childhood experiences of criticism and isolation but remembers feeling warm and secure during the hours he spent in front of the television engrossed in the idealistic world of the children of TV families. "I'd just shut out what was happening between my parents. I tried not to get involved. They were crazy. If they noticed me at all it was to blame me for everything, and sometimes I'd get beat up for it [by either parent]. So I'd get lost. I loved watching TV—and still do. It was my favorite activity. I'd get inside my own little world and get cozy.

"I knew my father drank. Never thought much about it. All the men I knew drank. It was part of being a man...In a way I couldn't wait to grow up so I could get out of the house. Not that I wanted to be an adult myself. I didn't like or trust adults. They acted like they knew it all, but they didn't...I had a hard time in school because I wanted to do things my way. Most authority figures are puffed-up fools, and I wanted to get as far away from them as possible. I wanted to be left alone. That's my idea of happiness...I used to find escape when I got high. Then nothing bothered me. And if it did, well, hell, I didn't remember it!"

According to Jean, the most meaningful time of her life was the day she met Ed: "For the first time I felt cared for and understood for who I am. I never felt 'real' before I met Ed." For Ed, the high point of his life was his wedding day: "It was the first time someone committed totally to me." In spite of feeling they had found a "soulmate," each felt the other was forever "pulling the rug out from under me." They describe their year-long courtship and 7-year-long marriage as emotionally intense and chaotic, with many separations lasting from a few days to several weeks.

At the time they met, Ed told Jean he was an alcoholic and a member of Alcoholics Anonymous (AA). He had begun using alcohol and marijuana in adolescence. Although he continued to use marijuana several times a week throughout his marriage, when he met Jean he had begun a period of abstinence from alcohol that would last until their third year of marriage. Jean was initially impressed with Ed's honesty, charm, and sensitivity to her as an individual. Later, however, she became intolerant of his forgetfulness, irresponsibility, verbal abusiveness, and anger— traits they both agreed were exacerbated while he was under the influence of alcohol or marijuana. She reported feeling emotionally intimidated by his criticism and angry shouting but had never feared for her physical safety; she had never known him to harm or threaten to harm either people or property.

Ed was initially attracted to Jean's warmth, shyness, and vulnerability. In her presence, he felt strong and cared for. "She needed me, and I liked that. I felt I was good for her." Later, he became exhausted by her criticism, tearfulness, and need to rehash past arguments. He also became threatened by her growing independence and afraid he was no longer "good enough" for her.

When emotions became particularly intense and chaotic, either Jean or Ed would effect a separation. Sometimes Ed would disappear emotionally into his protective world of drugs or TV. Sometimes Jean would tearfully and angrily demand that Ed leave the house. (She always felt their home was more hers than theirs, because she was the primary caretaker, both financially and physically.) Usually, however, Ed would be the one to initiate a separation by storming out in a rage shouting that he was in an "unsafe" relationship, "hounded, criticized, mistrusted, and unappreciated." Reconciliations typically resulted after Ed, drug-free, would contritely reapproach Jean, and she would apologize profusely for not being more "understanding." In time, however, this cycle of separation and reconciliation invariably would repeat itself.

Eventually, Jean initiated divorce action after she became convinced that she could no longer tolerate the emotional upheaval that characterized the relationship. She loved Ed, however, and missed the familiarity and even—as she confessed with chagrin—the chaos of their relationship. She also suffered periodic pangs of guilt, feeling that she might have created or at least had not helped Ed resolve those weaknesses that had driven her away. She felt responsible for his behavior and could not relinquish the idea that he would be a better husband if only she behaved differently toward him—an idea that Ed tended to share as well.

Ed took the divorce very hard. He felt completely rejected and abandoned and tried numerous times to reconcile. But for 2 years, Jean refused his romantic overtures.

During the period of separation, Ed drank heavily. As he described it, "I hit rock bottom. I'm an alcoholic, and I did what alcoholics do—pretended that I was in control when I wasn't. During that period, I finally accepted that by myself I was powerless and had to turn my life over to a higher power. I know how to play every mind game there is, but all it got me was a bankrupt existence. I loved Jean and I lost her. At first I hated her for leaving me. Then I got more involved in AA, stopped using alcohol and marijuana and knew that I could never use them again. I forgave myself for my past and wanted Jean to forgive me. I knew she had to do what was right for her and that I have to earn her trust. One of the Twelve Steps of AA is to apologize to those you've offended. And I hoped she'd listen."

Jean did listen but wasn't sure what she wanted to do. Jean wanted to recommit but feared that she could not trust Ed's promised reformation. She also began to wonder if sobriety alone was the answer to their problems. During the separation, neither Jean nor Ed had become romantically or sexually involved with others; each continued to fantasize about a better life together, but each also had fears about the other's ability to commit fully. Finally, Jean consented to live again with Ed but only if they entered couples therapy; Ed agreed.

FORMULATION

In Jean's and Ed's case, knowledge about family systems and the adult children of alcoholics provided the theoretical basis for assessment and intervention. Over the last few years, researchers have given more attention to members of this large group and their special problems in developing intimate adult relationships (Lawson et al., 1983; Norwood, 1985; Seixas and Youcha, 1985; Woititz, 1983).

Typically, children of alcoholics grow up in families with three covert, but powerful and damaging rules: don't feel, don't trust, and don't talk (Black, 1982). Although initially these rules serve to protect the hurting person, eventually they prolong the pain and make it more inaccessible to examination and resolution. These children often have issues surrounding visibility that evolve after years of being "invisible" within their families. They over-idealize intimacy and fear the sharing of anger because it is felt to damage and rarely, if ever, strengthen a relationship. In session, Jean and Ed both demonstrated this trait; whenever they argued, each was quick to reassure the other with statements of "I love you." Fearing rejection for their anger, both quickly terminated arguments with apologies and solicitous questions about the other's feelings.

Just as the alcoholic is obsessed with alcohol, the other family members—known as co-alcoholics—are obsessed with the alcoholic. To the extent that they remain part of the alcoholic family system, these co-alcoholics become enablers—helpmates in the perpetuation of the system. They often do so even unconsciously. Upon leaving the alcoholic family of origin, adult co-alcoholics frequently become intimately involved with other co-alcoholics or become alcoholics themselves. Jean and Ed took two different paths into adulthood, they found each other, and essentially recreated their families of origin.

Wegscheider (1981) describes a variety of roles assumed by children who grow up in alcoholic families, roles that provide them with ways to cope with stress and often are carried on into adulthood. Jean exhibited many of the characteristics of the "hero" that develop as a way of overcoming feelings of inadequacy and guilt. She was the "good girl," always willing to help and be super-responsible in hopes of being loved. Like many a "hero," she grew up to become a professional caretaker (pediatric nurse) and a lover of someone in need of "rescue."

During joint sessions with Ed, Jean seemed highly emotional, nervous, and painfully unsure of herself. She spoke hesitantly, circumstantially, and prefaced every statement with endless qualifiers. She clearly exhibited an impaired ability to maintain her individual integrity within her relationship with Ed. From a checklist of possible statements describing herself, she marked the following: "I constantly seek approval and affirmation"; "I overreact to personal criticism"; "I have trouble being assertive about my own needs"; "I feel excessive guilt"; "I judge myself without mercy"; "I have difficulty having fun"; and "I worry about being crazy." Underlying Jean's fears and anxieties was her basic belief that "I caused the alcoholism; therefore, I should do something about it."

Ed's profile was similar to the "scapegoat" and the "lost child," the one blamed for problems and of whom minimal achievement is expected. Feeling hurt and lonely and unimportant, he retreated into himself, fantasizing that someone would come along to alleviate his sense of helplessness and hopelessness. To deaden his chronic disappointment, he turned to alcohol and drugs. From a checklist of statements, Ed marked the following: "I fear failure, but sabotage my success"; "I have difficulty following projects through from beginning to end"; and "I look for immediate rather than deferred gratification." Just as he did in childhood, as an adult Ed continued to believe that "just like something outside myself is responsible for my pain, something outside myself will alleviate it."

Ed's charisma, charm, and highly developed social skills served to keep others attracted to and involved with him despite his repeated failures to keep promises. But Ed maintained that his sociability was a facade and that deep-down he did not feel truly connected. The person to whom he was least connected was himself. His insecurity led to a limited ability to negotiate, be flexible, and work within a dyad. Although Jean's insecurity led her to try (albeit with resentment) to become what Ed needed her to be, his insecurity was so profound that he felt incapable of becoming what she needed him to be.

Both Ed and Jean checked the following statements: "I fear rejection and abandonment, yet I am rejecting of others"; "I fear criticism and judgment, yet I criticize and judge others"; "I avoid conflict or aggravate it—rarely do I deal with it"; "I seek tension and crisis and then complain about the results"; and "I am either super-responsible [Jean] or super-irresponsible [Ed]."

COURSE OF TREATMENT

Although this was Jean's and Ed's first experience with joint therapy, each had extensive prior experience with psychiatric services. Twelve years earlier, Ed had participated in individual and group therapy during a 90-day mandatory rehabilitation program following an arrest for repeated drunk driving; at the time of the divorce, he had entered briefly into individual therapy to try to mitigate the abandonment he felt at the loss of his only significant one-to-one relationship. For 12 years, he had been involved intermittently in AA; during the past year he had become increasingly involved, often attending two meetings a day. The combined goals of Ed's therapies had been to become part of a compassionate support system, to gain insight into his substance abuse, and to stop using. At the start of couples therapy, he believed he'd reached each of these goals.

Jean had been participating in insight-oriented group and individual psychotherapy, including Al-Anon, for the past 5 years. Her goals, which she also believed she was reaching, were to gain increased awareness of her thoughts and feelings, increased self-acceptance, and membership in a supportive therapeutic network.

Both Ed and Jean stated they resented authority figures and avoided therapists who were directive and "tell us what we think and feel and what to do." Both appreciated therapists who were supportive, who guided them gently toward insight, and "who don't talk too much, as if they know what's going on and we don't." The couple's preferences dictated the need for a nondirective, supportive, insight-oriented, systems approach in conjoint sessions that would complement, not interfere with, their ongoing individual therapies. Additionally, their comments indicated a fear of the unknown concerning themselves and, despite an occasional wish for "divine interventions," a sensitivity to premature interpretations.

In the Beginning Phase, the couple anticipated a need for weekly therapy lasting 6 months to a year. Therapy began with history-taking interlaced with discussions of goals and expectations. The contract made mutually at the beginning was that the nonuse of all substances was supported and expected, that therapy would not be terminated if Ed resumed using, but that no session would be held while he was under the influence of marijuana or alcohol. The couple was given teaching aids—a poem and "I Am an Adult Who Grew Up in an Alcoholic Family"—to take home and read (see pages 459 to 461). Their inability to articulate specific goals was symptomatic of their relationship problems. But they did agree on the general outcome of reducing the emotional upheavals in their relationship and increasing the sense of security about their future together. In time, they also arrived at additional therapeutic goals: an increase in self-acceptance and self-esteem in both, a decrease in Jean's responsibility for Ed, and an increase in Ed's responsibility for himself. Their communication skills were already fairly well-developed and needed little more than fine-tuning. With much hesitation stemming from fear and guilt, each eventually was able to articulate specific needs and desires of the other as the first step in formal negotiation.

Jean wanted Ed to become more responsible for himself and less dependent upon her. Primarily, she wanted him to get a job and stay with it. But during the year of therapy, Ed went 6 months without working, entered a job-training program which he did not complete, and then changed jobs twice. Jean resented Ed sleeping, watching TV, playing cards with friends, or going to AA meetings while she worked and took care of all the household business and chores. She had taken on the responsibility for seeing that he got up on time for work, completed school assignments on time, remembered his therapist and doctor appointments, and so forth. The more she became Ed's maternal caretaker, the less sexual attraction she felt toward him. This decrease in Jean's sexual responsiveness had become a recent source of conflict between the couple and a loss for both Jean and Ed.

Jean found it very difficult not to feel responsible for Ed. Her perception of the boundary between them was sufficiently blurred so that his failures somehow became, in her view, her failures. Eventually, her sense of personal failure led to guilt and then anger as she realized her inability to control his behavior.

Although Ed was willing to give up responsibility for himself to Jean, he did not want to be controlled. The more she coaxed, cajoled, or coerced, the more resistive he became and the more unhappy they both grew. Ed told Jean he wanted her "to let me be...to accept me as I am. I take one day at a time, and I can't make promises about what I'm going to do tomorrow.... It makes me angry when you nag. I don't want to feel guilty when I can't work on your timetable. I don't like schedules dictating my life. Never have. I don't like being a bee buzzing around. I'd rather be the flower just swaying in the wind, hoping no one comes and picks at me.... I want to be responsible but not at your insistence. I can do only one thing at a time, and right now all my energy goes into AA and not drinking." Basically, he was giving Jean the message that his sobriety was a precious gift to her, and if she wasn't grateful enough not to ask for anything else at this time, he would withdraw this gift. But Jean did not want to choose between Ed's sobriety and other responsible behaviors; she wanted both. However, she continued to experience self-doubts whenever Ed did not respond to her needs and desires, and wondered if her additional demands of Ed were as selfish, insensitive, and wrong as he indicated.

Jean expressed anger over her role as the "good girl" and "hero." She felt overburdened and wanted out. A therapeutic breakthrough came one day with her agonized admission that not only did she want Ed to share responsibilities with her, but that she also wanted him to be strong enough for her to lean on when she was in need. Although Ed wanted to be strong, he painfully admitted that he could not allow Jean to lean on him at this time; however, he wanted Jean to stay with him anyway in the hope that someday he might. Thus were they in a quandary—Ed caught in the stranglehold of feeling helpless but promising to change, and Jean tormented by her confusion about how to handle the "carrot-on-the-stick" syndrome the couple was locked into.

During the sessions, Jean made some attempts to shift the responsibility for Ed from herself to me, the therapist. But when she sought to have me tell Ed what to do and to support her position, I shifted the negotiations back to them. This shift made Jean angry, and she threatened to terminate therapy. With my guidance, however, she began to realize that she was being hurt by her own doubts and self-criticism and that she need not depend on others to rescue her. Countertransference issues proved troublesome at this time, as I wrestled with my own pervasive desire to be perfect at all times and have my therapeutic efforts be successful and appreciated, not criticized.

While no definitive approaches exist for any therapy situation, clients and therapists who are adult children of alcoholics tend to believe they do, and desire to be "let in on" the secret. Since I am an adult child of an alcoholic, questions that arose in my mind—Am I responsible for the resolution of Jean's and Ed's difficulties? Should I be the authority and caretaker figure for them?—provoked transference and countertransference issues that alternately restricted and advanced Jean's and Ed's therapeutic progress.

As the Working Phase of therapy developed, the general goal became the elimination of the question mark in their relationship—whether or not they would stay together and actually remarry. Periodically, one or the other would seek my assurance that they would stay together. Although I would not offer a prediction, I did indicate that I thought they were going through a normal and expected phase in conflict resolution and advised them to bear with the temporary confusion.

During this phase, Ed enjoyed talking about "the relationship" and the similarities between himself and Jean. On the other hand, Jean intensely disliked discussing their relationship "as if it's a third person. I prefer to just talk about Ed or about me." While Ed was soothed by references to the relationship, Jean's individuality and independence were threatened by such talk. She was seeking differentiation from Ed and surcease from her frequent complaint of "I don't know who I am."

In the beginning, Jean's differentiation from Ed was very fragile. Her self-esteem had been dependent upon Ed's self-esteem and his ability to appreciate her strengths. But through her combined therapies, she eventually found a personal understanding and acceptance of herself that was as strong as what she had experienced through Ed at their first meeting. She no longer needed him to feel "real." Over time, she became even more confident and learned to rely upon her own views of self. But when Ed did not adjust to her evolving independence and remained threatened by it, Jean found herself at another crossroads.

During their year of therapy, Jean and Ed developed a greater capacity for acknowledging their own difficulties. Jean overcame the tendency to externalize the sources of and solutions to her problems to a greater extent than did Ed. In spite of his desire for self-improvement, Ed's belief in his capacity for change was low, and he continued to sabotage his successes. He feared that if he succeeded today, then he would be expected to succeed again tomorrow. This externalized expectation created a burden of responsibility that he believed himself incapable of fulfilling with any certainty. Ed's faith in his strengths and desire to exercise them remained lower than Jean was able to tolerate. His repeated remark "I am the way I am; and I can't change right now" provoked her frustration and anger. Having lived a life of excessive compromise, she now was jealous and resentful that Ed could be so willing to continue behaving in a way she found unacceptable. The more she became convinced that her changes were not effecting a change in Ed, the less hope she had for a compatible future with him. She now was prepared to make decisions based on the situation as it was and not as she wished it could or should be.

The Termination Phase of therapy began when Jean decided to terminate her relationship with Ed. Sensing her decision before she announced it, Ed began to miss appointments. Jean used Ed's absence to discuss what she was going to tell him and to examine her resolve. During these private sessions, Jean's demeanor was markedly different from when Ed was present. Her delivery was confident, calm, and straightforward. Although she felt less guilty about her feelings and needs and no longer believed that they were crazy or inappropriate, she wondered if she would maintain confidence in front of Ed. She also wondered whether she would find herself repeating the caretaker role in future relationships.

Ed accepted Jean's decision with some difficulty. Hurt and angry, he said he loved her and did not want the relationship to end but would respect her decision. They spent their final joint session negotiating the specifics of the separation—division of property and the how and when of future contact. At the session's end, they parted with words of concern to one another and tearfully hugged goodbye.

Both Ed and Jean were invited to one last individual session to terminate with me and to discuss their separate futures. Jean attended and dealt forthrightly with the termination. She had decided to continue with individual and group psychotherapy, including a group for adult children of alcoholics. Ed, who decided to continue with AA, said he would attend this session but did not appear or call to cancel. Previously, he had discussed his difficulty with terminations: "I don't like to say goodbye. I avoid the whole thing if I can.... I'm not sure I want to change."

SUMMARY

Ed and Jean entered therapy with the goal of determining whether their relationship was sufficiently stable and fulfilling to warrant remarriage. Through therapy, they met this goal deciding to terminate the relationship. A therapist is often tempted to feel disappointment when two people enter couples therapy through one door and leave through separate doors. But whether a relationship continues, changes, or ends, the most important therapeutic goals for both clients are to develop positive self-regard and to feel comfortable with their decisions.

REFERENCES

Black, C. *It Will Never Happen to Me!* Denver: MAC Printing and Publications Division, 1982.

Lawson, G., et al. *Alcoholism and the Family: A Guide to Treatment and Prevention.* Rockville, Md.: Aspen Systems Corp., 1983.

Norwood, R. *Women Who Love Too Much: When You Keep Wishing and Hoping He'll Change.* Los Angeles: Jeremy P. Tarcher, 1985.

Seixas, J.S., and Youcha, G. *Children of Alcoholism: A Survivor's Manual.* New York: Crown, 1985.

Wegscheider, S. *Another Chance: Hope and Health for the Alcoholic Family.* Palo Alto, Calif.: Science and Behavior Books, 1981.

Woititz, J.G. *Adult Children of Alcoholics.* Hollywood, Fla.: Health Communications, 1983.

SELECTED BIBLIOGRAPHY

A free catalog of publications is available from:

The National Council on Alcoholism
12 West 21st Street
New York, NY 10010
(212) 206-6770

After a while you learn the subtle difference
Between holding a hand and chaining a soul
And you learn that love doesn't mean leaning
And company doesn't mean security
And you begin to learn that kisses aren't contracts
And presents aren't promises
And you begin to accept defeats
With your head held up and your eyes open
With the grace of a person, not the grief of a child
And learn to build all your roads
On today, because tomorrow's ground
Is too uncertain for plans, and futures have
A way of falling down in mid-flight.
After a while you learn that even sunshine
Burns if you get too much.
So you plant your own garden and decorate
Your own soul instead of waiting
For someone to bring you flowers.
And you learn that you really can endure
That you really are strong
And you really do have worth
And you learn and you learn...
With every good-bye you learn.

       —Anonymous
       Alcoholism Center for Women
       Los Angeles

I AM AN ADULT WHO GREW UP IN AN ALCOHOLIC FAMILY

Once I thought I was unique, different and alone. Certainly, the disease of alcoholism kept me ignorant and isolated. The disease told me not to wash my family's linen in public. I obeyed, and so suffered in silence. I survived the disease of my parents only to acquire it myself.

Knowing only that I was affected by alcoholism, I began my recovery, sometimes in Al-Anon, sometimes in Alcoholics Anonymous. For a long time, there was this nagging awareness that once I had dealt with the problem of the moment, I would have to deal with the alcoholism of my family of origin, and its effects on my character. In spite of the progress I had made in my recovery, I was still getting in trouble, still having difficulty with other people. Peace of mind seemed to last only until I created the next crisis.

Some of the answers were sought in therapy. Sometimes I was told I was sick, sometimes that I was just wrong. Mostly I was told that the answers were to be found within myself. I insisted that I did not know the answers. I wasn't even sure how to ask the questions. It never occurred to "them" that I might be truly ignorant rather than neurotic or crazy.

Then I began to discover other Adult Sons and Daughters of Alcoholics. Slowly at first, we shared our experiences, feelings, and behaviors. I discovered in ourselves a common history, despite having been raised generations and miles apart. I was no longer alone!

As my trust began to build, the walls came down, if only for a short time. I learned again to feel the hurt and cry where before I could not. Some of my behaviors had turned into habits and were causing me difficulty in my job and in my family life. I came to understand that my past and my present formed a pattern. Once I had identified my feelings and my behaviors, I began to understand myself better. I resolved to change myself whenever I could, knowing that it would not be easy to alter the habits of a lifetime.

Here are some of the things I found out about myself and that I am now beginning to change:

1. *I guess at what normal is.*
2. *I have difficulty following projects through from beginning to end. If I end the project, someone can judge it.*
3. *I lie when it would be just as easy to tell the truth.*
4. *I judge myself without mercy.*
5. *I have difficulty having fun.*
6. *I take myself very seriously.*
7. *I have difficulty with intimate relationships.*

8. *I overreact to changes over which I have no control.*
9. *I feel different from other people.*
10. *I constantly seek approval and affirmation.*
11. *I am either super responsible or super irresponsible.*
12. *I am extremely loyal even in the face of evidence that the loyalty is undeserved.*
13. *I look for immediate as opposed to deferred gratification.*
14. *I lock myself into a course of action without giving serious consideration to alternate behaviors or possible consequences.*
15. *I seek tension and crisis and then complain about the results.*
16. *I avoid conflict or aggravate it; rarely do I deal with it.*
17. *I fear rejection and abandonment, yet I am rejecting of others.*
18. *I fear failure, but sabotage my success.*
19. *I fear criticism and judgment, yet I criticize and judge others.*
20. *I manage my time poorly and do not set my priorities in a way that works well for me.*

In order to change, I cannot use my history as an excuse for continuing my behaviors. I have no regrets for what might have been, for my experiences have shaped my talents as well as my defects of character. It is my responsibility to discover these talents, to build my self-esteem and to repair any damage done. I will allow myself to feel my feelings, to accept them, and learn to express them appropriately. When I have begun these tasks, I will try to let go of my past and get on with the business of managing my life.

I have survived against impossible odds until today. With the help of God and my friends, I shall survive the next twenty-four hours. I am no longer alone.

Reprinted by permission, Thomas W. Perrin, Inc., P.O. Box 190, Rutherford, N.J. 07070, 1-201-460-7912.

Anthony:
Individual and Family Treatment for Chronic Mental Illness

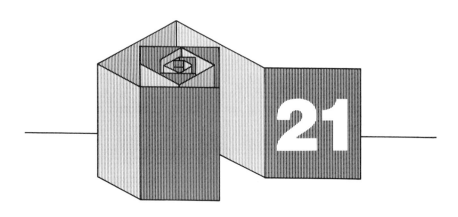

Diane L. Grimaldi, MS, RN, CS

Many clients suffering from chronic psychiatric disorders require long-term outpatient treatment, which is frequently provided by community mental health centers. Such treatment is planned and delivered by a multidisciplinary group of mental health professionals united in the cause of providing services for a population that is typically under-served.

The following case study illustrates the evolution of a long-term treatment plan for a family with a member suffering from a chronic mental illness. Nursing diagnoses represented in this case include:
- Ineffective family coping: compromised, related to inter-family conflict secondary to reaction to son's chronic illness.
- Altered thought processes related to auditory hallucinations and paranoid delusions secondary to schizophrenia.
- Anticipatory grieving related to disappointment and unfulfilled dreams secondary to chronic illness.

CASE STUDY

Anthony DeLuca, a 29-year-old single, white male, was the youngest of two children (and the only son) in a first-generation Italian-American family. His only sibling, a sister, was a physician with a well-established internal medicine practice in California.

Anthony graduated from a local music institute in 1979 at the age of 23, but was unemployed and collecting social security disability insurance at the time of this psychiatric contact. His history included 14 psychiatric hospitalizations of both short- and long-term duration. Anthony was well known in the mental health system due to his recurrent psychotic episodes and subsequent hospitalizations, which initially took place at private psychiatric facilities but ultimately, due to exorbitant medical costs, occurred at the state mental institution.

During these hospitalizations, Anthony consistently had been diagnosed as having chronic paranoid schizophrenia. He was discharged from each hospitalization with a strong recommendation for outpatient treatment that included individual therapy, family therapy, and antipsychotic medication. But Anthony refused to comply with those treatment recommendations, denying the need for treatment by explaining that his hospitalization occurred only because his father wanted to punish him after an argument.

Mr. and Mrs. DeLuca started family treatment in 1979, when Anthony had become acutely psychotic shortly after his graduation from music school and required yet another psychiatric inpatient stay. Before they began therapy, they were very skeptical about psychiatric treatment, in particular about family therapy without the presence of the "identified patient," Anthony. They feared that they would be blamed by mental health professionals for Anthony's problems and perceived questions about social, developmental, and family history as an attack on their parental devotion and their genetic constitution.

As Mr. and Mrs. DeLuca continued in treatment, Anthony's hospitalizations increased in frequency and duration. This trend seemed to correspond with Mr. and Mrs. DeLuca's progress toward establishing some ego boundaries and beginning the formidable work of setting limits on Anthony's inappropriate and/or psychotic behaviors and demands. As Mr. and Mrs. DeLuca progressed in treatment, they became able to respond to Anthony more effectively. This radically altered the family equilibrium. Anthony was no longer able to engage in behavior such as dictating menus and seating arrangements at dinner or screening and monitoring his parents' phone calls—behavior that his parents previously had responded to submissively for fear of precipitating a violent outburst. They replaced submission with firm limit-setting and a willingness to ask Anthony to leave the house if he could not comply with their limits and a willingness to call the police if he became threatening or displayed symptoms of tenuous control.

As a result of this shift in family dynamics, Anthony was no longer able to live at home due to his parents' intolerance for his behavior that they previously accepted. Following several episodes of family violence and hospitalizations, Anthony agreed to move into an apartment of his own and finally to accept outpatient treatment.

My first contact with the DeLuca family occurred in 1983. By that time, Mr. and Mrs. DeLuca had been in treatment with a psychiatrist, Dr. Kauffman, for approximately 4 years. Dr. Kauffman and I planned to meet with them and Anthony to discuss the family crisis and formulate a treatment plan.

Anthony was unwilling to meet us on unfamiliar territory, and so the meeting took place at his newly acquired apartment. This gave us the added bonus of being able to assess Anthony's functional abilities and disabilities in his home environment. Dr. Kauffman and I were met outside of Anthony's apartment by Mr. and Mrs. DeLuca, who warned us of the maze of clutter, filth, and disarray we were about to encounter. They also indicated that Anthony was psychotic and ambivalent about meeting us.

Within minutes of our introduction to Anthony, we were struck by his obvious acute psychosis with predominantly paranoid features. He was extremely bizarre and unkempt in appearance and paced while he spoke incoherently about his thoughts being controlled by another planet. He was disoriented to the day and date and was tangential and circumstantial. His thoughts were grossly disorganized, and he frequently experienced thought-blocking. He was initially unable to comprehend repeated attempts to identify ourselves and the intended purpose of our visit.

The confusion was enhanced by Mr. and Mrs. DeLuca's compulsion to challenge and debate Anthony's paranoid delusions, which resulted in an escalation of tension and disorder. Once this process was interrupted, we were able to elicit a relevant history.

We learned that Anthony had moved out of his parents' home and into this apartment 6 weeks previously. Even so, unpacked boxes were strewn all over the apartment. He had been wearing the same clothes each day since he moved, because his other clothing was still packed away. Anthony's parents had offered to help him with the work of getting settled in his apartment, but he refused their help. He was only willing to accept money and meals prepared and served at his parents' home. If they bought him groceries, he would throw them out. If they brought prepared meals and put them in his refrigerator, he would pull out the plug, causing the food to spoil.

Clearly, Anthony's psychotic episode was precipitated by his move out of his parents' home. This was compounded by the fact that Anthony's sister had recently married and moved to California to start a practice in internal medicine. This loss was significant, since Anthony always felt that his sister understood him better than anyone. (In fact, he affectionately referred to her as his "alter ego.")

Since moving to his new apartment, Anthony had become increasingly withdrawn to the point where he ultimately did not go out at all. Unable to interact with others due to his paranoid ideation, he had been asked to leave several coffee shops due to boisterous and inappropriate behavior and had even lost a part-time job he'd had for years at a pizza and sandwich shop, folding pizza boxes in exchange for lunch or dinner. Consequently, he felt "backed into" his apartment by the limits and expectations imposed by his parents and society. He did not perceive any logical association between his own behavior and the limits imposed by others. Instead, his perceptions about the reactions of other people were based on bizarre delusions with persecutory content.

Anthony felt desperate in this dilemma, and desired to respond to it by returning to the protective haven of his parents' home. For the first time, however, Mr. and Mrs. DeLuca were unwilling to absorb the projection of Anthony's psychotic terror in the service of making him feel safe. They were able to understand that, in reality, Anthony would be safe only if he was not allowed to make inappropriate and unrealistic demands on others or to behave in threatening or violent ways.

Anthony was able to understand that he would be affected by his parents' new attitude. Since he would not be allowed to return home at times like these, he would have to find other ways of defending against his acute psychotic terror. Mr. and Mrs. DeLuca repeatedly explained to him that they would help him only if he would participate in treatment. Anthony's response to such explanations initially took the form of primary process. His tentative agreement to participate in the family meetings was ascribed to his need for help in adjusting to his new apartment and living separate from his parents. Anthony reluctantly agreed at this point to take Prolixin Decanoate injections on a biweekly basis, since his compliance with oral antipsychotic medications had been very poor in the past.

Anthony's medical history was unremarkable, with no hospitalizations or treatments for serious acute or chronic medical problems. He contracted the usual childhood illnesses without complications and had no known allergies. He had no history of drug or alcohol abuse, but had smoked two to three packs of cigarettes per day for the past 8 years. He reported some shortness of breath on exertion.

The DeLuca family immigrated to the United States from Sicily in 1963, when Anthony was age 5 and his sister, Lisa, age 7. The move was prompted by the desire to establish a prosperous business here. Mr. and Mrs. DeLuca both worked as tailors and manufactured woven goods in what was to become a profitable though demanding business. They invested much of their early profits in real estate, which ended up being the primary source of the family's wealth.

History revealed that Mr. and Mrs. DeLuca treated Lisa as the favored child. They described her as bright, attractive, articulate, conformable, thoughtful, sensitive, and helpful, with no behavioral problems at home or at school. She was well-liked by teachers and classmates, and never had trouble making friends. She attended classes for the academically talented and was targeted for higher education in the finest universities.

Anthony was born when his mother was age 37 and his father age 42. His parents were firm in their decision not to have any other children, and so Anthony was born into the role of the youngest child and the only son—a role that came with certain expectations, namely inheriting and assuming responsibility for the family business and marrying and reproducing progeny to carry on the family name. Anthony, therefore, experienced certain pressures that were not a part of Lisa's relationship with her parents.

Anthony's childhood memories lacked a great deal of detail. He did recall constantly feeling scrutinized and criticized by both of his parents. He portrayed his father as a perfectionistic man who was tyrannical in his efforts to elicit perfect behavior from Anthony, and who denounced any less-than-perfect behavior as worthless and interpreted it as evidence that Anthony would never be capable of carrying on the family business.

According to Anthony, his mother's criticisms took the form of a constant barrage of observations about his personal hygiene and grooming. She was extremely intrusive and would become outraged when Anthony refused to take her suggestions about his hairstyle or clothes. She frequently bought him clothes and insisted he wear them, regardless of his bitter protests.

Generally, Mr. and Mrs. DeLuca did not openly display affection toward each other or their children. Lisa received a fair amount of positive attention for her academic performance and general sense of competence, but Anthony tended to receive negative attention that usually focused on his poor grades and reports from school about his inability to concentrate. Such reports typically precipitated an escalation of Mr. DeLuca's tyrannical behavior and Mrs. DeLuca's intrusiveness.

In retrospect, Mr. and Mrs. DeLuca interpreted and responded to

Anthony's symptoms associated with childhood schizophrenia as willful disobedience and rebelliousness. They believed that if they "laid down the law," he would improve his grades and become more interested in socializing with his classmates. For instance, they frequently chided him for spending hours alone in his room listening to music rather than participating in sports. Over the years, they made a concerted effort to channel his behavior towards ways of a son bound for personal fulfillment and academic success. They regarded behavior that did not meet such expectations as a conscious attempt to betray and disappoint them.

But despite his parents' protests, Anthony's interest in music and preference for solitude increased during his adolescent years. In turn, his parents became increasingly alarmed by his behavior, especially as it contrasted with the social and academic success of his older sister.

During his senior year in high school, Anthony was accepted for enrollment at a local music institute. His parents, although never impressed with Anthony's diversified musical talents, reluctantly agreed to pay his tuition even as they argued that a degree in music was not very practical. Their concession was ultimately based on the fantasy that Anthony might teach music one day.

Anthony's adolescent and early adulthood years were difficult and were marked by recurrent acute psychotic episodes. Initially, he seemed to resume his usual level of functioning following such an episode. However, as time went on, each psychotic episode further diminished his functional capacity.

On our initial meeting, Anthony presented as a tall, somewhat disheveled, large-framed man who appeared slightly younger than his stated age. His hair was long and matted, and he was unshaven and unbathed. Throughout the initial assessment interview, he rocked back and forth in his chair and deeply inhaled cigarette smoke while occasionally scanning the room. He made only fleeting eye contact. He rarely initiated topics for discussion, instead waiting attentively until addressed and then carefully choosing the words for calculated responses.

During the initial assessment, Anthony exhibited affect ranging from blunted and inappropriate to content, to sad or angry and appropriate to content. He described a chronic and well-defined delusional system that varied only in terms of the degree to which it preoccupied his consciousness.

He perceived the world as a dangerous place in which people formed relationships on the premise of caring but eventually revealed their true sadistic and egocentric ulterior motives. He was, therefore, distrustful and vulnerable in his relationships with others, and generally expressed such characteristics in the context of symptoms such as social isolation, persecutory auditory hallucinations, and paranoid ideation (others being able to control his thoughts).

Anthony's IQ was in the bright-normal range, and he spoke articulately. His attention span and ability to concentrate were, at times, diminished by thought-blocking, loose associations, and thought intrusion. His capacity for abstraction and insight were fair, and his judgment ranged from poor to fair, depending upon the prominence of psychotic symptomatology at the time.

FORMULATION

Anthony was born into an atmosphere of general unhappiness at a time when his parents were struggling financially. His birth was met with parental expectations regarding his role as the family's only son.

Historically, Anthony was unable to derive a sense of security from his interfamilial relationships. The maternal-child relationship was fraught with tension stemming from his mother's intrusive domination and attitude of disapproval. When Alanen (1958) studied the mothers of 100 schizophrenic clients, he found that the majority of these women had severe personality disorders; many were schizoidal or near-psychotic. He identified a maternal attitude known as a schizoid pattern of interpersonal relationship, characterized "especially by a tendency to domination, which does not have any understanding for the child's own needs and feelings; but often at the same time also to powerful possessiveness, which is quite particularly likely to suppress the child's possibilities to develop into an independent person and to tie him up to an authority which is inimical to his own self."

In the paternal-child relationship, Anthony had experienced a pervasive sense of failure and an apparent inability to adequately fulfill his father's expectations or to win his approval. In Anthony's case, this may be a function of his mother's dominance and intrusiveness. Such expectations were generally related to Anthony's identity as a man and called for a demonstration of behaviors which his father perceived as evidence of masculinity. Each successive failure seemed to reinforce the prophetic notion that Anthony would never achieve the ultimate goals his father held for him—getting married, raising a family, and running the family business.

In a study of fathers of schizophrenic clients, Lidz (1957) and his associates described these men as having "poor self-esteem and marked insecurity regarding masculinity resulting in a need for an abundance of admiration from others. Paranoia and paranoid-like irrational behavior was common, and they were impervious to the feelings and needs of others." Anthony's description of his father's perfectionistic behavior may have been a symptom of the poor self-esteem Lidz (1957) describes.

During his childhood, Anthony developed a prepsychotic schizoid personality. As described by Arieti (1974), the schizoid appears aloof, detached, and less emotional, concerned, and involved than the average person. Actually, at an unconscious level, he continues to be very sensitive, but he has learned to avoid anxiety and anger in two ways: by putting physical distance between himself and situations that are apt to arouse these feelings, and by repressing all emotions. According to Arieti, "the schizoid personality defends the self from the distressing others who constitute the family and the world. It is a set of defenses built as reaction to chronic danger, not to immediate fear; it provides tepid responses to poorly expressed states of anxiety and anger. By detaching himself emotionally, the patient will avoid the pain connected with the attacks on self-esteem."

Throughout his life, Anthony has maintained the defense of isolation for the sake of preserving the self. His social interactions were marginal at best and absent at worst. His self-perception as a defective person was reinforced by others responding to his unkempt physical appearance and his somewhat strange to frankly bizarre behavior.

COURSE OF TREATMENT

The family treatment provided for the parents in this case was an essential prerequisite for Anthony's individual treatment. Through years of family treatment, Mr. and Mrs. DeLuca were able to begin defining boundaries and setting limits on Anthony's potentially violent or otherwise inappropriate behavior. This shift in family dynamics placed Anthony in the position of needing to adjust to the threat of separation imposed by these new boundaries and limits.

The recommendation for Anthony's treatment included weekly individual psychotherapy sessions, biweekly family therapy sessions, and antipsychotic medication (Prolixin Decanoate) administered intramuscularly on a biweekly basis at the end of individual sessions.

Anthony's decision to accept treatment represented an adaptive response to his inability to find a livable environment either with or separate from his parents. He initially presented requesting help with the adjustment to his new living situation. Anthony agreed, with some reluctance, to attend family meetings in order to establish the ways in which his parents would be allowed and would not be allowed to help with the task of organizing his belongings and apartment. He also agreed to begin individual sessions, which he could only tolerate for 10 minutes on a weekly basis.

In the Beginning Phase of treatment, family meetings focused on the concrete tasks associated with helping Anthony to get settled in his new living situation. It was decided that Anthony would allow his parents to perform certain tasks and that he would assume responsibility for others. The family's ability or inability to follow through on these prescriptions was then discussed and explored.

In the meantime, Anthony began attending his brief individual sessions, during which he spent most of his time talking about his fear of being controlled by external forces. But 6 months after individual treatment began, after the Working Phase had been established, he was able to tolerate 30-minute sessions and to at times discuss content based on reality and the tasks of everyday life. And after more than a year in treatment, his sessions were 50 minutes in duration and the content increasingly focused on the ways in which his parents attempted to control his life and his emotional and behavioral reactions to such attempts.

Consistent collaboration between the individual therapist and the family therapist proved necessary. For, although Anthony was raising concerns about his father pressuring him to go out and find a job teaching music during his individual sessions, he was terrified with the prospect of addressing that issue in the family meetings. Therefore, the individual therapist periodically attended family meetings in order to facilitate such discussions and to provide Anthony with the security afforded by the presence of a perceived ally.

The major focus of the individual therapy dealt with Anthony's grief and profound disappointment about his unfulfilled dreams. As his content during the individual sessions became less psychotic and more coherent, Anthony was able to describe how he envisioned his life without the limitations imposed by his illness.

Anthony's course of treatment was interspersed with brief psychotic episodes that corresponded with feelings of depression and intense anger toward his parents for their lack of confidence in him, as demonstrated by their failure to acknowledge his accomplishments and talents. These episodes did not require hospitalization and were described by Anthony as "escapes from his mundane life."

Anthony's development of the ability to grieve over the loss of lifestyle he would never achieve finally allowed him to begin to pursue more realistic goals and to gradually become more functional. He was able to begin day treatment and consequently became less isolated due to the structure afforded by the program. While still feeling trapped in a "mundane life," he was able to take some pleasure in the relationships he developed through participation in day treatment and displayed pride in his new-found ability to maintain a living arrangement separate from his parents.

SUMMARY

In summary, this case study illustrates the evolution of long-term out-patient treatment for a family with a schizophrenic member. The treatment involved the parents of the "identified patient" for a period of 4 years before the client perceived any need for treatment himself.

The parallels between individual therapy and family therapy were facilitated by collaboration and a team approach derived from the basic tenets of community psychiatry. The family work focused on dealing with issues regarding ego boundaries, individuation, and separation. Individual therapy focused on those same issues and the impact of Anthony's illness on his life. Given some definition of boundaries, and the beginning of grieving and resolving the loss of the life he might have had without schizophrenia, Anthony was finally able to find certain adaptive ways of improving his functional capacity.

REFERENCES

Alanen, Y.O. "The Mothers of Schizophrenic Patients," *Acta Psychiatrica et Neurologica Scandinavica,* Supplement No. 124, Helsinki, 1958.

Arieti, S. *Interpretation of Schizophrenia.* New York: Basic Books, 1974.

Lidz, T. "The Intrafamilial Environment of the Schizophrenic Patient: The Father," *Psychiatry* 20:329, 1957.

SELECTED BIBLIOGRAPHY

Brown, B. "Influence of Family Life on the Course of Schizophrenic Disorders: A Replication," *British Journal of Psychiatry* 121:241, 1978.

Goldman, H.H. "Mental Illness and Family Burden: A Public Health Perspective," *Hospital and Community Psychiatry* 33(7):557-60, 1982.

Hoskins, P.P. "The Chronically Mentally Ill in the Community," in *Comprehensive Psychiatric Nursing,* 3rd ed. Edited by Haber, J., et al. New York: McGraw-Hill Book Co., 1987.

Krauss, J.B., and Slavinsky, A.T. *The Chronically Ill Psychiatric Patient and the Community.* Boston: Blackwell Scientific Publications, 1982.

Nicholi, A. *The Harvard Guide to Modern Psychiatry.* Cambridge, Mass.: The Belknap Press of Harvard University Press, 1978.

Vaughn, C., and Leff, J. "The Influence of Family and Social Factors on the Course of Psychiatric-Illness: A Comparison of Schizophrenic and Depressed Neurotic Patients," 129:125, 1976.

Christina:
Dysthymic Disorder

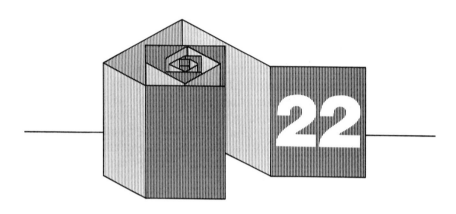

Ann Cousins, MSN, RN, CS

A client who complains of feeling sad and depressed over an extended period, while not always meeting the formal criteria for major depression, nevertheless may share many symptoms of this diagnosis. This case study presents the nursing care plan developed by a clinical nurse specialist for such a client, based on the following nursing diagnoses:

• Sleep pattern disturbance related to inadequate duration secondary to anxiety in relationship with boyfriend.

• Ineffective individual coping related to superficial relationships secondary to dysthymic disorder.

CASE STUDY

Christina, a 38-year-old, single, white female, presented to a local mental health center with the complaint of "My relationship with my boyfriend is upsetting me; I'm tense and I'm feeling worse and worse." At the time of contact, she was a part-time creative writing teacher living alone in a city close to the health center.

Christina dated the onset of this tenseness to 8 months before, when she met her boyfriend Phil. From the start, Christina and Phil shared an intense relationship, spending hours discussing their various individual dilemmas and conflicts. They quickly became sexually involved—which Christina later regretted, as she experienced difficulty with the sexual relationship. She described Phil as being "unusually interested" in her, which caused her to experience anxiety when with him to such an extent that her muscles became tense. Her discomfort with Phil rapidly accelerated after he enrolled in a self-development course and tried to persuade her to do so as well.

When asked specifically about depressive symptoms, Christina reported sleeping an average of only 3 hours a night when with Phil (as compared to 7 or 8 hours a night when not with him). Her appetite was good but her energy level was low, and she constantly ruminated and brooded about her inadequacies and experienced difficulties both in teaching and in writing because of poor concentration. Additionally, she was pessimistic about the future; 3 years of individual therapy prior to this contact, while providing her with some "insights," did nothing to alleviate her feelings of being "down, sad, and blue."

Christina described no overt symptoms of psychosis, and denied any alcohol or drug use. She described intrusive thoughts about "how I think I look." When asked to elaborate, she stated that she pictured herself possessing "a sunken, fatigued face." She described no recent developmental crises, such as a new job or home. She had been in long-term individual psychotherapy for the previous 3 years, but had terminated 2 months prior to this contact.

Christina experienced symptoms of a major depression at age 33, shortly after she terminated a 4-year-long relationship with a man with whom she had lived for 3½ years. At that time, she felt "down in the dumps." Associated with her depressed mood was difficulty in sleeping. She slept for only 3 to 5 hours a night, often awakening up to 2 hours early "in a snit." Her appetite was minimal, and she lost 20 pounds over a period of 2 months. Her energy level was low, and she doubted her competence as a writer. Once an ardent play and movie buff, she could no longer retain her interest. Additionally, she avoided supermarkets and department stores because she couldn't make decisions, and she secretly hoped for a "quick terminal illness." About 2 months prior to the onset of symptoms, Christina had switched to a higher-dose oral contraceptive pill because of breakthrough bleeding. Even though Christina's symptoms persisted for a period of 7 months, she did not seek help. Finally, her symptoms abated. But rather than remitting completely, they merely decreased to their level at the time of this contact. She had not experienced an asymptomatic period (psychological or physical) in the past 5 years.

Christina first sought psychotherapy 3 years previously to try to "restore some semblance of happiness" to her life. But although this therapy gave her some "insight" into her "low self-confidence," she continued to "feel gloomy."

Christina experienced the usual childhood diseases, with no hospitalizations or operations. She did sustain a head injury with loss of consciousness at age 7, after being hit by a swing, but with no headaches or neurological symptoms associated with paroxysmal psychiatric symptoms either then or now.

Christina's family history was positive for ovarian cancer and hypertension. Her mother died of cancer when Christina was age 17½. Two maternal aunts had ovarian cancer, and one maternal aunt had cancer of the pancreas. Her father suffered from high blood pressure. Christina described him as having a "strong temper"; "not able to show his feelings"; "critical and judgmental." "He always sheltered me to the point that I don't have confidence in my abilities, especially in making decisions. He has a natural, subtle sense of humor. He shows his love for me by doing things for me, and, in a way, we share similar views and interests. He is cautious, careful, and fearful of taking risks...quite sensitive and always elicits warm feelings for others, as he is most sweet and kind to others outside my family...an incredible pessimist who often focuses on the negative aspects of others' suggestions...doesn't know how to enjoy himself or relax...nervous most of the time...has taken sleeping pills for insomnia for the past 25 years."

Christina described her mother, Norma, as "always keeping up a good front, often lively, articulate, and chatty. Inside, she was obviously riddled with resentment about her situation of being married to a writer and being one herself. She suppressed her own abilities to support his. I think she did it because she felt it was only right for a wife to give herself up to her husband's needs. I think she was so delighted she married, she did this with a vengeance. She didn't consider herself pretty, so she might have been overwhelmed at her luck at finding someone. Actually, she didn't take good care of herself, and she neglected her appearance. Also, she was a rather poor housekeeper.

"Mother embarrassed my sister and me by describing us in hyperbole...about how wonderful and creative we were. She pushed us to do things of all types, from stomach exercises for weight loss to sunbathing for our acne. Both she and dad were strangely concerned about our personal appearance, even though she neglected her own.

"Mom was very intelligent, well-read, and, of anyone in the family, the most willing to show affection. She was a talented writer but stopped writing at some point because she felt less gifted than dad. She also liked to write in my father's style.

"Mom's worst act was her 'silent treatment.' She would get angry at me and not talk to me for hours or days. I would beg and plead, but she would walk around like a stone wall. It was just horrible. My sister insists mother was depressed. I'm not sure if she was depressed or just neurotic.

"The last sequence of my mother's life was her death from cancer. She got cancer and didn't tell anyone for months. Her tumor was so big that she appeared pregnant. At the insistence of dad, she went to a couple of doctors. One suggested immediate surgery, and the other said to wait. Of course, she believed the latter doctor. So her tumor got bigger, and she just let it grow until her intestines became blocked. They operated then, but it was too late. She was bedridden at the end. All through this, she hid her feelings and went on being a wife and mother. Dad didn't talk about it either. Everything was hush-hush.

"I always confided in mother. She was my judge and jury of what I might have done, right or wrong, in my social interactions. She also helped me endlessly with my schoolwork."

Christina described her sister Olivia, the editor of a publication for a major scientific firm, as "emotionally closed, seemingly self-assured, strong and competent career-wise.... Olivia is nervous; she picks her blemishes, has bouts of insomnia, and anxiety attacks. She's a workaholic who has no idea how to relax. She seems driven. She is super-intelligent, verbal, and has lots of friends. She divorced her husband and has no relationships with men, since she is convinced that most men are unable to meet her needs. She has a 10-year-old daughter whom I enjoy even though I hardly see her.

"My sister told me a long time ago that she was unable to be close to me because she didn't trust me. Basically, we do 'get along' when we see each other; however, a lack of trust is always there.

"Olivia dresses well, but she always looks anxiety-ridden and tired. She really is, and always was, pretty. She relies entirely on her female friends for closeness. She can be fun with a dry sense of humor, although she has a critical air and makes quick judgments about people.

"Olivia fought my parents more than I. She excluded me from many activities. I used to follow her around. She has very definite ideas about me and my problems. She always devalued people as a child and still does. She laughed at my pals and admits this now.

"Olivia was always very popular, and she received excellent grades. She had many friends, was very successful and smart. She received a four-year scholarship to a prestigious women's college."

Christina was the product of a normal labor and delivery. As far as she knew, she met her early developmental milestones on time. Her earliest memories were "sharing the same room with my sister, trying to fall asleep while she bit her nails" and "following my sister around a lot; she didn't like it." Christina didn't attend kindergarten, as there was none available in her small southern country town. Her first year in school was uneventful, as she had prepared for it by "playing school" constantly before actually attending. She had lots of friends throughout school, who she described as "equally as quiet as me." They played "dolls and house." During her school years, she proved to be particularly good in English; she struggled with math, however. Her mother helped her with her homework "endlessly."

When Christina was in junior high school, her family moved to another southern state, where her father was hired and later tenured at a prestigious state school. Christina slowly made the adjustment to the junior high school in her new town. Christina's memory of her high school years was sketchy; her mother's struggle with cancer and death dominated her recollections of that period. Christina graduated high school with honors and attended a university in a neighboring state. Her adjustment to the university was more difficult than it had been in high school. She studied constantly and had "precious few friends" because she felt "outrageously unconfident." This feeling was supported by a short story that Christina had written during this period, in which she poignantly described this "unconfidence" as painful self-consciousness.

Christina had worked as an English teacher since her graduation from college. She sold a number of short stories during this period, and continued to write prolifically; however, she was less likely to submit a story for publication since her depression at age 33. At that time, she changed to a part-time job at a private girls school, and her father has subsidized her income.

Christina went out on only one date while in high school. She began meeting men during her sophomore year in college and became sexually active in her junior year. Initially, she found sexual relations enjoyable. But the onset of the period of depression marked a decrease in her capacity to experience pleasure. By the time of contact, Christina rarely experienced orgasm; in her words, she was "just too nervous."

Christina had a number of long-term relationships over the years, the longest lasting 4 years with a man 5 years her junior. She met him on a bus after previously noticing him on the numerous bus trips they shared. Approximately 2 months after they started dating, he joined a religious commune; 4 months later, Christina moved in with him, although she never became a full religious member. She left the commune when the leader became, in her view, psychotic. She left her boyfriend behind; he remained fully committed in his devotion to the leader. Shortly after, she terminated the relationship, having become terrified by his fanatical devotion. (Sometime later, her boyfriend left the commune; eventually, he became a drug addict.)

After this breakup and before beginning her relationship with Phil, Christina dated extensively and had several relationships averaging about 6 months' duration. At the time of initial contact, Christina and Phil were in couples therapy with a private therapist. Christina insisted that the therapist favored Phil.

During her initial evaluation interview, Christina presented as an attractive, artistic-appearing person who appeared somewhat younger than her stated age. She made good eye contact; however, sitting with Christina left the interviewer feeling hazy. Something about her, perhaps her ruminations, caused her to appear as less than fully present. She described feeling "down" and to some extent appeared this way. She reported difficulty in sleeping associated with extreme tension with her boyfriend Phil; however, closer questioning revealed no change in her sleep pattern when she's alone. She described three symptoms of depression at the moderate level, as well as pessimism, that pervade her perceptions. She displayed no overt symptoms of psychosis. She expressed feeling tormented by her belief that her face appears "sunken and fatigued," but described this symptom as a stimulus to sharing her worries with Phil, who enjoyed "ardently" reviewing her difficulties with her. Christina denied any suicidal or homicidal ideation. But sometimes, she confided, she wished Phil would "give up on his interest in me." She expressed a strong desire for a permanent relationship that would lead to marriage and children. She would like to be a mother but, at the same time, feared she herself needed too much mothering.

Formal mental status testing indicated that Christina had orientation in four spheres. She remembered four words in 5 minutes and again in 20 minutes. She exhibited a good fund of knowledge and responded abstractly to proverbs and similarities. She recited serial sevens accurately, and responded correctly to seven numbers forward and six numbers backward. Her judgment appeared good. She displayed no symptoms suggestive of neurological disorders.

During the examination, Christina denied current medical symptoms or difficulties. Her menses came every 28 days, and she described no changes in this area. She denied the use of any medication, including birth control pills.

The evaluation spanned two 1-hour sessions. After the first session, Christina called the therapist and insisted "I don't want therapy; I really need medications." During the second session, she screamed her request for medication, adding, "I have trouble asking for what I want—please listen to me."

FORMULATION

Initial impressions derived from the data gathered led the clinician to believe that Christina was suffering from a dysthymic disorder (rule-out subaffective vs. characterological). Numerous possibilities arose in formulating an initial understanding of Christina's current difficulties. Biological, psychodynamic, family, and behavioral contributions were all relevant and could be culled from her history.

Christina experienced symptoms of a major depression at age 33—symptoms that never fully remitted. The duration of residual symptoms for more than 2 years points to a diagnosis of dysthymic disorder. In a naturalistic study of depression, Keller and Shapiro (1982) found women in their thirties who have experienced depressions like Christina's are at risk for only partial recovery, with sustained symptoms of a minor depression. Akiskal and Webb (1983) have delineated such subtypes of depression as falling into the category of dysthymic disorder. Christina's history and her own constellation of symptoms raised questions regarding possible biological and dynamic contributions to her current symptoms and difficulties.

The onset of depression prior to age 40, as well as the correlation with an increased dose of oral contraceptives along with questionably depressed behavior of her parents, suggested a biological component to Christina's depression. However, one cannot ignore the likelihood of Christina's having a powerless and depressed maternal (and paternal) introject, similar to women her current age who have achieved independence and mastery of career. Having the powerless maternal introject she demonstrated in her current love relationship, Christina needed to integrate the two disparate views of herself. Additionally, she demonstrated intrapsychic developmental lags in the areas of separation and individuation—problems common to children of depressed parents.

Relationships were always difficult for Christina in terms of choice and closeness. She had chosen generally younger, less stable men. And once stability was achieved, Christina retreated from closeness by writing excessively or developing symptoms of depression. This behavior, combined with her sister's resignation to having no further male-female relationships, raised questions about the quality of her parents' relationship. Barrigan (1976) describes a family dynamic of "good child" vs. "bad child" and heightened sibling conflict in families with unacknowledged marital discord. Christina's sister's focus on a lack of trust may have been a remnant of this type of family dynamic, or it may have been suggesting a pattern in Christina's behavior indicative of long-term personality adjustment secondary to developmental lags.

Christina expressed intrusive thoughts that her face looks "sunken." These thoughts, barely dystonic at worst, seemed to provide the stimulus for her ardent review of the dynamics of her relationship with her boyfriend. While her intrusive thoughts may have seemed indicative of an obsessive-compulsive syndrome that behaviorists view as serendipitously learned, Christina's misperception of facial features was likely melancholic. These thoughts may have been the "tip of the iceberg" of the delayed and conflicted grief she felt for her mother. One wonders what Christina's mother's face looked like, given her long bout with cancer.

Developmental periods challenge people's adaptation, especially when one has negative introjects. In such a context, Christina's current difficulty with her boyfriend took on added pressure. For, like many other women in their thirties, Christina would like to marry and have children.

COURSE OF TREATMENT

Although the clinic staff was tempted at first to offer Christina a 15-week developmental women's group, they eventually realized that her difficulty with closeness would likely limit her ability to establish relationships in the short term. Thus, a long-term (1–1½-year) group was recommended. The longer period of time was seen as essential in helping Christina develop a capacity for closeness. In addition, the less-focused nature of this group was thought to be more suited to helping Christina tolerate intimacy and maintain her personal sense of power, and its "here and now" focus would limit her need to continuously reflect inward.

Shortly after starting therapy, Christina requested antidepressant medication. We also decided, after consultation with the mental health team psychiatrist, to offer Christina a trial of antidepressant medication as an empirical attempt to treat the long-term symptoms of her dysthymic disorder.

Christina did not wish long-term individual psychotherapy, since she had just recently terminated a 3-year course. But short-term therapy was not negotiated, since Christina experienced difficulty maintaining her focus in the weekly sessions during the evaluative period. And so, somewhat fearfully, Christina agreed that a long-term group would best address her struggle with relationships and explore her style of psychological withdrawal.

In preparation for the long-term group, Christina was asked to think about her specific difficulties in relationships. She was also asked to try to anticipate patterns and blocks from her previous experience in non-therapy groups. Christina thought she would do well in the beginning. She noted that her "haziness" tended to develop "when I worry if people will like me." However, she was "worried about being tense." We discussed how she might engage the group to help her to not withdraw in the face of closeness, with the intermediate goal of establishing relationships. We hoped that once she was able to establish relationships with the group members, her "outside" relationships would benefit, especially if she felt stronger in her ability to identify her feelings and determine her own needs.

While waiting for admission to the long-term group, Christina was evaluated for antidepressant medication. She delayed the medication trial by deciding to visit relatives the day after the prescription was written. After her return, she was started on 25 mg of imipramine orally. She called 2 days later, reporting dry mouth and nervousness. Subsequently, she stated that she preferred to not take the medication.

Eventually, Christina entered a long-term group with seven other clients. Before long, she began to withdraw, almost to the point of invisibility. Most members of the group barely noticed her withdrawal, but more active members attempted to include Christina. When they did so, however, Christina would become quite tense and would tend to ruminate over her various conflicts and negative self-perception. While this initially seemed obsessive in nature, it actually served her narcissism by distancing her from the group.

During group sessions, Christina had difficulty incorporating feedback from others. Initially, she would listen carefully and return the next week feeling accused. She would then give sharp feedback to others about their problems. This feedback was projective in style and included barely cloaked envy of others. Although Christina made gains in the group, she terminated early, explaining that she had found a new boyfriend. She explained that she had left Phil because he had become "disinterested" and that she found her new boyfriend more attentive. She rationalized leaving the group because the therapist didn't "do encouragement."

SUMMARY

During the course of therapy, Christina actively pursued evaluation for antidepressant medication but quickly rejected the medication trial once expected side effects became evident. She actively participated in her pregroup preparation to anticipate patterns that might hold her back. Although her defensive structure initially seemed obsessively similar to some depressives, her personal sense of vulnerability was far more severe than that commonly found in such clients. Her ruminations—a distancing technique—spoke to her narcissistic defenses, which included the use of projection and projective identification. Although she received little negative feedback, Christina was exquisitely sensitive. She often remarked sharply about others' problems. Throughout group sessions, Christina carefully watched the therapist. She seemed reluctant to either challenge or join others, including the therapist, around issues of leadership and membership roles in the group.

Christina's termination from the group concerned the therapist. Her feelings of abandonment as a teenager, and perhaps her early termination from the group, spoke to theories of loss. A drive to master loss was evident in the process of her leaving. She left the group before the group left her. Staving off potential abandonment, Christina chose to leave first rather than risk evoking feelings associated with previous losses that left her so vulnerable.

REFERENCES

Akiskal, H., and Webb, W. "Affective Disorders I. Recent Advances in Clinical Conceptualization," *Hospital and Community Psychiatry* 34:695-701, 1983.

Barrigan, M. "The Child Centered Family," in *Family Therapy: Theory and Practice*. Edited by Guerin, P. New York: Gardner Press, 1976.

Keller, M., et al. "Recovery in Major Depressive Disorder," *Archives of General Psychiatry* 39: 1982.

SELECTED BIBLIOGRAPHY

Akiskal, H.S., and McKinney, W.T. "Overview of Recent Research on Depression: Integration of 10 Conceptual Models into a Comprehensive Clinical Frame," *Archives of General Psychiatry* 32:285-305, 1975.

American Psychiatric Association. *Diagnostic and Statistical Manual of Mental Disorders*, 3rd ed. Washington, D.C.: American Psychiatric Association, 1980.

Beck, A. *Cognitive Therapy and the Emotional Disorders*. New York: New American Library, 1976.

Daley, B., and Koppenaal, G. "The Treatment of Women in Short-Term Women's Groups," *Forms of Brief Therapy*. Edited by Budman, S. New York: Guilford Press, 1981.

Freud, S. "Mourning and Melancholia," in *Complete Psychological Works of Sigmund Freud,* vol. 14. London: Hogarth Press, 1924.

National Institutes of Mental Health. *Depressive Disorders: Causes and Treatments.* Washington, D.C.: U.S. Government Printing Office, 1982.

Paykel, E., et al. "Life Events and Depression: A Controlled Study," *Archives of General Psychiatry* 21:753-60, 1969.

Pelletier, L.R., and Cousins, A. "Depression Update," *Journal of Emergency Nursing* 10(6):315-18, 1984.

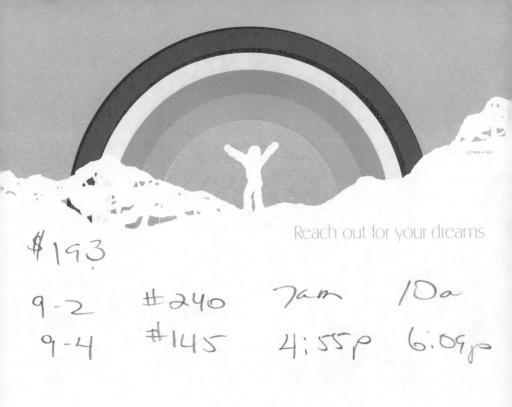

Reach out for your dreams

$193

9-2   #240   7am   10a
9-4   #145   4:55p 6:09p